Management of Chronic Lower Limb Ischemia

Management of Chronic Lower Limb Ischemia

Edited by

JOSEPH L MILLS SR MD
Professor of Surgery, Chief of Vascular Surgery,
University of Arizona Health Sciences Center, Tucson,
Arizona, USA

A member of the Hodder Headline Group
LONDON
Co-published in the United States of America by
Oxford University Press Inc., New York

First published in Great Britain in 2000 by
Arnold, a member of the Hodder Headline Group,
338 Euston Road, London NW1 3BH

http://www.arnoldpublishers.com

Co-published in the United States of America by
Oxford University Press Inc.,
198 Madison Avenue, New York, NY10016
Oxford is a registered trademark of Oxford University Press

Whilst the advice and information in this book are believed to be
true and accurate at the date of going to press, neither the authors
nor the publisher can accept any legal responsibility or liability for
any errors or omissions that may be made. In particular (but without
limiting the generality of the preceding disclaimer) every effort has
been made to check drug dosages; however it is still possible that
errors have been missed. Furthermore, dosage schedules are
constantly being revised and new side-effects recognized. For these
reasons the reader is strongly urged to consult the drug companies'
printed instructions before administering any of the drugs
recommended in this book.

British Library Cataloguing in Publication Data
A catalogue record for this book is available from the British Library

Library of Congress Cataloging-in-Publication Data
A catalog record for this book is available from the Library of
Congress

ISBN 0 340 75956 9 (hb)

1 2 3 4 5 6 7 8 9 10

Commissioning Editor: Nick Dunton
Project Editor: Sarah de Souza
Production Editor: Rada Radojicic
Production Controller: James Rabson
Cover Design: Terry Griffiths

Typeset in 10/12 pt Minion by Phoenix Photosetting, Chatham, Kent
Printed and bound in Great Britain by The Bath Press

What do you think about this book? Or any other Arnold title?
Please send your comments to feedback.arnold@hodder.co.uk

To my parents, for their encouragement and teaching me to love learning

To my wife, Margaret, and three sons, Andrew, Daniel and Joe Jr., for their support and teaching me to love life

Contents

Contributors

Michael Belkin MD
Associate Professor of Surgery, Division of Vascular Surgery,
Brigham and Women's Hospital, Harvard Medical School,
Boston, Massachusetts, USA

Scott S Berman MD
Assistant Professor of Clinical Surgery, Chief of Vascular
Surgery, St Mary's Carondelet Hospital, Tucson, Arizona, USA

Victor M Bernhard MD
Clinical Professor of Surgery, Division of Vascular Surgery,
Northwestern University, Chicago, Illinois, USA

Andrew W Bradbury
Professor of Vascular Surgery, Heartlands Hospital, University
of Birmingham, UK

Ronald L Dalman MD
Associate Professor of Surgery, Division of Vascular Surgery,
Stanford University School of Medicine, Stanford, California,
USA

Andrew T Gentile MD, RVF
Vascular Surgeon, St Mary's Carondelet Hospital, Tucson,
Arizona, USA

E John Harris Jr MD
Associate Professor of Surgery, Division of Vascular Surgery,
Stanford University School of Medicine, Stanford, California,
USA

John D Hughes MD
Associate Professor of Clinical Surgery, Department of
Vascular Surgery, University of Arizona Health Sciences
Center, Tucson, Arizona, USA

James B Knox MD
Vascular Fellow, Division of Vascular Surgery, Brigham and
Women's Hospital, Harvard Medical School, Boston,
Massachusetts, USA

John M Marek MD
Assistant Professor of Surgery, University of New Mexico,
Department of Vascular Surgery, Albuquerque, New Mexico, USA

Joseph L Mills Sr MD
Professor of Surgery, Chief of Vascular Surgery, University of
Arizona Health Sciences Center, Tucson, Arizona, USA

Gregory L Moneta MD
Professor of Surgery, Division of Vascular Surgery, Oregon
Health Sciences University, Portland, Oregon, USA

John M Porter MD
Professor of Surgery, Chief, Division of Vascular Surgery,
Oregon Health Sciences University, Portland, Oregon, USA

Klaus See-Tho MD
Fellow, Division of Vascular Surgery, Stanford University
School of Medicine, Stanford, California, USA

Andres E Tovar-Pardo MD
Department of Vascular Surgery, Hospital Santa Teresa,
La Coruna, Spain

Alex Westerband MD
Assistant Professor of Clinical Surgery, Department of
Vascular Surgery, University of Arizona Health Sciences
Center and Southern Arizona Veterans Affairs Health Care
Systems, Tucson, Arizona, USA

Christopher L Wixon MD
Clinical Fellow, Vascular Surgery Section, University of
Arizona Health Sciences Center, Tucson, Arizona, USA

John HN Wolfe MS, FRCS
Consultant Vascular Surgeon, St Mary's Hospital, London, UK

Julie M Zaetta MD
Assistant Professor of Radiology, Division of Vascular and
Interventional Radiology, University of Arizona Health
Sciences Center, Tucson, Arizona, USA

Preface

Vascular surgery is a speciality whose birth and subsequent rapid evolution have occurred only in the twentieth century. While in the early 1900s the very issue of whether or not it was feasible to successfully repair or reconstruct arteries was in doubt, nearly every large community now in the western world is blessed with well-trained vascular surgical specialists who routinely reconstruct blood vessels for a variety of traumatic, degenerative, occlusive and aneurysmal conditions. The most significant advances in the last decade, however, have taken place in the area of lower extremity arterial reconstruction. Patients with advanced chronic limb ischemia, particularly diabetics and the very elderly, are no longer condemned to inevitable major limb amputation. In fact, the dramatic improvements in the surgical treatment of lower limb occlusive disease have helped elevate vascular surgery into a recognized entity and distinct subspeciality.

When initially approached about preparing a vascular surgical textbook, my first question was whether or not another textbook was really necessary. Medical and surgical journals, as well as textbooks, seem to abound. However, upon reflection, it became obvious that there was a need for a concise, well-constructed text focusing on lower extremity arterial reconstruction. I sought to emphasize the development and evolution of currently available techniques, present expected outcomes of modern lower extremity arterial reconstruction clearly, and discuss ongoing technological advances and their potential future application.

It is my impression that, despite the increasing frequency with which lower extremity arterial reconstruction is being performed and its generalized resounding success when performed by competent well-trained vascular surgeons, vascular surgery has done itself a disservice by failing to disseminate to the broader medical community the appropriate diagnostic evaluation, available management options and expected outcomes of lower limb arterial reconstruction. This point was brought home to me recently when I received a communication from a prominent physician in our medical community with broad experience in cardiovascular disease, who referred a patient with rest pain and long-standing, non-healing multiple ischemic toe ulcers. This patient, in fact, had been refused bypass elsewhere because he was thought to be too frail and, based on angiographic studies, was also deemed unreconstructible. The patient had good-quality saphenous vein and repeat arteriography demonstrated an excellent dorsalis pedis vessel, allowing us to perform a successful femoral to dorsalis pedis bypass. A follow-up note from the referring physician stated '... it sounds like the operation went very well. I cannot imagine a graft from the right femoral to the dorsalis pedis vessel'. His surprise at this operation, which most experienced vascular surgeons view as routine, astounded me. It made me realize that perhaps vascular surgery has made the mistake of talking only to itself within the confines of its subspeciality and of not communicating to the medical community at large the advances made over the last decade in the care of patients with chronic lower limb ischemia.

I, therefore, undertook the task of preparing a text focused on lower limb arterial reconstruction. The intended audience for this textbook includes both resident and attending physicians and surgeons who manage as part of their medical or surgical practices the increasing proportion of our aging population affected by chronic arterial occlusive disease. There has been a paucity of textbooks on lower extremity arterial reconstruction and most of them have been confined to presentations of purely technical matters of principal concern only to vascular surgeons. In an effort to provide a state of the art textbook, aimed not only at vascular surgeons but also at a broader community of physicians and surgeons, I gathered multiple colleagues with whom I have been associated in the last decade of my practise in vascular surgery. These colleagues come from across the United States and the United Kingdom. All are practicing vascular specialists who have as a component of their practise a significant commitment to the care of patients with lower limb arterial occlusive disease. The contributors have been selected specifically because they are in the active phases of busy medical and surgical careers, and their words represent those 'in the trenches'. These chapters are not written by distant academics. This approach has resulted in a concise presentation of current state of the art care of patients with chronic lower limb arterial occlusive disease. I believe there is sufficient, well-summarized technical detail to be of use to practicing general and vascular surgeons, as well as a broader scope of chapters covering preoperative evaluation, noninvasive testing, arteriographic findings, and management of the diabetic foot. In addition, detailed presentations of expected outcome results analyzed by proper life table methods are provided which all practicing physicians and surgeons who take care of atherosclerotic patients should find of use.

I would like to thank Arnold for their staunch support in making this textbook possible. I appreciate the efforts of the numerous contributors who have succeeded in producing a thorough, yet concise, review of lower limb arterial reconstruction in the last decade of the twentieth century, as we approach the centennial of the birth of vascular surgery. Finally, I would like to thank my mentor and colleague, John M. Porter, MD, who attempted to teach me the art of critical thinking, appropriate application of carefully designed surgery in properly selected patients, and an aggressive approach to maintenance of functional limb salvage in patients threatened by diabetes, infection and chronic progressive lower extremity arterial occlusive disease. The ability to salvage such limbs, in frequently critically ill patients, to allow them to resume or maintain an independent lifestyle, is truly one of the greatest advances that surgery has produced in this century.

Joseph L Mills

The history of infrainguinal bypass

CHRISTOPHER L WIXON AND JOSEPH L MILLS

The twisting paths from the past, beginning as unmarked trails in a jungle of ignorance, leading past many false sidetracks, built with imagination and courage but also with toil and tears, emerge upon the plateau of today, a broad and illuminated avenue teeming with surgical travelers (W. Andrew Dale, MD)

INTRODUCTION

Most texts credit the first infrainguinal bypass to Jean Kunlin, who in 1948 performed a reversed saphenous vein bypass from the common femoral to the popliteal artery in a man with ischemic pain and tissue loss.[1] It is fitting for such an event to have occurred in Paris, as Ambrose Paré, Alexis Carrel, Mathieu Jaboulay and René Leriche were also native to France. Yet, as innovative as this event appears, 40 years had elapsed since Carrel's first description of the venous autograft. Why had such a long time elapsed since Carrel's first reports and what obstacles had first to be overcome?

This chapter will attempt to address the numerous contributions leading up to Kunlin's historic procedure. In order to present historic concepts, events are presented without strict adherence to a timeline. Nonetheless, because it is sometimes useful to view developments as a continuum, a timeline is provided (Fig. 1.1).

EARLY FOUNDATIONS OF VASCULAR SURGERY

The foundations of vascular surgery are rich and can be traced back Galen's description of a patient's pulse and Antyllus' application of the ligature. However, the early promise of the Hellenistic period was soon lost as Europe became enveloped by the Dark Ages. During this period, Europe was ravaged by the Black Plague, which left three-quarters of its population dead. Medicine was of little help and people clung to superstitions, magic and potions. The barber-surgeons of the time could be found traveling from town to town, publicly performing surgical procedures as onlookers watched the spectacle with macabre anticipation. Predictably, procedures performed under such deplorable conditions frequently aggravated the patient's affliction and the patient's family often ran the barber-surgeon out of town. Consequently, the medical community shunned the barber's procedure-oriented practice and surgery was considered an inferior branch of medicine.

As Europe attempted to resurrect itself from the throes of the medieval age, so too a young French barber-surgeon emerged by the name of Ambrose Paré who attempted to redefine the practice of surgery. Having been trained in the usual manner of the time, he had been taught the medieval practice of treating traumatic wounds with boiling oil. Soon after embarking on a military career, his troops engaged in a costly battle and Paré was confronted with a multitude of injured men. While treating the men, he fortuitously ran out of boiling oil. He was familiar with Galen's teachings of ligation and applied these techniques to his soldiers' injuries, and then dressed the open wounds with egg yolk, rose oil and turpentine. The next morning he feared that the men would be ill with the sepsis of uncoagulated tissue, and he hesitantly examined the men. Surprisingly, the men treated with the substitutive dressings were well, they experienced less pain and their wounds healed rapidly.[2]

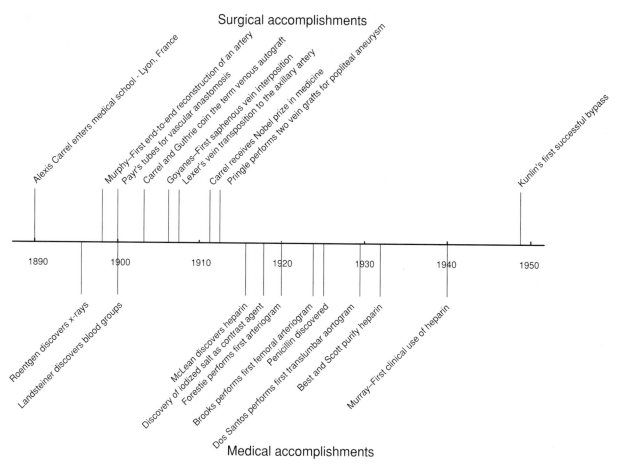

Figure 1.1 *Timeline of medical and surgical accomplishments. There is a notable lack of surgical progress during the first half of the 1900s.*

He carefully noted these observations and never used boiling oil again.

Paré's influence on the future practice of surgery cannot be overestimated as it represents the rebirth of scientific surgical thought and the power of observation. Paré, however, remained humble, understating his ingeniousness: 'I dressed him, but God cured him'.

Another significant figure to emerge during this period was the great anatomist, Andreas Vesalius. Unlike his contemporaries who were studying the historical writings of Galen, Vesalius performed his own dissections of human cadavers. In doing so, he faced considerable scrutiny from authoritative religious leaders as desecration of the human body was poorly accepted. Frequently, it was necessary to steal freshly executed corpses from the Cemetery of the Innocents (an above ground burial site for criminals) and perform his meticulous dissections in seclusion. Because Vesalius' work was often in direct contradistinction to Galen's more primitive anatomic descriptions, he also lacked support from the emerging, but fiercely dogmatic, scientific community.

However, European scholars could not turn a blind eye to Vesalius' persistence for long. As the great thinkers

of Europe opened their minds during the Age of Awakening, the importance of Vesalius' work became increasingly clear. Soon, anatomy schools cropped up throughout Europe and there was further speculation on the concept of circulation. An Englishman, William Harvey, had a most profound impact on the future of medicine and vascular surgery. He proposed that blood moves in a circle, the arteries carrying blood away from the heart, and the veins returning it back. In *De Motu Cordis*, he further specified the pressure gradients that exist in these vessels.

It was from these European schools of anatomy that a curious and unconventional Scot emerged, Sir John Hunter. His motto, 'Why ask the question, do the experiment', helped to establish the essential foundations of modern vascular surgery. In addition to his numerous contributions to comparative anatomy, he described collateral blood flow, the muscularity and elasticity of arteries, and provided a better understanding of aneurysms.

While he never contemplated a surgical bypass, he should be credited for the first attempt at limb salvage. During this period in eighteenth-century England, popliteal aneurysms were common among coachmen as a result of their frequent crouching position and repeated trauma to the popliteal artery while driving. Hunter despised the surgical mutilation of the patient, as contemporary management remained amputation. Based on his previous observation of collateral blood flow, he proposed to ligate the popliteal artery proximal and distal to the aneurysm sac. He successfully performed this procedure in 1785 on a 45-year-old man who survived the operation, remained functional and was gainfully employed after the procedure. After the man's death, Hunter performed an autopsy of the man and carefully preserved the specimen. It serves as a symbol of the beginning of the modern vascular surgical era and can be viewed today in the Hunterian Museum in London.

It was Hunter's ability to correlate practice with comparative anatomy and physiologic experiment that makes him so important, as he provided a scientific basis for the practice of modern surgery.

EARLY ANASTOMOTIC TECHNIQUE

The first recorded direct repair of a lacerated artery came almost 200 years after Paré's rediscovery of the ligature. At this time in mid-eighteenth-century Europe, surgeons had only recently been officially separated from barbers, and the technique of antecubital venesection for phlebotomy remained common practice. On 15 June 1759, one such attempt at venesection resulted in the laceration of the brachial artery.[3] A Yorkshire surgeon by the name of Hallowell was summoned. It was his previous experience with the generally poor functional outcome after ligation of such injuries that caused him to consider an alternative treatment. He placed thin slivers of wood through the lacerated arterial margins, everted the lacerated edges, and then coapted them with a suture that was wrapped in a figure-of-eight around the wooden slivers (Fig. 1.2). This historical event marks the first attempt at vascular reconstruction for limb salvage.

Unfortunately, the experimental application of Hallowell's technique in canines by Asman, resulted in either infection or thrombosis, and led to the premature conclusion that arterial repair always resulted in thrombosis.[4] Remarkably, no progress was made for the next century and the prevailing treatment of arterial lacerations and aneurysms remained ligation.

The first reported vascular anastomosis was performed in 1877, by a Russian surgeon named Nickolai Eck.[5] Ironically, his intent was to study the metabolic effect of blood shunted from the portal vein to the inferior vena cava. The technique utilized a continuous side-to-side suturing of the vein walls using silk suture. Only after the suture line was created were the walls of the vein opened using a special pair of scissors. Six of his eight dogs survived the operation and necropsy confirmed anastomotic patency. Unfortunately, the event did not attract significant attention, as the focus of the experi-

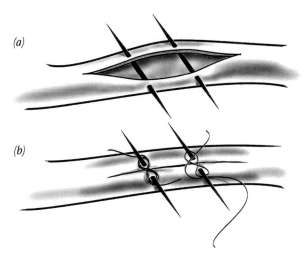

Figure 1.2 *Hallowell's repair of a lacerated brachial artery. (a) Two slivers of wood are placed though the lacerated arterial margins. (b) The walls of the artery are coapted by wrapping the slivers with silk suture.*

ment was metabolic changes in the liver. Nonetheless, it represents the first successful vascular anastomosis.

Almost 20 years after Eck's report, the potential benefit of successful vascular anastomosis was recognized, and a variety of primitive techniques were reported from both Europe and America. Early reports by Abbe described an hour-glass-shaped tube, over which the two ends of the severed vessel could be tied (the first prosthetic bypass!) (Fig. 1.3).[6] Owing to the thrombogenicity of the tube, however, these attempts routinely failed. To eliminate the contact of blood with the tube, Payr devised an absorbable magnesium tube, over which the proximal end of the artery could be everted. The unit was then inserted into the more distal end of the vessel, and secured with a suture (Fig. 1.4).[7] This also failed as it created a cul-de-sac which caused eventual thrombosis.

Other reports focused on direct end-to-end suture technique. Jassinowsky and Jaboulay utilized interrupted sutures of fine silk, aseptic technique and sutures confined to the adventitia and media, but the results were

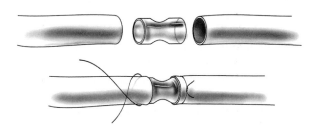

Figure 1.3 *Abbe's end-to-end anastomosis over an hour-glass-shaped tube. Both ends were secured using a silk suture.*

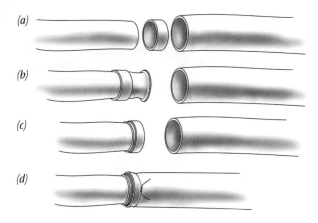

Figure 1.4 *(a) Payr's absorbable magnesium tube. (b) The proximal end is everted over the edge of the tube. The unit is advanced into the distal end (c) and secured with a silk suture (d).*

only intermittently successful.[8,9] The well-known surgeon from Chicago, J.B. Murphy (known for popularizing appendectomy), described end-to-end anastomoses by invaginating the proximal end into the distal end and securing the repair with fine sutures.[10] Again, success was limited, as suture line breakdown, hemorrhage and thrombosis continued to be more common than successful reconstruction.

In 1890, a young man entered medical school who was destined to change the course of vascular surgery. Alexis Carrel studied medicine at the University of Lyon, where he was influenced by Mathieu Jaboulay's work with vascular reconstruction. Later in 1894, he was deeply influenced by the assassination of the French President, Sadi Carnot. The President had exanguinated from an injury to the portal vein. Carrel failed to understand why the vessel could not be repaired and he openly questioned his mentor's technical ineptitude.

Carrel's controversial nature caused him to be rejected by his French colleagues and he sought refuge on the other side of the Atlantic. It was in the USA that he continued his vascular experiments and formed a mutually beneficial alliance with Charles Guthrie at the Hull Research Foundation, in Chicago. Together, they performed the seminal work in vascular anastomotic technique, much of which remains pertinent to the modern training of vascular surgeons.

Carrel recognized the superficial veins to be expendable, and he described venous transplantation using either uniterminal or biterminal technique. Anastomotic technique was greatly facilitated by 'triangulation' of the blood vessel and he stressed techniques that minimized trauma to the blood vessel wall.[11] He emphasized strict adherence to aseptic technique, the apposition of endothelial surfaces and the use of specialized instruments, fine suture and sharp, rounded needles. His prodigious contributions to vascular surgery were recog-

nized immediately and he was awarded the Nobel Prize in Physiology and Medicine in 1912.

Yet, Carrel remained a controversial figure. On one occasion he proclaimed, 'I am the creator of techniques; it is for others to use them'. Indeed, the surgical community inexplicably would wait nearly 40 years before his techniques were widely applied. It was first necessary to develop an understanding of vascular occlusive disease, suitable imaging techniques and clinically useful anticoagulation.

ESSENTIAL MEDICAL DEVELOPMENTS

Arteriography

Paramount to the development of the venous autograft was the development of reliable angiographic techniques that would localize the diseased segments and identify adequate inflow and outflow vessels. On 8 November 1895, Wilhelm Konrad Roentgen first observed 'Roentgen rays'. For this discovery, he was awarded the Nobel Prize in medicine in 1901 and these techniques remain a cornerstone of our diagnostic armamentarium. Only 3 months after Roentgen's discovery, the first arteriograms were performed by Haschek and Lindenthal on a previously amputated arm.[12] Twenty years later, Cameron discovered the utility and safety of iodized salts as a suitable contrast agent. These new agents were applied clinically by Barney Brooks, in 1923, who performed the first femoropopliteal imaging.[13] Significant contributions soon followed: the first cerebral arterial imaging by Egas Moniz[14] and the first translumbar aortography by Reynaldo Dos Santos.[15] Thus the field of interventional radiology was born out of surgery.

Heparin

One of the final developments necessary for successful infrainguinal bypass was that of a suitable agent to prevent thrombosis while the bypass graft was being constructed. In 1916, Jay McLean, then a medical student working in the laboratory of W.H. Howell, discovered heparin.[16] However, because of impurities it could not be used clinically. By 1933, Best and Scott had developed a suitable purification method.[17] The first clinical use came over 20 years after its discovery, when Gordon Murray first employed heparin in 1938 after an embolectomy procedure.[18]

CONDITIONALLY ESSENTIAL MEDICAL DEVELOPMENTS

If the development of suitable radiographic techniques and anticoagulants were *essential* to the successful development of the bypass, then the development of anesthesia, asepsis and transfusion must be considered *conditionally essential*.

Lister's work on antisepsis was originally published in 1870. Despite convincing data, his methods were generally met with bland indifference and occasionally, frank hostility. By the early twentieth century, however, antiseptic surgery was well accepted. The previous practice of atmospheric decontamination gave way to more specific methods of wound and instrument cleansing.

Likewise, during the early twentieth century, the field of anesthesia was under rapid development. Approximately 50 years had passed since Morton first articulated under the ether dome of the Massachusetts General Hospital, 'Sir, your patient is ready' (referring to the first clinical administration of a general anesthetic in 1846). Conquering pain during surgical procedures was a significant development as it alleviated anxiety both on the part of the patient and the surgeon. As a result, the surgeon could act more carefully and deliberately, thus increasing the safety and efficacy of the procedure.

Finally, the early 1900s saw Crile's early experiments of transfusion between animals and Landsteiner's description of blood groups. These developments laid the groundwork for the clinical application of blood transfusion, and soon the surgeon had whole blood, plasma and banked blood at his disposal.

The combination of antisepsis, anesthetic support and the potential for blood transfusion provided the vascular surgeon with reassuring confidence, and led to a willingness to accept operations of greater magnitude. It also permitted the application of meticulous techniques necessary for infrainguinal bypass.

EARLY EXPERIENCE WITH INFRAINGUINAL BYPASS

In reality, Kunlin was not the first to employ the venous autograft as an arterial conduit. In 1906, Jose Goyanes, of Madrid, used a segment of popliteal vein as a bypass graft after resection of a syphilitic popliteal aneurysm in a 41-year-old candymaker.[19] Similarly, Lexer performed a greater saphenous vein interposition graft after resection of a large axillary pseudoaneurysm.[20] Other anecdotal reports by Stitch and Pringle were performed after resection of aneurysms or tumors, but these also received little attention from the medical community.[21]

As significant as these first procedures were, of equal significance was the decided lack of progress that occurred over the next 30–40 years. In spite of Carrel's descriptions in the early 1900s there remained an almost deliberate lack of progress. This is particularly striking as it occurred in the face of tremendous need for technical progress, as Europe was devastated by two World Wars.

During battle it was common military practice for 'daisy cutter' machine guns to strike at the limbs of their attacking enemies as it was clear that nonfatal limb injuries required the expenditure of significant resources and were demoralizing to uninjured soldiers. On the battlefield, sepsis was inevitable and attempts at limb salvage through revascularization were rare. In 1925, Weglowski reported attempts at revascularization in only 51 patients during World War I.[22]

An ironic side note returns us to Alexis Carrel. Because Carrel never sought US citizenship, the French government recalled him when World War I began. Resentful of his success in the USA, the Nobel Prize winner was given the menial task of caring for minor injuries in a railroad yard! Through his political connections in the USA and with funds raised through the Rockefeller Institute, however, he was given permission to establish a hospital facility 8 miles from the front. It was here that he witnessed the devastation of war and recognized the inadequacy of current methods of wound care. He quickly allied himself with the English chemist, Henry Dakin, and the two of them developed Carrel–Dakin solution as a method of preventing wound sepsis without causing wound inflammation. Ironically, the Nobel Prize winner for vascular reconstruction saved the lives of many men who would have otherwise died of sepsis by advocating debridement, early amputation and wound care.

By the early 1940s little progress had been achieved, as illustrated by DeBakey's review of 2471 arterial injuries identified during World War II. Attempt at reconstruction was made in only 54 patients and the success rate was dismal.[23] The fear of infection precluded attempts at vascular repair, and debridement and amputation remained the primary form of treatment.

By the end of World War II, however, the time was ripe for concerted attempts at lower extremity revascularization. The necessary tools of arteriography, anticoagulants, anesthesia and suture technique were readily available, and it was only necessary to assemble the pieces. A persuasive stimulus to do so was unwittingly provided by the French surgeon René Leriche.

Leriche's first experience with arterial surgery came as a medical student in Lyon during his interactions with his chief resident, Alexis Carrel. Later, he served as an infantry surgeon who was in charge of a large receiving hospital. This was the era of France's motorized ambulance brigade, and frequently large numbers of injured men were triaged. Again, the treatment of large bleeding vessels remained ligation, and this spawned Leriche's interest in ischemia, the development of collaterals and the role of sympathectomy.

Leriche is best known for his recognition of aorto-iliac occlusive disease, and he correctly described the associated clinical triad of leg fatigue, impotence and diminished femoral pulses, the syndrome of which still bears his name.[24] He was able to recruit Reynaldo Dos Santos from Lisbon to study these occlusive lesions arterio-graphically.

Later, it was Leriche who provided the stimulus to perform a bypass procedure. In a discussion with Kunlin, he said 'It would be a good thing if we could reunite the ends of the arterial section with a graft'.[25] However, Leriche never mentioned it again, and he remained committed to the technique of arteriectomy and sympathectomy as a means of reversing the arterial ischemia.

At the center of these developments was Jean Kunlin, a young French surgeon who was influenced by his countryman's success with the suturing of blood vessels, the experience of Reynaldo Dos Santos with angiography, and the clinical acumen of Dr Leriche. In the summer of 1948, Leriche performed sympathectomy and femoral arteriectomy on a 54-year-old man with ischemic rest pain and tissue loss. After the operation, he entrusted Kunlin with the care of his patient, as Leriche traveled to present his experience with sympathectomy.

Kunlin noted that the benefit from Leriche's operation was transient; the rest pain returned and the ulcers failed to heal. Kunlin found himself in a precarious position: either to recommend amputation, or to attempt an innovative procedure. On 3 June 1948, he elected the latter, and returned the patient to the operating theater. His initial plan was for an end-to-end anastomosis but the reoperative dissection was difficult, and for safety concerns he decided to perform both proximal and distal anastomoses in an end-to-side fashion. The conduit utilized was a 26 cm segment of reversed greater saphenous vein and was performed from the common femoral artery to the popliteal artery. After the operation, Kunlin observed reactive hyperemia, immediate and longstanding resolution of ischemic symptoms, and subsequent healing of the ulcerations.

Upon Leriche's return to Paris, he was outwardly pleased with the result and later reported the results of the first eight patients treated by this technique to the Academy of Sciences. However, according to Kunlin, the irony of having left town to discuss the merits of sympathectomy while the first successful bypass was performed left Leriche deeply disturbed. Nonetheless, Kunlin remained indebted to Leriche, claiming that the bypass could not have been performed without the enormous influence of his mentor and friend, Professor René Leriche (Fig. 1.5).

EARLY EXPERIENCE IN THE USA

Halsted recognized the clinical significance of venous autograft near the turn of the century. He encouraged one of his residents, Bertram Bernheim, to study Carrel's techniques within the confines of the newly developed Hunterian Laboratory at the Johns Hopkins Hospital.

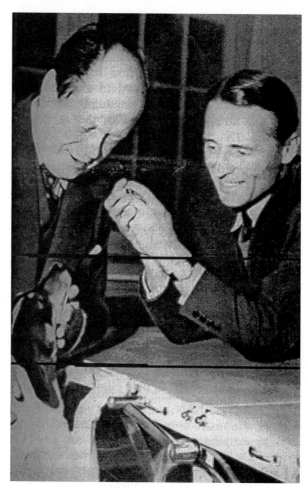

Figure 1.5 *Professor René Leriche and Jean Kunlin in the surgical laboratory of the Clinique Chirurgicale.*

After several months, Bernheim was given his clinical opportunity. In 1906, Dr Halsted summoned Bernheim after a successful resection of a popliteal sarcoma in which it had been necessary to resect the popliteal artery. Bernheim expertly harvested a piece of contralateral greater saphenous vein, reversed it and performed a beautiful proximal anastomosis to the above the knee popliteal artery. When performing the distal anastomosis, however, he chose the distal popliteal vein and created a perfect arteriovenous fistula! As expected, the graft failed to restore distal circulation and thrombosed several hours later. Undaunted, Bernheim persisted in the study of vascular surgery and published a book of techniques of vascular surgery in 1913.[27] The book was published 2 years prior to Bernheim's first successful anastomosis.

In 1949, 35 years after Bernheim's attempt, the first successful bypass in this country was performed by William Holden, on a man with a 5-year history of chronic lower extremity ischemia. Holden conceded that, although the operation seemed radical, it was no more radical than amputating the man's leg.

LATE DEVELOPMENTS

By 1951, Kunlin reported on 17 such cases with continued patency[28] and the utility of the greater saphenous vein conduit became firmly established (Table 1.1). Afterward, explosive growth ensued as surgeons aspired to extend the indications, improve patency and facilitate implantation of the venous autograft.

Table 1.1 *Early series of infrainguinal bypasses*

1951	Fontaine	28 cases
1952	Julian	19 cases
1957	Lord and Stone	21 cases
1959	Dale and DeWeese	31 cases

By the late 1950s several reports appeared that described an anteromedial approach to the infrageniculate popliteal artery. This approach had several advantages over traditional posterior or posteromedial approach: no division of muscles or tendons, simultaneous access to the femoral and the popliteal artery, and little to no trauma to collateral vessels around the knee.[29,30] As a result, the approach facilitated infrageniculate popliteal artery reconstruction and this approach remains the favored approach to the infrageniculate popliteal artery.

As angiography reliably improved the ability to delineate distal vascular anatomy, a groundswell of enthusiasm arose to extend the surgical indications. As early as 1960, anastomoses were reliably performed to tibial vessels utilizing simple magnification and manual suture techniques. Initial critics of the technique argued that revascularization to a single tibial vessel would not maintain limb viability, but this skepticism soon gave way to successful surgical reports.[31]

A stimulus to explore alternative techniques was provided by the mismatch created by attempts to perform reversed saphenous vein bypasses to increasingly smaller distal vessels. There was further speculation that one could reduce vein manipulation and preserve vein blood supply by using an *in situ* technique. It is therefore not surprising that the *in situ* technique was developed simultaneously in two independent centers either by direct excision of the valve leaflets or by introduction of a valvulotome.[32]

Darling's attempts to apply the technique in this country were less successful secondary to associated valvulotome trauma. The *in situ* technique was generally abandoned until it was rediscovered by Leather in 1979. Today, the relative merits of reversed versus *in situ* saphenous vein remain a subject of contention.

CONCLUSIONS

The development of the infrainguinal bypass can be likened to a sleeping giant. Although there were early attempts to arouse the giant, the stimuli were not strong enough and the environment was not ripe. While Carrel provided the technical expertise to perform the procedure 40 years earlier, it was first necessary to develop an understanding of peripheral vascular occlusive disease, methods of proper imaging and anticoagulation, and the proper use of anesthesia, antisepsis and transfusion. With the completion of Kunlin's successful bypass, the giant arose with a fury. In the short time since this historic procedure, the field has progressed at an almost exponential rate as surgeons continue to apply increasingly aggressive approaches to limb salvage.

What will the future hold for such a giant? Will the giant continue to rage as surgeons explore alternative conduits, minimally invasive bypass techniques and attempts to inhibit myointimal hyperplasia, or will the giant be laid to rest by the promise of balloon angioplasty or the development of gene therapy for the prevention of atherosclerosis?

For the present, there is little doubt that the giant is alive and well, and that the future of infrainguinal bypass remains bright. Our challenge as vascular surgeons of the twenty-first century will be to focus our efforts properly by responsibly selecting patients in whom bypass will be most effective. As it becomes clearer that healthcare resources are limited, so too our giant's endurance is finite. Purposeless activity, in terms of ill-advised procedures, may cause ineffectiveness, fatigue and susceptibility to other emerging giants.

REFERENCES

1 Kunlin J. Le traitment de Farterite obliterante par la greffe veineuse. *Arch Mal Coeur* 1949, **42**: 371.

2 Hamby, WB. *The case reports and autopsy reports of Ambrose Paré*. Charles C. Thomas, 1960.

3 Eastcott HHG. *Arterial surgery*. Philadelphia: J.B. Lippincott Co, 1969.

4 Smith S. Studies in experimental vascular surgery. *Surgery* 1945, **18**: 627.

5 Eck N. Ligature of the portal vein. *Voen Med Zh* 1877, **1**: 120.

6 Abbe R. The surgery of the hand. *NY Med J* 1894.

7 Payr E. Beitrage zur Technik der Blutgefässe und nervennaht nebst Mittheilungen uber die verwendung eines resorbirbaren metalles in der Chirurgie. *Arch Klin Chir* 1900, **62**: 67.

8 Jaboulay M, Briau E. Recherches experimentales sur la suture et la greffe arterielle. *Lyon Med* 1896, **81**: 97.

9 Jassinowsky A. Ein Beitrag zur Lehre von der Gefässnaht. *Arch Klin Chir* 1891; **42**: 816.

10 Murphy JB. Resection of arteries and veins injured in continuing end-end suture experimental and clinical research. *Med Rec* 1897, **51**: 73.

11 Carrel A, Guthrie CC. Uniterminal and biterminal transplantation of veins. *Am J Med Sci* 1906, **132**: 415.

12 Haschek E, Lindenthal OT. Ein Beitrag zur praktischen Verwerthung der Photographie nach Roentgen. *Wein Klin Wochenschr* 1896, **9**: 63.

13 Brooks B. Intra-arterial injection of sodium iodide. Preliminary report. *JAMA* 1924, **82**: 1016–19.

14 Moniz E. Uencephalographique arterielle; son importance dans la localization des turneurs cerebrales. *Rev Neurol* 1927, **2**: 172.

15 Dos Santos R, Lanas A, Pereirgi CJ. L'arteriographie des membres de l'aorte et ses branches abdominales. *Bull Soc Nat Chir* 1929, **55**: 587.

16 Howell WH. Two new factors in blood coagulation – heparin and proantithrombin. *Am J Physiol* 1918, **47**: 328.

17 Best CH, Scott C. The purification of heparin. *J Biol Chem* 1933; **102**: 425.

18 Murray G. Heparin in the surgical treatment of blood vessels. *Arch Surg* 1940, **40**: 307.

19 Goyanes J. Neuvos trabajos de chirurgia vascular: substiucion plastica de las arterias por las venas, o arterioplastica venosa, aplicado como neuvo metodo, al traitamiento de los aneurismas. *El Sigo Med* 1906, **53**: 561.

20 Lexer E. Die ideale Operation des arteriellen und des arteriellvenosen Aneurysma. *Arch Klin Chir* 1907, **83**: 458.

21 Pringle JH. Two cases of vein grafting for the maintenance of direct arterial circulation. *Lancet* 1913, **1**: 1795.

22 Weglowski R. Uber die Gefass Transplantation. *Zentralbl Chir* 1925, **52**: 2241.

23 DeBakey ME, Simeone FA. Battle injuries of the arteries in World War II. *Ann Surg* 1946, **123**: 534.

24 Leriche R. De la resection du carrefour aortico-ialaque avec double sympathectornie lombaire pour thrombose arteritique de l'aorte; le syndrome de Fobliteration. *Presse Med* 1940, **48**: 601–4.

25 Kieny R. Rene Leriche and his work, as time goes by. *Ann Vasc Surg* 1990, **2**: 105–11.

26 Kunlin J. Le traitement de l'ischemic arteritique par la greffe veineuse longue. *Rev Chir Paris* 1951; **70**: 206–36.

27 Bernheim BM. *Surgery of the vascular system*. Philadelphia: JB Lippincott Co., 1913.

28 Kunlin J. Treatment of arterial ischemia by long vein grafts. *Rev Chir* 1951, **70**: 206.

29 McCaughan JJ. Surgical exposure of the distal popliteal artery. *Surgery* 1958; **44**: 536–9.

30 Morris GC, DeBakey ME, Cooley DA, Crawford ES. Arterial bypass below the knee. *Surg Gyn Obs* 1959; **108**: 321–32.

31 Tyson RR, DeLaurentis DA. Femrotibial bypass. *Circulation Suppl* 1966; **1**: 1183–88.

32 Hall VK. The greater saphenous vein used in situ as an arterial shunt after extripation of the vein valves. *Surgery* 1962; **51**: 492–5.

2

Noninvasive evaluation of lower extremity ischemia

ANDREW T GENTILE, GREGORY L MONETA AND JOHN M PORTER

INTRODUCTION

Because the differential diagnosis of chronic leg pain is quite broad, the ability to confirm the presence of arterial obstruction and quantify the hemodynamic and physiologic significance of detected lesions is of paramount importance. The noninvasive vascular laboratory has a critical role as an essential adjunct to the history and physical examination in providing an objective, quantitative diagnosis of lower extremity arterial occlusive disease and the functional abnormalities resulting from a decrease in limb blood flow.

HISTORY AND PHYSICAL EXAMINATION

The clinical history provides valuable information in the evaluation of patients with chronic lower extremity pain. In most patients, the clinical history, including questioning for coexistent atherosclerotic risk factors, coupled with the physical examination is all that is necessary to establish the diagnosis firmly of exercise-induced muscular ischemia, intermittent claudication (IC) or ischemic extremity pain at rest.

Patients with exercise-induced leg or buttock pain should be specifically asked the location of the pain, its relationship to walking, the duration and severity of symptoms, the time required for relief of symptoms and symptomatic progression over time. Only exercise-induced muscular pain of the calf, thigh or buttock,

relieved within a few minutes of rest and reliably reproduced by further walking can confidently be improved by lower extremity revascularization. Almost all patients with IC have diminished or absent lower-extremity palpable pulses. Occasionally, however, a patient may give a classic history of vasculogenic claudication yet have palpable pedal pulses at rest. Under these circumstances, exercise testing with postexercise Doppler-measured ankle–brachial systolic blood pressure ratios is critical to confirm the diagnosis of IC (see below).

Ischemic rest pain should be suspected when a patient complains of pain and/or numbness in the forefoot, toes or instep. Rest pain is typically aggravated by elevating the leg and improved by placing the leg in a dependent position. It is usually worsened by exercise. Nocturnal leg cramps, which are frequently associated with lower extremity arterial occlusive disease, are themselves not manifestations of rest pain. However, true ischemic rest pain is frequently worse at night. Afflicted patients will often describe the need to sleep in a chair in order to keep the involved foot dependent, a position that provides some relief from ischemic pain because of gravitational-induced increase in leg blood flow. Because of the need to maintain the foot in a dependent position, many patients with chronic ischemic pain develop significant edema of the symptomatic extremity. It is important to note that edema is not a classic feature of arterial insufficiency but rather reflects prolonged dependency of the ischemic extremity.

In addition to an absence of pedal pulses, patients with rest pain will frequently have thin, atrophic skin of the foot and lower leg, often with dependent rubor and pallor on elevation, and ultimately, areas of cutaneous gangrene and ulceration. If the findings on physical examination are not consistent with atherosclerotic ischemic pain, the physician should carefully inquire about a history of diabetes mellitus or alcoholism, both of which can produce neuropathy with nocturnal foot dysesthetic discomfort similar to ischemic rest pain.

While the history and physical examination are clearly important in establishing the diagnosis of lower extremity arterial insufficiency, the information obtained is by nature subjective and dependent on the skill of the observer. The location and hemodynamic significance of various atherosclerotic lesions can only be grossly approximated by history and physical examination alone. This is clearly inadequate for monitoring individual lesions, and for predicting the magnitude and complexity of any revascularization procedure. For these reasons, together with an increasing appreciation of the importance of arterial hemodynamics in determining and following the outcome of reconstructive procedures, the noninvasive vascular laboratory has assumed a pivotal role in the modern practice of peripheral arterial surgery.

PERIPHERAL VASCULAR LABORATORY

The objectives of modern noninvasive testing of patients with lower extremity arterial occlusive disease are to confirm the presence of arterial ischemia, to provide quantitative, reproducible physiologic data concerning its severity, and to document the location and hemodynamic significance of individual arterial lesions. Two broad categories of noninvasive techniques are used to evaluate lower extremity arterial disease: plethysmography, and various applications of Doppler ultrasound. Each technique has advantages, disadvantages and limitations, an understanding of which is required for the optimal and cost-effective use of the vascular laboratory.

PLETHYSMOGRAPHY

Plethysmography preceded ultrasonography in the evaluation of lower extremity ischemia. Plethysmography is based on the detection of volume changes in the limb in response to arterial inflow. In addition to volume flow, the basic technology can be modified to produce pulse waveforms and determine digital systolic pressures. Mercury strain gauge, air plethysmography (pulse volume recordings), and photoplethysmography have all been used clinically.

VOLUME FLOW

Calf or foot blood flow can be conveniently recorded with a mercury-in-silastic strain gauge. Measurements are based on the detection of minute changes in the electric resistance of the mercury column, which depends on its length. Unfortunately, neither calf nor foot blood flow at rest differ between normal subjects and patients with even severe degrees of arterial insufficiency.[1] Hyperemic flow may be decreased in patients with arterial ischemia when compared with normal subjects, but these changes in volume flow are not routinely used to quantify precise differences in severity of arterial occlusive lesions.[2] For these reasons, measurements of volume flow have not proved useful in the evaluation of chronic lower extremity ischemia.

PULSE VOLUME RECORDINGS

Air plethysmography can be used clinically to demonstrate pulse volume waveforms.[3] These pulse volume recordings are obtained with partially inflated segmental blood pressure cuffs that detect volume changes sequentially down limbs. Volume changes beneath the cuffs resulting from systole and diastole cause small pressure changes within the cuffs, which, with the use of appropriate transducers, can be displayed as arterial waveforms. A normal pulse volume waveform is characterized by a sharp systolic upstroke and peak, and a prominent dicrotic notch on the downward portion of the curve. Such a waveform reflects normal arterial inflow to the portion of the extremity under the cuff. With increasing proximal arterial occlusion, the dicrotic notch is lost and the pulse wave peak becomes rounded with loss of amplitude, and there are nearly equal upstroke and downstroke times. With very severe proximal occlusive disease, the pulse wave may be completely absent.[4] Pulse volume waveforms are generally evaluated in a qualitative fashion based on the shape of the curve with flat, dampened curves considered severely abnormal. Although quantitative interpretative criteria have been proposed, these criteria, which are based on amplitude and contour changes of the pulse volume curves, have not been widely utilized clinically.[5] The lack of reliable, reproducible, quantitative data in pulse volume recordings limits the utility of air plethysmography in the modern practice of vascular surgery.

DIGITAL MEASUREMENTS

Perhaps the greatest current role for plethysmography is in the evaluation of digital pressures and waveforms. Air and strain-gauge, as well as photoplethysmography, can all be adapted for this purpose. Strictly speaking, photoplethysmography is not a method to record volume change; rather a photoelectrode is used to detect changes in cutaneous blood flow. This allows the technique to be readily used in combination with pneumatic cuffs to

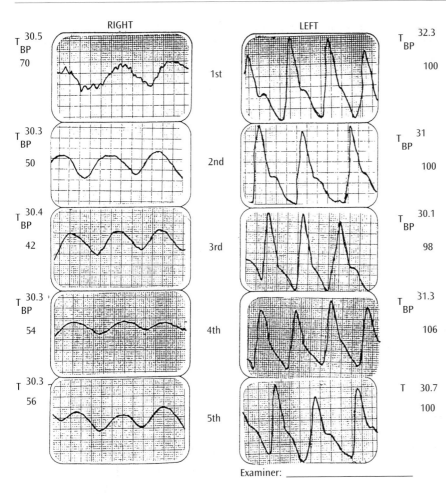

Figure 2.1 *Plethysmographic digital waveforms with individual digit temperature and occlusive pressure. Waveforms on the left extremity are normal. All waveforms on the right extremity reveal flattening consistent with digital artery occlusions.*

detect digital systolic pressures. These techniques are particularly useful in patients with pedal artery occlusive disease or highly calcified vessels, in whom Doppler-derived ankle blood pressures may not accurately reflect true intraluminal arterial pressure because of the relative incompressibility of the arterial walls. The presence of normal digital waveforms in patients with calcified proximal vessels indicates minimal restriction to blood flow despite the calcific arterial disease. Conversely, an obstructive digital waveform in the presence of normal ankle pulses frequently indicates pedal artery occlusive disease, a situation frequently encountered in diabetics or patients with distal atheroembolism (Fig. 2.1).

DOPPLER ULTRASOUND TECHNIQUES

Ultrasound has proved to be the single most important modality in the noninvasive evaluation of lower extremity ischemia. Ultrasound techniques are based on the principle that sound waves emitted from a transducer are reflected at the interface of two surfaces. By coupling the transducer with a receiver, and knowing the transmitting frequency and the acoustical characteristics of the transmitting medium, the reflected ultrasound waves

can be analysed for energy loss and frequency shift by the receiver. With appropriate technology, these reflected waves can then be processed to produce a picture (B-mode image) or a velocity waveform. The generation of velocity waveforms is based on the observation that an ultrasound wave undergoes a frequency shift proportional to the velocity of any moving object (e.g. red blood cells) encountered, the Doppler principle. The reflected waves can be processed into audible signals (continuous-wave Doppler) or displayed as an analog waveform similar to plethysmographically derived waveforms. If the angle between the transmitting ultrasound beam and the flowing blood is known, quantitative measurements of systolic and diastolic blood flow velocities can be derived from the analog waveforms by using the Doppler equation.

ANKLE–BRACHIAL SYSTOLIC BLOOD PRESSURE INDEX

The ankle to brachial systolic pressure ratio is the simplest application of Doppler ultrasound to the noninvasive vascular laboratory and is perhaps also the most useful. With the patient supine, a pneumatic pressure cuff placed just above the ankle is inflated to suprasystolic levels. As the cuff is deflated, a hand-held Doppler probe positioned over the posterior tibial or dorsalis pedis artery distal to the cuff is used to determine the systolic pressure, the cuff pressure at which distal blood flow is first heard using the Doppler probe. The ankle pressure is then divided by the *higher* Doppler-determined brachial artery systolic pressure yielding an ankle–brachial index (ABI). Changes in systolic pressure are used both because they are more sensitive to the presence of arterial occlusive disease than changes in diastolic or mean pressure and because only systolic pressures can be accurately determined with the hand-held Doppler probe. By comparing ankle systolic pressure with brachial artery systolic pressure, the test is independent of day-to-day variations in arterial blood pressure, permitting quantitative comparison by serial examinations.

The ABI serves as an excellent indicator of the overall arterial supply of each lower extremity. A normal ABI is 1.0 to 1.1, with progressively lower values corresponding to worsening arterial disease (Table 2.1). This test, however, has definite limitations. Significant bilateral subclavian or axillary artery occlusive disease may result in a falsely elevated ABI. In addition, patients with long-standing renal failure or diabetes may have medial calcinosis of the popliteal and tibial arteries. These calcified arteries may be inadequately compressed by the ankle pressure cuff resulting in a falsely elevated (suprasystolic) ankle pressure/ABI. Under these circumstances, qualitative analysis of Doppler-derived analog or plethysmographic waveforms or measurement of digital systolic pressures (see above) is more appropriate. Finally, in the presence of severe arterial occlusive disease, no arterial Doppler signal may be audible at the ankle. Under such circumstances, venous signals may be confused with arterial flow signals.

Table 2.1 *Correlation between ankle–brachial index (ABI) and severity of arterial ischemia*

ABI	Clinical status
1.1 ± 0.1	Normal
0.6 ± 0.2	Intermittent claudication
0.3 ± 0.1	Ischemic rest pain
0.1 ± 0.1	Impending tissue necrosis

SEGMENTAL LIMB PRESSURES

Multiple pneumatic cuffs may be used on the leg to determine the arterial blood pressure in different segments of the limb. These segmental leg pressures are compared to each other and to the higher brachial artery systolic pressure. Most laboratories prefer a four-cuff technique. Cuffs

are placed: (1) as far proximal on the thigh as possible; (2) immediately above the knee; (3) just below the knee; and (4) just proximal to the malleoli. Theoretically, each cuff width should be 20 per cent greater than the diameter of the limb at the point of application.[6] This would in most cases necessitate a single, wide, thigh cuff. Use of two cuffs above the knee permits a determination of iliac artery inflow, as well as superficial femoral artery disease. Narrower cuffs may be associated with the measurement of artifactually high pressures and do not permit more accurate disease localization. An awareness of this problem will help avoid confusion in the interpretation of segmental limb pressures.

The examination is performed by using the hand-held Doppler probe to detect the most prominent Doppler signal at the ankle. The high-thigh cuff is inflated first until the Doppler signal at the ankle is no longer audible. The cuff is then deflated and the cuff pressure at which there is return of the Doppler signal at the ankle is the high thigh pressure. The above-knee, below-knee and ankle pressures are determined in a similar fashion. If no Doppler signal is audible at the ankle, the popliteal artery is examined with the Doppler probe. Under such circumstances, only high-thigh and above-knee pressures can be determined. By comparing the pressures at various levels in the leg, one can detect with reasonable accuracy the location of arterial occlusive lesions (Fig. 2.2).

There are a number of potential problems and significant limitations in the interpretation of segmental limb pressures. In addition to cuff-induced artifacts, the high-thigh pressure is subject to particular difficulties in interpretation. Ideally, the high-thigh pressure should reflect iliac artery inflow to the groin. A diminished high-thigh pressure should indicate a pressure-reducing stenosis in the ipsilateral common or external iliac artery. A diminished high-thigh pressure, however, may also reflect a significant common femoral artery stenosis or tandem pressure-reducing lesions in both the profunda femoris and the proximal superficial femoral artery. As noted, calcified arteries may also result in artificially elevated pressures. In patients with multilevel disease, diminished proximal pressures may mask gradients that exist farther down the leg. Finally, segmental pressure gradients give no information as to the nature of the pressure-reducing lesion. No differentiation is possible between short and long-segment occlusions, or between occluded versus patent but highly stenotic arteries.

EXERCISE TESTING

Measurement of Doppler-determined pressures can be combined with treadmill exercise testing, assuming the patient does not have a significant medical contraindication to exercise. After determination of supine resting ankle pressures and ABI, the patient is asked to walk con-

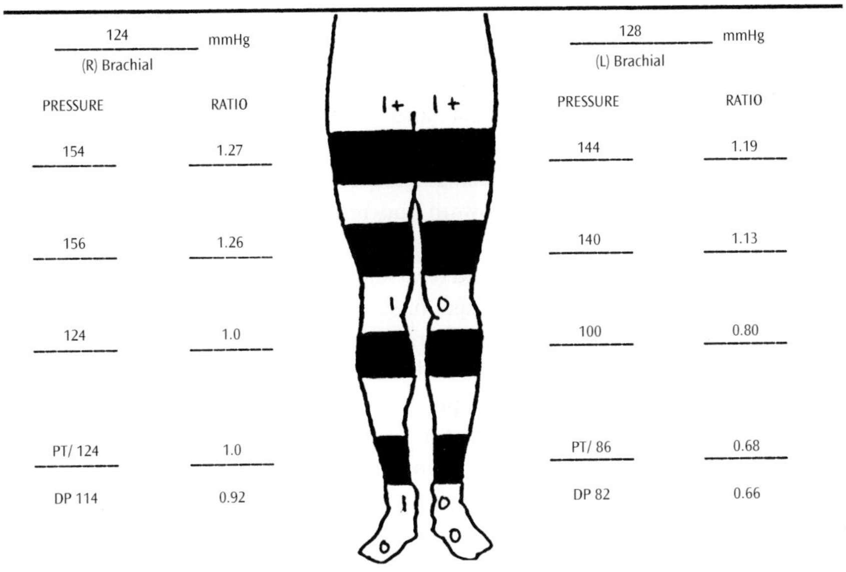

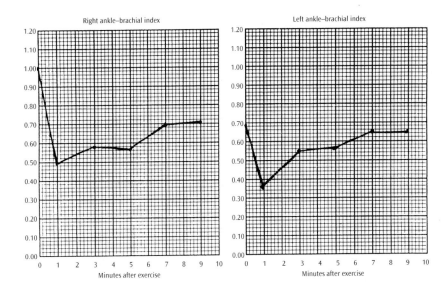

	124	mmHg		128	mmHg
	(R) Brachial			(L) Brachial	
	PRESSURE	RATIO		PRESSURE	RATIO
	154	1.27		144	1.19
	156	1.26		140	1.13
	124	1.0		100	0.80
	PT/ 124	1.0		PT/ 86	0.68
	DP 114	0.92		DP 82	0.66

Figure 2.2 *Vascular laboratory peripheral arterial examination demonstrating Doppler ultrasound-derived segmental limb pressures and ankle–brachial indices in a patient with left calf claudication and left-sided femoral and infrapopliteal occlusive disease.*

tinuously on a treadmill with a 10 per cent incline at a predetermined rate, usually 1.5 mph. The test lasts for 5 minutes or until the patient is forced to stop because of claudication symptoms. The time to onset of symptoms, as well as the location of symptoms, is recorded. At the completion of the test the patient is immediately placed supine and ABIs are determined. If the ABI has dropped from the resting measurement, ABIs are determined every half-minute until they return to normal. The greater the drop in ABI with exercise, and the longer the time required to return to baseline, the worse the patient's arterial occlusive disease (Fig. 2.3).

Whereas many laboratories perform exercise testing in all patients with suspected lower-limb vascular insufficiency, the examination in most patients serves only to confirm the diagnosis suspected by history and physical examination. A patient with classic symptoms of claudication and absent peripheral pulses, combined with a

diminished ABI in the appropriate lower extremity, does not require routine exercise testing for the determination of ABI decrease and recovery. However, exercise testing is indicated in preoperative patients, as the postexercise recovery time of ankle pressure provides an objective assessment of potential postoperative benefit.

Exercise testing is particularly useful in the occasional patient with symptoms of claudication but palpable pedal pulses at rest with a normal or near-normal ABI. Patients with claudication secondary to arterial insufficiency will show a significant decrease in the ABI post-exercise. In our vascular laboratory, the criteria for a positive exercise treadmill test are generally a decrease in the absolute ankle pressure of 20 mmHg or 20 per cent, or a decrease in the ABI of 0.2 in the symptomatic extremity postexercise testing.

With the exception of the rare patient with buttock claudication secondary to isolated internal iliac disease,

Figure 2.3 *Exercise treadmill test curves in a patient evaluated for left leg claudication. Resting pressures are normal on the right side. Postexercise blood pressures reveal a positive dynamic response in both lower extremities with slow recovery of pedal pressures, indicating hemodynamically significant arterial stenosis involving both lower extremities.*

failure of the ABI to decrease 20 per cent with exercise in association with a normal resting ABI substantially rules out arterial insufficiency as the cause of the patient's leg pain. The infrequently encountered condition of spinal stenosis and neurogenic claudication may be confused with arterial ischemia. These patients typically present with symptoms of exercise-induced calf pain, but careful questioning reveals atypical characteristics including occurrence of the pain with standing, occasional pain relief by leaning forward, worsening with coughing and prolonged time requirement for pain abatement after exercise. In these patients, exercise testing reveals normal ankle pressures that do not decrease with exercise despite the onset of the symptoms. Failure of ankle pressures to decrease with exercise may also be a clue to the presence of other uncommon conditions, such as venous claudication and chronic exercise-induced compartment syndromes.

DOPPLER ANALOG WAVEFORM ANALYSIS

Doppler analog waveforms may be obtained using a continuous-wave Doppler probe and analysed in a qualitative fashion analogous to plethysmographic waveforms. Normal lower-extremity Doppler waveforms are triphasic with a reverse flow component in early diastole and low end-diastolic forward flow. The reverse flow component and low overall diastolic velocities reflect a relatively high end-organ resistance to blood flow in the resting extremity. With increasing proximal stenosis, the shape of the waveform changes. Initially, the reverse flow component is lost. With more severe degrees of stenosis, the rate of rise of the systolic upstroke is decreased, the amplitude of the waveform is diminished and diastolic flow increases relative to systolic flow (Fig. 2.4).

The primary clinical application of qualitative Doppler waveform analysis has been in assessing the adequacy of iliac artery inflow to the common femoral artery. An attenuated waveform recorded from the common femoral artery indicates proximal disease. Unfortunately, the technique cannot quantify stenosis or distinguish between iliac stenosis and occlusion. In addition, attenuated waveforms may be caused by superficial femoral artery disease or a combination of inflow and outflow disease.

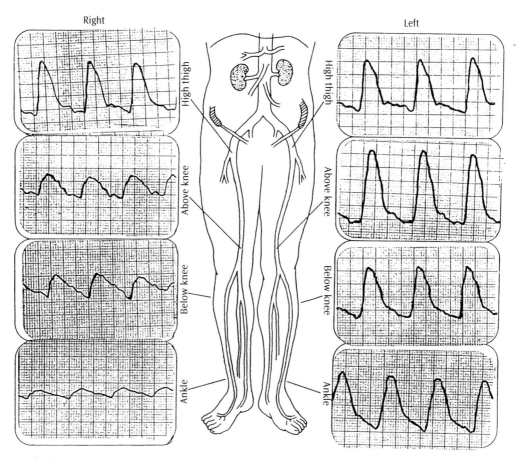

Figure 2.4 *Doppler-derived analog waveforms demonstrating normal triphasic left lower extremity arterial waveforms and flattening of the right-sided waveforms consistent with right side femoropopliteal artery occlusive disease.*

DUPLEX SCANNING

Duplex scanning of the peripheral arteries is the newest development in the noninvasive assessment of lower extremity ischemia. While duplex scanning has been used for many years in the examination of the carotid artery, recent engineering improvements have permitted the development of transducers that permit examination of the peripheral arteries from the aorta through the tibial vessels.

Duplex scanning utilizes both B-mode and pulsed Doppler ultrasound. Hemodynamically significant soft plaques with the same acoustic properties as blood may not be detected with B-mode imaging, but associated flow disturbances are readily detected with the Doppler technique. B-mode imaging does, however, allow visualization of the artery and precise placement of the Doppler sample volume at a known angle to the arterial segment being examined. Knowledge of this angle allows quantitative determinations of frequency shifts (see above). These frequency shifts can then be used to quantify blood flow velocities in normal vessels and to determine the degree of stenosis of individual arterial lesions (Table 2.2). Prospective, blinded evaluation of the classification system detailed in Table 2.2 indicates the duplex examination has an overall sensitivity of 82 per cent, a specificity of 92 per cent, a positive predictive value of 80 per cent, and a negative predictive value of 93 per cent in the determination of a hemodynamically significant peripheral arterial stenosis of >50 per cent diameter reduction.

Equipment and personnel

Color-flow duplex systems greatly aid in the performance of peripheral artery duplex scanning. While not an absolutely necessary component of peripheral artery duplex scanning, the use of color-flow decreases the time required to perform the examination by facilitating identification of the arteries to be examined. This is particularly important when examining the iliac arteries and the popliteal trifurcation. Color-flow can also indicate the length of arterial occlusions and the site of reconstitution of the vessel below its point of occlusion.

Other than characterizing occluded arteries, we do not use color-flow changes alone to predict the degree of stenosis in a peripheral artery. Subocclusive levels of stenosis are determined primarily by velocity waveform analysis.

Because arteries supplying the lower extremity are located at varying distances from the skin surface, peripheral artery duplex scanning requires a selection of transducers. For examining the iliac vessels, a 2 or 3 MHz probe is usually required. The remainder of the examination, down to and including the tibial vessels, can usually be performed with a 5 MHz probe. Occasionally, lower megahertz transducers will also be needed to examine the superficial femoral artery in patients with large thigh diameters.

The use of 'angle-corrected' velocity recordings is a practical necessity in peripheral artery duplex scanning. Because patients vary in their body habitus and the depth of their vessels from the skin surface, it is not possible with current technology to insonate specific vessels at the same angle in all patients. In most current duplex devices, the angle of insonation of the vessel with respect to the sound beam, the so-called Doppler angle, is automatically determined with placement of the cursor by the technologist. The velocity waveform displayed is then based on this angle. While 60° is often sited as the ideal angle of insonation,[7] angles between 30° and 70° are practical for examination of the peripheral arteries and are probably sufficiently accurate for clinical purposes.[8,9]

A complete peripheral artery duplex examination in our laboratory includes the distal aorta, common and external iliac arteries, common femoral artery, origin of the profunda femoris, proximal, mid and distal superficial femoral artery and the popliteal artery. Virtually all patients are also examined below the knee, from the level of the popliteal trifurcation to the ankle. Before aortic examination, whenever possible, patients are examined after fasting for 8–12 hours to reduce abdominal gas. The entire examination is performed with the patient supine, with exception of the popliteal artery, where the patient is examined either prone or in a lateral position. Examination of the tibial arteries is frequently facilitated by beginning near the ankle and following individual vessels proximally. Velocities are recorded from several sites in each vessel and from any site where a flow dis-

Table 2.2 *Duplex ultrasound blood-flow velocities (mean ± standard deviation) of normal lower-extremity arterial segments*[10]

Artery	Peak systolic velocity (cm/s)	Peak reverse flow velocity (cm/s)	Peak diastolic velocity (cm/s)
External iliac	119 ± 21	42 ± 11	18 ± 8
Common femoral	114 ± 25	41 ± 9	16 ± 6
Superficial femoral	91 ± 14	36 ± 8	15 ± 7
Popliteal	69 ± 14	28 ± 9	10 ± 6

turbance is identified. In particular, the technologist should note areas of high peak systolic velocity suggestive of a hemodynamically significant stenosis or areas of marked velocity decrease indicating a more proximal stenosis or occlusion.

Currently, a complete bilateral lower extremity examination in our laboratory using a color-flow scanner with angle correction requires $1–1^1/_2$ hours. Follow-up examinations are often limited to specific arterial segments and require less time. The examination is made more efficient by preduplex physical examination and determination of segmental pressures and exercise testing. Peripheral artery duplex scanning is usually not indicated if the physical examination combined with segmental pressures and exercise testing is normal. However, abnormalities in the physical examination and segmental Doppler pressures can direct the technologist to examine specific areas more intensely with the duplex scanner.

Velocity patterns and classification of stenosis

The normal resting peripheral artery waveform is triphasic with a short reverse-flow component at the beginning of diastole (Fig. 2.5). Because of the high end-organ resistance of the extremity circulation, there is virtually no flow at the end of diastole. Peak systolic velocities steadily decrease from the level of the iliac arteries to the tibial vessels; however, the triphasic waveform is generally maintained for the length of the leg.[10]

The best information concerning the hemodynamic significance of individual lesions in vessels proximal to the popliteal trifurcation is obtained from analysis of blood-flow velocity waveforms. Particular attention is given to the magnitude of peak systolic velocities and the presence or absence of a reverse-flow component. Markedly elevated peak systolic velocities (>100 per cent of the immediate proximal arterial segment) suggests a greater than 50 per cent stenosis at that examination site. Significantly depressed peak systolic velocities and/or the absence of the reverse-flow component implies a pressure and flow-reducing lesion proximal to the examination site.

The original duplex-derived classification of peripheral artery lesions developed at the University of Washington also utilizes spectral broadening in an attempt to discriminate between lesions of 1–19 per cent angiographic stenosis and those with 20–49 per cent angiographic stenosis, as well as higher degrees of arterial stenosis[11] (Table 2.3). While it is clear that such distinctions can be made, it must be remembered that assessment of spectral broadening requires reference to a set of standards developed at a constant Doppler angle.[12] Because maintaining a constant Doppler angle is frequently not possible in peripheral artery duplex scanning, the analysis of varying degrees of spectral broadening is often impractical in routine clinical peripheral artery duplex examinations.

It is important to note the relatively high standard deviations of the mean velocities obtained in normal individuals. Velocities and waveforms vary somewhat with cardiac output, arterial inflow and outflow resistance. Each patient must be considered independently and waveforms carefully analysed immediately proximal and distal to an area suspicious for a flow-reducing lesion.

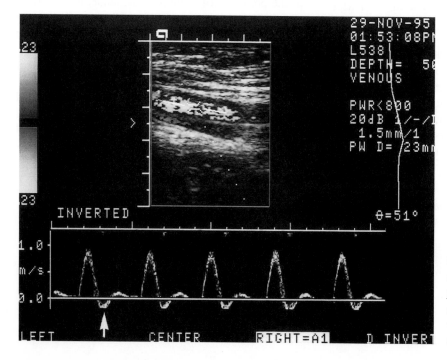

Figure 2.5 *Duplex ultrasound-derived image and velocity waveforms from a normal common femoral artery. Note the normal triphasic waveform with reverse flow in early diastole (arrow).*

Table 2.3 *University of Washington duplex criteria for determination of peripheral arterial stenosis*[10]

Degree of stenosis (%)	Criteria
0	Normal waveform and velocities
1–19	Normal waveform and velocities with spectral broadening
20–49	Marked spectral broadening, 30% increase in peak systolic velocity
50–99	Marked spectral broadening, 100% increase in peak systolic velocity, loss of reverse diastolic flow component of waveform
Occluded	No detectable flow signal in well-visualized artery

We currently image and evaluate tibial arteries in only a semiquantitative fashion. Examination of these vessels can be quite difficult, especially if there is significant proximal disease. Under these circumstances, velocities in angiographically normal tibial arteries may be < 10 cm/s and the vessels are difficult to follow even with a color-flow scanner.

The principal advantage of duplex scanning over other noninvasive methods of assessment of peripheral arterial occlusive disease is that it allows direct point-by-point examination of the artery under study. It is therefore possible to map the location of hemodynamically significant lesions precisely and noninvasively. In addition, the technique allows discrimination between stenotic and occlusive lesions. The development of color-flow imaging combined with Doppler permits rapid and accurate mapping of the lengths of arterial occlusions.[13] Although not currently in widespread use, peripheral artery duplex scanning has a number of potentially important clinical applications. Duplex scanning of peripheral arteries permits direct evaluation of the sites of endovascular procedures, such as transluminal angioplasty, thereby providing objective, noninvasive evaluation of the efficacy and durability of such procedures. In addition, it may be possible to screen patients with symptomatic lower-extremity arterial disease for the presence of obstructive lesions that can be readily treated by a local surgical procedure or transluminal angioplasty. Duplex scanning may eventually be able to calculate pressure gradients across iliac artery stenosis, which may be important in predicting the extent of arterial reconstruction required to relieve lower extremity ischemic symptoms.

Color-flow scanning also provides the potential for tibial artery mapping, but this has not been systematically evaluated to date. Presently, angiography remains essential for the definition of arterial anatomy in the distal part of the leg in sufficient detail to permit optimal surgical planning.

SUMMARY

The noninvasive vascular laboratory provides critically important objective and cost-effective information to supplement a careful history and physical examination in the evaluation of patients with chronic lower extremity ischemia. Optimal cost-effective ordering and interpretation of vascular tests will always depend on a sophisticated knowledge of vascular disease and detailed knowledge of the individual patient. A keen awareness of the limitations of each form of testing and potential sources of error is mandatory. Noninvasive vascular testing allows quantitative, physiologic assessment of lower extremity ischemia and provides the scientific basis for modern therapeutic approaches to the care of patients with arterial occlusive disease. Clearly, the vascular laboratory provides the objective diagnostic foundation on which the modern practice of vascular surgery is built.

REFERENCES

1 Yao JST, Nedham TN, Gourmos C *et al*. A comparative study of strain gauge plethysmography and Doppler ultrasound in the assessment of occlusive arterial disease of the lower extremities. *Surgery* 1972; **71**: 4–9.

2 Yao JST, Flinn WR. Plethysomgraphy. In: Kempczinski RF, Yao JST eds *Practical noninvasive vascular diagnosis*, 2nd edn. Chicago: Yearbook Medical Publishers, 1987: 80–94.

3 Darling RC, Raines JK, Brener BF *et al*. Quantitative segmental pulse volume recorder: a clinical tool. *Surgery* 1972; **72**: 873–87.

4 Strandness DE Jr. *Peripheral arterial disease: a physiologic approach*. Boston: Little Brown Publishers, 1969: 112–30.

5 Kempczinski RF. Segmental volume plethysomgraphy: the pulse volume recorder. In: Kempczinski RF, Yao JST eds *Practical noninvasive vascular diagnosis*. Chicago,: Yearbook Medical Publishers, 1987: 140–53.

6 Krikendall WM, Burton AC, Epstein FH *et al*. Recommendations for human blood pressure determination by sphygomanometers: Report of a subcommittee of the postgraduate education committee, American Heart Association. *Circulation* 1967; **36**: 980–8.

7 Beach KW, Lawrence R, Phillips DJ, Primozich J, Strandness DE Jr. The systolic velocity criterion for diagnosing significant internal carotid artery stenosis. *J Vasc Tech* 1990; **13**: 65–8.

8 Rizzo RJ, Sandanger G, Astelford P *et al*. Mesenteric flow velocity variations as a function of angle of insonation. *J Vasc Surg* 1990; **11**: 688–94.

9 Thiele BL, Strandness DE Jr. Duplex scanning and ultrasonic arteriography in the detection of carotid disease. In: Kempczinski RF, Yao JST eds *Practical noninvasive vascular diagnosis*, 2nd edn. Chicago: Yearbook Medical Publishers, 1987: 339–63.

10 Jager KA, Phillips DJ, Martin RL *et al*. Noninvasive mapping of the lower limb arterial lesions. *Ultrasound Med Biol* 1985; **11**: 515–21.

11 Jager KA, Ricketts HJ, Strandness DE Jr. Duplex scanning for evaluation of lower limb arterial disease. In: Bernstein EF ed. *Noninvasive diagnostic techniques in vascular disease*. St Louis: CV Mosby, 1985: 619–31.

12 Beach KW, Strandness DE Jr. Carotid artery velocity waveform analysis. In: Bernstein EF ed. *Noninvasive diagnostic techniques in vascular disease*. St Louis, CV Mosby, 1985: 409–22.

13 Cossman DV, Ellison JE, Wagner WH *et al*. Comparison of contrast arteriography to arterial mapping with color-flow duplex imaging in the lower extremities. *J Vasc Surg* 1989; **10**: 522–9.

3

Preoperative vascular imaging

JULIE M ZAETTA

INTRODUCTION

Lower extremity (LE) arteriography remains the gold standard for evaluation of patients with symptomatic peripheral vascular disease. In the past, the primary goal of LE arteriography was to provide high-quality diagnostic images. However, in the past several decades, percutaneous interventions have become more common and there has been a growing trend in the surgical arena away from primary amputations toward limb salvage procedures.[1–3] To construct a successful distal bypass, the surgeon needs a highly accurate preoperative depiction of the arterial anatomy. Although the contribution of pedal arch patency with respect to long-term graft patency is controversial, accurate delineation of pedal arteries is critically important since such vessels may serve as outflow for distal bypasses, especially in diabetic patients. Furthermore, it has been suggested that outcome of both percutaneous endovascular and surgical procedures are greatly affected by the presence or absence of distal pedal outflow.[4–7] Failure to identify a status amendable to recanalization properly may result in unnecessary amputations; failure to diagnose poor pedal outflow may result in unnecessary interventions or suboptimal procedures with high failure rates.

Today's angiographer must be familiar with techniques used to improve distal arterial visualization and must be able to tailor the examination to each individual patient. A thorough pre-angiographic clinical assessment becomes a necessity. The interventionalist will then be able to address the needs of the patient, plan for any possible therapeutic interventions and provide an accurate arterial road-map to the vascular surgeon. A well-performed, LE arteriogram will limit the need for intra-operative diagnostic studies, improve endovascular and surgical procedural outcomes and hopefully prevent unnecessary amputations.

PRE-ANGIOGRAPHIC EVALUATION

The importance of preprocedural assessment cannot be overemphasized. Performing a thorough evaluation makes it much less likely that an inappropriate angiogram or therapeutic procedure will be performed.[8] The clinical assessment of a patient with peripheral vascular disease can be broken down into the history, physical examination, laboratory tests and the vascular laboratory findings. Since atherosclerosis is the most common cause of LE arterial occlusive disease, knowledge of the risk factors (Table 3.1) predisposing a patient to atherosclerosis is essential. In addition, a history of the patient's symptoms and previous pertinent surgical procedures, such as bypass graft placement, should also be obtained. Once the ischemic process has been clinically characterized, the anatomic level of disease and the severity of the ischemia should be delineated by a physical examination, which includes assessment of the peripheral pulses. This will determine if a conventional common femoral artery approach is possible or if alternative arterial access must be pursued.

The patient's hematologic and renal status should be reviewed prior to the angiogram. Laboratory testing has been a common aspect of the preprocedural evaluation

Table 3.1 *Risk factors for atherosclerotic peripheral vascular disease*

Cigarette smoking
Hypertension
Diabetes mellitus
Lipid abnormalities
Male gender
Vascular disease in other beds
    Cerebrovascular
    Coronary

Modified from Bierman EL. Disorders of the vascular system. In: Isselbacher KJ *et al.* eds *Harrison's principles of internal medicine*, 13th edn. New York: McGraw-Hill Inc., 1994: 1106–11.

of patients undergoing vascular radiology procedures.[9] However, in the present cost-restrictive healthcare environment, the use of routine preprocedure testing has been called into question. Many studies show that routine laboratory testing is not the most effective way of evaluating patients. Although laboratory testing can aid in optimizing the patient's condition once a disease is suspected or diagnosed, it is ineffective in screening for asymptomatic disease.[10,11]

A baseline assessment of renal function may be important prior to LE angiography. Routine screening is rarely indicated because the clinical history will suggest the need for further evaluation. However, patients with a history of pre-existing renal insufficiency or diabetes will require blood urea nitrogen and creatinine tests. These patients are at increased risk for developing acute renal failure following the administration of iodinated contrast agents.[12,13]

Although often ordered prior to arteriography, routine studies of hemostatic function are probably unnecessary for vascular procedures such as angiography and angioplasty, with the exception of thrombolytic procedures. Thrombolytic procedures are more complicated. The risk of major bleeding is higher, reported at 3–23 per cent.[14] Bleeding is most frequently from the puncture sites but it may occur remotely and hidden from view. Because thrombolytic procedures are associated with an increased risk of bleeding complications that may be difficult to recognize rapidly, and due to the potentially life-threatening nature of such complications, routine screening with baseline hemoglobin, hematocrit, platelet count, prothrombin time (PT), and partial prothrombin time (PTT) is warranted. The best preprocedural screen to predict bleeding is a carefully conducted history, including previous dental, surgical, drug and family history.[15] Any suggestion of a bleeding disorder should be evaluated with a bleeding time, platelet count, PT, and PTT. As a rule of thumb, arteriography should be avoided if the international normalized ratio (INR) is greater than 1.5 or if the platelet count is less than 50 000 platelets/mm^3 (see ref. 16).

The vascular laboratory examination, often referred to as 'noninvasive' evaluation, is an essential part of the preprocedure assessment. Peripheral vascular laboratory (PVL) testing, provides objective, reproducible data for the initial and postprocedural hemodynamic evaluation of patients with peripheral vascular disease. Pulse volume recordings, Doppler waveform analysis and segmental limb pressures are all excellent physiologic modalities for assessing arterial insufficiency.[17] Exercise testing is also an important component of peripheral vascular arterial studies, particularly in the assessment of patients with claudication. The ability to reproduce clinical symptomatology associated with a significant fall in ankle–brachial index allows confirmation of a vascular etiology of the symptoms.[18] Finally, familiarity with the PVL results allows the interventionalist to formulate a treatment plan, and to inform patients of therapeutic options and their potential for success.

DIAGNOSTIC ANGIOGRAPHY

Over the past decade there has been a technical evolution in the manner in which diagnostic angiography is performed in this country. Conventional screen-film angiography has given way to computer-generated digital subtraction angiography (DSA).[19] When originally developed, DSA used intravenously injected contrast medium.[20] This technique has virtually disappeared from most departments, being replaced by the less problematic intra-arterial DSA.[21] In patients with renal insufficiency or an allergy to iodinated contrast medium, alternative contrast agents, such as carbon dioxide and gadolinium, are now being utilized. Finally, the trend towards less invasive procedures has provided the impetus for the use of magnetic resonance angiography (MRA) as a diagnostic method for peripheral vascular disease (PVD).

CONVENTIONAL FILM ANGIOGRAPHY

While still available in many departments, conventional film angiography is rapidly yielding to DSA. Conventional films may be individual film sheets or continuous rolls placed in rapid film changers. These devices permit up to six films per second to be obtained. During LE arteriography, moving step tables can be used to shift the patient position over a single injection, thereby chasing the bolus of contrast as it flows through the vascular bed.

Doses of contrast media and their rates of injection vary considerably with the procedure being performed but, in general, are greater when compared with newer DSA techniques. Selective catheter placement ensures the best opacification of vessels while allowing the least amount of contrast to be used. Once the vessel of interest is selected, a test injection of contrast is made to gauge the flow, which in turn dictates the injection rate. Too rapid an injection rate will result in contrast reflux into nontarget areas with diminished opacification of the region under investigation. The duration of the injection is tailored to the size of the vascular bed and the lesion under investigation. The total dose of contrast medium should ideally not exceed 3–5 ml/kg of body weight, and it should be kept to a minimum in patients with renal insufficiency, cardiac dysfunction or myeloma.[12,13,22]

Once the catheter is positioned in the appropriate vessel, a scout film is obtained to evaluate film technique and patient position. The catheter is then attached to a power injector and the injection parameters are set. Ideally, filming rates must take into account the normal variations within the body, since total flow and circulation rates vary with the target organ's functions and demands. In areas of rapid flow, film rates of 2–3 films per second are normally used. Alternatively in regions of sluggish flow, such as in atherosclerotic lower extremity vessels, filming for periods of 45 seconds or longer may be necessary.

In most cases a single projection is adequate for diagnosis. However, in the workup of abdominal aortic aneurysms, trauma or complex atherosclerotic stenoses, orthogonal oblique, or anteroposterior (AP) and lateral views may be necessary to avoid overlooking posterior wall lesions (Fig. 3.1).[23,24] This requires separate injections for each additional view, which adds contrast, cost and time to the examination.

Advantages of conventional screen-film angiography include high-spatial resolution and, because of the short exposure times and nondependence on subtraction, problems of patient motion are reduced, particularly when imaging the abdomen. The major disadvantages are that all the films must be developed and reviewed before additional contrast injections or views are obtained. This adds considerable time to the examination. In addition, the nature of filming lends itself to a large number of superfluous films being exposed and therefore higher costs.

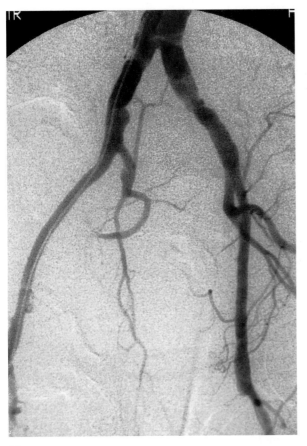

(a)

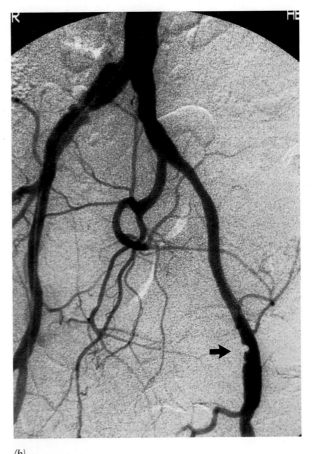

(b)

Figure 3.1 *(a) Right posterior oblique projection: occlusion of right superficial femoral artery at its origin with apparent patency of the CFA and the profunda origin. (b) Left posterior oblique projection: posterior plaque of the right common femoral artery is uncovered (arrow).*

DIGITAL ANGIOGRAPHY

Advances in technology and computer applications have made digital angiography the current technique of choice for diagnostic angiography in most radiology departments. Refinements have occurred mainly in the areas of data acquisition, postprocessing manipulation and film storage. Subtraction angiography is a technique in which the first contrast-free image of an angiographic series is used as a mask that is superimposed on a subsequent image of a contrast-filled blood vessel, effectively eliminating the background image and leaving only the contrasted vessel visible. DSA is a computerized version of this technique (Fig. 3.2).[25] Advantages include the ability to review the images immediately, and electronically manipulate them to change the contrast and window levels, integrate frames, and compensate for a certain amount of patient motion (Fig. 3.3).[26] Originally described using the intravenous injection of contrast, DSA today is performed almost exclusively using intra-arterial contrast injection. Intra-arterial DSA surmounts many of the problems associated with intravenous DSA. Specifically, intra-arterial studies are less subject to patient motion, utilize smaller doses of contrast medium and are less dependent on cardiac output.[21,27] While intravenous DSA has virtually disappeared from most departments, it remains a viable option if no arterial access site is readily available. On occasion, such as with aortic occlusion, intravenous DSA actually provides better images since *all* of the collaterals are filled, as opposed to only those below the intra-arterial catheter position.[20]

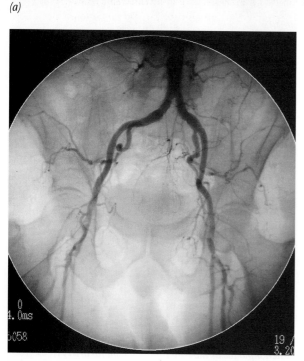

(a)

(b)

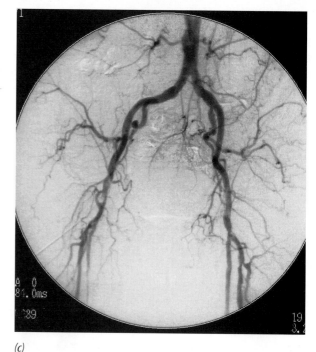

(c)

Figure 3.2 *Subtraction angiography. (a) Mask film: pelvis radiograph without angiographic contrast medium. (b) Pelvic angiogram with contrast medium. (c) Subtraction angiogram: (a) + (b) background subtracted leaving only contrasted vessels visible.*

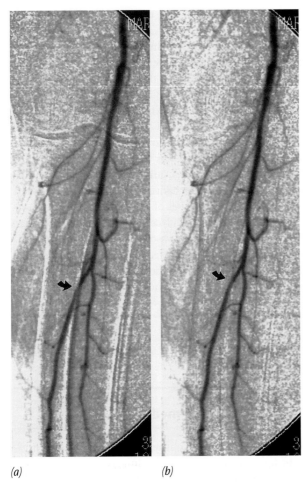

(a)   (b)

Figure 3.3 *(a) Trifurcation angiogram demonstrates occlusion of the anterior tibial artery at its origin, with run-off being through the peroneal and posterior tibial (PT) arteries. Patient motion obscures the proximal pt artery (arrow). (b) Patient motion eliminated with computer-assisted pixal shifting. Proximal PT artery is free of significant disease (arrow).*

LOWER EXTREMITY INTRA-ARTERIAL DSA: A TAILORED APPROACH

Optimizing the lower extremity arteriogram requires knowledge of various techniques to augment visualization, as well as the ability to apply them to the individual patient. These methods begin with the preprocedure assessment, which dictates the choice of puncture site and the type of arteriogram to be performed. Augmentation techniques include increasing the amount of delivered contrast.

In general, the status of the iliac arteries, which has been determined by the preprocedure assessment, dictates the access site. In patients with aortoiliac disease, in most cases, an approach ipsilateral to mort symptomatic side is desired: (1) anticipating the need for measurement of pressures; (2) anticipating the possible need for

percutaneous transluminal angioplasty (PTA); and (3) and avoiding puncture of healthy leg. In the case of a nonpalpable femoral artery pulse, bony landmarks or ultrasound guidance may be useful to facilitate access. Measurement of aortoiliac pressure gradients at rest and after vasodilator injection is important, particularly in patients with claudication or prior to infrainguinal bypass graft placement. The drop in peripheral vascular resistance with vasodilatation distal to a stenotic lesion results in increased capacitance below the site of narrowing and increased flow demand. This is manifested by a pressure gradient sometimes not evident without exercise or vasodilatation. If patient assessment has revealed infrainguinal disease, a contralateral femoral access on the asymptomatic side is often preferred, although the option of antegrade puncture remains.

Increased visualization of the distal vessels can be achieved by increasing the amount of contrast medium delivered to the vessel in question. This can be accomplished in several ways. Most angiographers simply increase the volume of contrast material injected or perform a more selective arteriogram. Another available technique is to perform inflow balloon occlusion angiography. Pharmacoangiography with nitroglycerine or papaverine can also be utilized to induce peripheral vasodilatation.

For standard, bilateral, lower extremity arteriogram, a pigtail catheter is placed at the iliac bifurcation, and contrast is power injected and visualized as it flows through the vascular bed. The volume of contrast injected will depend on the degree of vascular disease that is suspected from preprocedural assessment.[28,29] The contrast volume should be sufficient to visualize the lower extremity arteries to the level of the metatarsals. An unopacified artery should not be considered occluded unless there is adequate opacification of adjacent collaterals (Fig. 3.4).[30] It has been shown that using larger volumes of contrast medium will lead to better opacification.[31] Therefore, just increasing the contrast volume often yields better visualization. However, the rate of injection should not be increased as this can result in unnecessary reflux. Larger contrast volumes result in increased patient discomfort if ionic contrast agents are used. Therefore, use of a low osmolality or iso-osmolar agent is recommended since they produce less subjective patient discomfort.[32] An additional advantage associated with less patient discomfort is less patient motion.

A second method to increase distal opacification is to inject the contrast material more selectively. In patients with asymmetric vascular disease, contrast will flow preferentially down the extremity with less disease. For example, an injection performed at the iliac bifurcation will result in better opacification of the less diseased extremity. Selective catheter injection can avoid this problem. Specifically, the catheter should be selectively positioned in the affected extremity external iliac artery

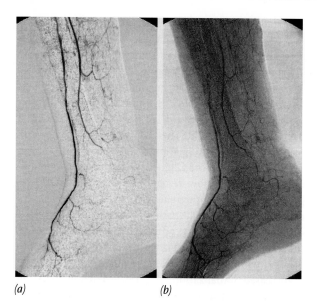

(a)   *(b)*

Figure 3.4 *(a) Inadequate contrast enhancement. Lack of arterial opacification beyond the ankle joint makes it impossible to determine the patency of the plantar arch. (b) Satisfactory contrast enhancement. Filling of collaterals along the hindfoot confirms posterior tibial artery occlusion.*

or distally if possible. This will result in better opacification of the affected extremity.[31,33] Occasionally, when there is an ipsilateral common or external iliac occlusion and poor collateralization from the contralateral pelvis, it may be necessary to perform an ipsilateral common femoral arterial puncture. This will allow optimal opacification of the distal vessels, which may not otherwise be well opacified.

An infrequently used technique, balloon occlusion angiography, can also increase opacification of the distal blood vessels. First described in 1974 by Morettin,[34] this technique involves placing an occlusion balloon in the affected extremity external iliac artery and injecting contrast distal to the balloon. This in effect results in less contrast dilution from inflowing arterial blood. While some authors have indicated that this technique results in superior distal opacification, a more recent study suggests the increased opacification is due to the selective position of the catheter.[31,34,35]

Another method to augment contrast flow to the distal arteries is to use reactive hyperemia or vasodilators, such as nitroglycerine, tolazoline, prostaglandin E1 and papaverine. To induce reactive hyperemia, a blood pressure cuff is placed on the distal thigh and inflated to 50 mmHg above the systolic level for a period of 3–5 minutes. Maximal vasodilatation occurs approximately 10 seconds following release of the cuff in response to the accumulation of metabolites in the bloodstream. The contrast medium is injected at this point and greatly increases the circulation rate in the area of interest. At

least one study found that reactive hyperemia was far superior to pharmacologic methods.[36] Tolazoline is a potent vasodilator with a duration of action of several minutes. For bilateral lower extremity arteriography, usually 25 mg of tolazoline diluted in 10 ml of saline is injected slowly through the catheter immediately prior to filming. If only a single extremity is being imaged, the dose should be reduced to 12.5 mg.[37] Full knowledge of the patient's overall cardiovascular status is recommended, for this drug has the potential of inducing hypotension, tachycardia, arrhythmias and myocardial infarction.[33] A safe alternative vasodilator is nitroglycerine. Administered in doses of 100 mg, some investigators have reported that nitroglycerine is more effective than tolazoline in producing vasodilatation and is approximately equivalent to the effects of reactive hyperemia.[38] Probably the most inexpensive and underutilized method of distal vasodilatation is warming of the lower extremity.[33] Clearly, this approach is somewhat cumbersome.

CONTRAST MEDIA

Iodinated contrast media

During angiography, contrast media is injected intra-arterially to render visible images of the lumen. Contrast-mediated associated nephrotoxcity (CM-AN) is a well-documented complication after the administration of contrast media.[39] Chronic renal insufficiency has been identified in numerous studies to be the most important risk factor predisposing to CM-AN. This is a well-documented risk factor, even in the absence of diabetes mellitus. The reported incidence varies widely but appears to be directly proportional to the severity of renal insufficiency.[40] However, several studies demonstrated that patients with chronic renal insufficiency, especially if mild and if under proper preparation and management, can safely undergo intravascular contrast media studies.[40]

Diabetes mellitus is a frequently cited risk factor for CM-AN. However, more detailed analysis shows that most or all of the increased risk results from associated chronic renal insufficiency. Some studies have indicated that diabetics without renal insufficiency are at little or no increased risk. On the other hand, the association of diabetes mellitus with chronic renal insufficiency poses a substantial risk of contrast-induced nephropathy ranging from 10 to 40 per cent in those with mild to moderate renal failure and 50 to 90 per cent in diabetics with severe chronic renal failure.[12,39]

Over the past decade, low osmolality and iso-osmolar (Visipaque) contrast agents have become available. These newer agents, by virtue of their lower osmolality, cause fewer physiologic alterations during injection, produce less pain or discomfort, and are associated with fewer adverse reactions than conventional ionic contrast media. In addition, a recent meta-analysis concluded that lower osmolality contrast agents are less nephrotoxic in patients with azotemia than high-osmolality contrast media.[41]

Previous studies in the literature have reported variable results with regard to the efficacy of mannitol or furosemide administration to prevent CM-AN. In a recent prospective clinical trial, Solomon et al.[42] compared the prophylactic value of saline hydration alone with that of saline plus mannitol and saline plus furosemide in 78 patients with chronic renal insufficiency, undergoing cardiac angiography. All patients received 0.45 per cent saline for 12 hours before and 12 hours after angiography. Mannitol and furosemide were given just before angiography. Results showed that patients receiving saline alone had a lower incidence of CM-AN when compared to those patients receiving mannitol or furosemide. Since this represents the best, unbiased trial data currently available, it is recommended that high-risk patients be adequately hydrated prior to contrast angiography.

CARBON DIOXIDE DIGITAL SUBTRACTION ANGIOGRAPHY

Carbon dioxide (CO_2) as an imaging agent was originally used for the visualization of the abdominal viscera.[43] With the development of DSA, stacking software, tilting tables and reliable delivery systems, it has become a viable alternative imaging agent for patients with azotemia or an allergy to iodinated contrast agents.[44]

Carbon dioxide is a nontoxic, invisible gas that is highly compressible, nonviscous and buoyant. Most importantly, CO_2, as an intravascular imaging agent, lacks both allergic potential and renal toxicity. Unlike iodinated contrast, CO_2 does not mix with blood but displaces it to produce an image. When injected, the buoyancy of CO_2 causes it to rise to the anterior, nondependent portion of the vessel. Consequently, a potential deficiency arises in imaging larger diameter vessels (aorta and iliac arteries); if an insufficient volume is injected, there is incomplete displacement of blood, diminished contrast and potentially a spurious image. Normal vessels may appear smaller then their true caliber. To overcome this problem, either a larger amount of CO_2 must be administered or, using the buoyancy principle, the area of interest should be placed in the nondependent position.[45,46]

CO_2 has been used primarily in patients with iodinated contrast allergy and renal failure; however, its gaseous characteristics and low viscosity permit detection of small collaterals in lower extremity arterial ischemic disease. Furthermore, there is no maximum dose if less than 100 ml is injected every 2–4 minutes, since CO_2 dissipates rapidly as carboxyhemoglobin.[45,46]

Because CO_2 is invisible, it is susceptible to contamination without detection. Therefore, a pure medical-grade source and a disposable CO_2 cylinder are mandatory. Furthermore, a closed delivery system is imperative to eliminate the additional possibility of room contamination. Currently, there is only one safe delivery mechanism approved for use in the USA.[47] A rare, yet potential complication is 'trapping'. This occurs when an excessive volume of CO_2 is delivered. Because of buoyancy, it usually occurs in the nondependent portion of a vessel. As a result, a bolus of gas can cause a vapor lock, which can potentially restrict blood flow and cause ischemia. Abdominal aortic aneurysms, pulmonary outflow tracts, and celiac, superior mesenteric and inferior mesenteric arteries are most susceptible because of their nondependent location. If trapping does occur, it can be reduced by positional maneuvers. As a precaution for trapping, fluoroscopy of susceptible sites can be performed between CO_2 injections. If persistent gas is visualized or, if the patient experiences abdominal pain, positional changes can be instituted.[48,49]

GADOLINIUM DIGITAL SUBTRACTION ANGIOGRAPHY

Another alternative contrast agent that has been used with increasing frequency in recent years is gadolinium (Gd). Initial experience with the use of intra-arterial Gd in doses up to 0.3 mmol/kg suggest that Gd may be less nephrotoxic than iodinated contrast in patients with renal insufficiency.[50] Disadvantages include the low concentration of gadolinium (0.5 mmol/ml), which makes it difficult to visualize during fluoroscopy, and its toxicity, which constrains the study of larger vessels. Therefore, the use of full-strength Gd and high-quality DSA is mandatory (Fig. 3.5). Selective extremity Gd-DSA can be performed using the same injection rates and doses that would be used if iodinated contrast medium were being injected. Diligent selective catheterization affords the most optimal images.[51]

PERIPHERAL MAGNETIC RESONANCE ANGIOGRAPHY

There is considerable interest in developing noninvasive techniques for the preoperative evaluation of the pedal vessels, especially since the accuracy of standard preoperative angiography for assessing patency of distal infrainguinal vessels has been questioned.[52] Recent studies have shown that MRA provided information not found with conventional DSA in up to 22 per cent of cases.[53,54] In one clinical study, this altered clinical management in 17 per cent of cases. Successful bypass operations, which would not otherwise have been considered feasible, were performed.[54]

A comprehensive description of the physics of MRA is beyond the scope of this chapter. In short, MRA capitalizes on the high signal of inflowing nonsaturated (not exposed to the magnetic field) blood on gradient echo images causing flowing blood to be the highest intensity object. By suppressing background stationary tissue and only focusing on the high signal of flowing blood, one can obtain an image, which depicts only vascular structures. The most commonly used MRA pulse sequence for evaluating lower extremity arteries is two-dimensional time-of-flight (2D TOF) (Fig. 3.6). This sequence is ideally suited to depict the slow, unidirectional, nonpulsatile flow in reconstituted vessels distal to severe stenoses or occlusions.

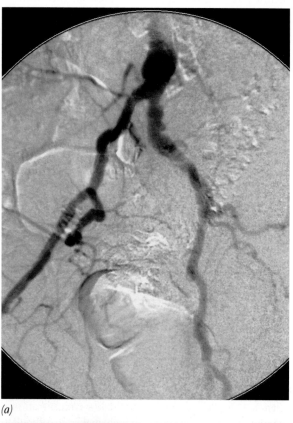

(a)

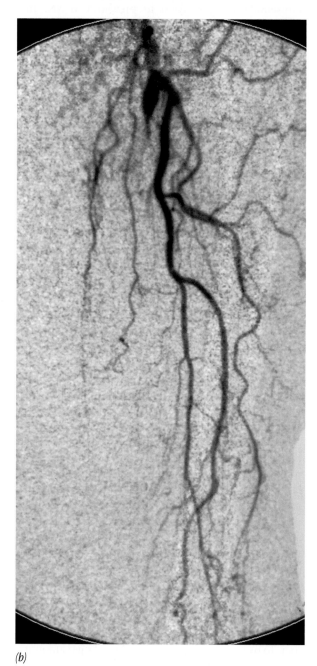

(b)

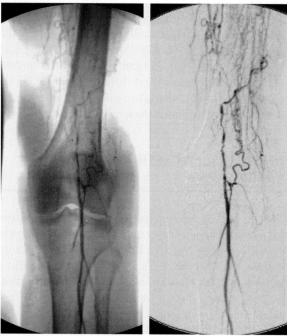

(c)

Figure 3.5 *(a–c) Gadolinium digital subtraction angiography reveals left SFA occlusion with reconstitution of the above-knee popliteal artery.*

Although there are multiple reports in the literature attempting to compare MRA to contrast angiography, the studies are inconclusive because of differing techniques, parameters of evaluation, equipment and diagnostic experience. In the most current studies using up-to-date software and optimizing scan parameters, MRA was fairly accurate in demonstrating occlusions (Fig. 3.7), distinguishing short- from long-segment disease, and correctly identifying the level of reconstitution

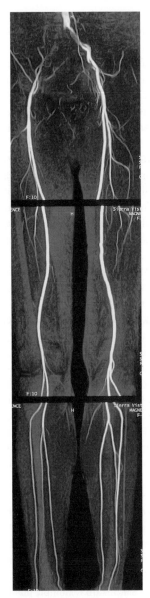

Figure 3.6 *Coronal maximum intensity projection (MIP) of TD TOF magnetic resonance angiogram of the lower extremities.*

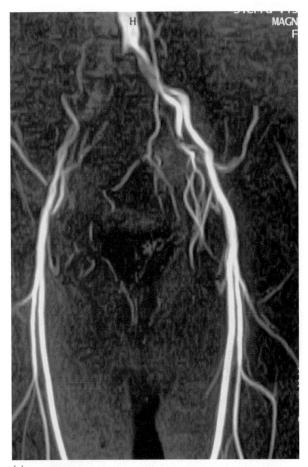

(a)

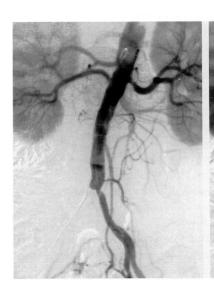
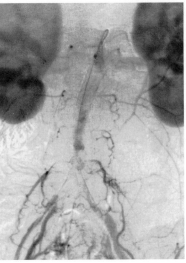

Figure 3.7 *(a) Coronal MIP reconstruction obtained with 2D TOF MRA shows occlusion of the right common iliac artery. (b) Aortopelvic digital subtraction angiography confirms right common iliac artery occlusion.*

(b)

of occluded segments.[55–59] However, in the discrimination of hemodynamically significant from insignificant stenoses, the results were less encouraging. MRA usually overestimated the severity of disease.[55,57–59] At present, for the majority of patients who do not have significant risk factors for angiography, 2D TOF MRA is not a satisfactory replacement. However, 2D TOF MRA may be used to direct therapy or limit angiography in those patients who have substantial risk factors, such as renal insufficiency or a significant allergy to iodinated contrast.

Recent improvements in magnetic resonance imaging have occurred with the use of intravascular MRA contrast agents. These agents minimize signal loss due to saturation effects, such as turbulent blood flow. Recent reports by Quinn and others demonstrated that conventional 2D TOF for evaluation of infrainguinal arteries combined with gadolinium-enhanced three-dimensional MRA for the study of the aorta and arteries above the inguinal ligaments correlates closely with conventional angiography.[60] This combined approach may limit the pitfalls and artifacts experienced with conventional 2D TOF and make MRA a more practical imaging method for many institutions.[61]

REFERENCES

1 Taylor LM Jr, Hamre D, Dalman RL, Porter JM. Limb salvage vs. amputation for critical ischemia: the role of vascular surgery. *Arch Surg* 1991; **126**: 1251–58.

2 Marks J, King TA, Baele H, Rubin J, Marmen C. Popiteal-to-distal bypass for limb threatening ischemia. *J Vasc Surg* 1992; **15**: 755–60.

3 Hallett JW. Trends in revascularization of the lower extremity. *Mayo Clin Proc* 1986; **61**: 369–76.

4 Jeans WK, Armstrong S, Cole SEA, Horrocks M, Baird RN. Fate of patients undergoing transluminal angioplasty for lower-limb ischemia. *Radiology* 1990; **177**: 559–64.

5 Johnston KW. Femoral and popliteal arteries: reanalysis of results of balloon angioplasty. *Radiology* 1992; **183**: 767–71.

6 Karacagil S, Almgren B, Bowald S, Enksson I. A new method of angiographic runoff evaluation in femorodistal reconstructions: significant correlation with early graft patency. *Arch Surg* 1990; **125**: 1055–8.

7 O'Mara CS, Flinn WR, Nieman HL, Bergan JJ, Yao JST. Correlation of foot arterial anatomy with early tibial bypass patency. *Surgery* 1981; **89**: 743–52.

8 Gocke J. The clinical assessment of peripheral arterial disease. *J Vasc Technol* 1994; **18**: 231–4.

9 Murphy TP, Dorfman GS, Becker J. Use of preprocedural tests by interventional radiologists. *Radiology* 1993; **186**: 213–20.

10 Macpherson DS. Preoperative laboratory testing: should any tests be 'routine' before surgery. *Med Clin North Am* 1993; **77**: 289–308.

11 Kaplan EB, Sheiner LB, Boeckmann AJ *et al.* The usefulness of preoperative laboratory screening. *JAMA* 1985; **253**: 3576–81.

12 Parfrey PS, Griffiths SM, Barrett BJ *et al.* Contrast material-induced renal failure in patients with diabetes mellitus, renal insufficiency, or both. *N Engl J Med* 1989; **320**: 143–9.

13 Lautin EM, Freeman NJ, Schoenfeld AH *et al.* Radiocontrast-associated renal dysfunction: incidence and risk factors. *Am J Radiol* 1991; **157**: 49–58.

14 Koltum WA, Gardiner GA, Jr, Harrington DP *et al.* Thrombolysis in the treatment of peripheral arterial vascular occlusions. *Arch Surg* 1987; **122**: 901–5.

15 Felin FM, Murphys S. Perioperative evaluation of patients with hematologic disorders. In: Merli GJ, Wertz HH eds *Medical management of the surgical patient*. Philadelphia: WB Saunders, 1992: 84–115.

16 AbuRahma AF, Robinson PA, Boland JP. Safety of arteriography by direct puncture of a vascular prosthesis. *Am J Surg* 1992; **164**: 233–6.

17 Burnham CB. Segmental pressures and doppler velocity waveforms in the evaluation of peripheral arterial occlusive disease. *J Vasc Technol* 1994; **18**: 249–55.

18 De Masi RJ, Gregory RT, Wheeler JR. Exercise testing: diagnosis and follow-up. *J Vasc Technol* 1994; **18**: 257–62.

19 Mistrelta CA, Crummy AB, Strother CM. Digital angiography: a perspective. *Radiology* 1981; **139**: 273–6.

20 Kinnison M, Perler BA, White RI Jr *et al.* Tailored approach for evaluation of peripheral vascular disease: intravenous digital subtraction angiography. *Am J Radiol* 1984; **142**: 1205–9.

21 Kaufman SL, Chang R, Kadir S, Mitchell SE, White RI Jr. Intraarterial digital subtraction angiography in diagnostic arteriography. *Radiology* 1984; **151**: 323–7.

22 Miller DL, Chang R, Wells WT *et al.* Contrast media for angiography: effect of dose on renal function. *Radiology* 1988; **167**: 607–11.

23 Sethi GK, Scott SM, Takaro T. Multiple plane angiography for more precise evaluation of aortoiliac disease. *Surgery* 1975; **78**: 154–9.

24 Crummy AB, Rankin RS, Turnipseed WD, Berkoff HA. Biplane arteriography in ischemia of the lower extremity. *Radiology* 1981; **141**: 33–7.

25 Crummy AB, Strother CM, Lieberman RP *et al.* Digital video subtraction angiography for evaluation of peripheral vascular disease. *Radiology* 1981; **141**: 33–7.

26 Guthaner DF, Wexler L, Enzmann DR *et al.* Evaluation of peripheral vascular disease using digital subtraction angiography. *Radiology* 1983; **147**: 393–8.

27 Crummy AB, Stieghorst MF, Turski PA. Digital subtraction angiography: current status and use of intra-arterial injection. *Radiology* 1982; **145**: 303–7.

28 Kader S. Arteriography of the lower extremity vessels. In: Kader S ed. *Diagnostic angiography*. Philadelphia: WB Saunders, 1986: 254–307.

29 Bron KM. Femoral arteriography. In: Abrams HL ed. *Abrams angiography: vascular and interventional radiology*, 3rd edn. Boston: Little, Brown, 1983: 1835–75.

30 Alson MD, Lang EV, Kaufman JA. Pedal arterial imaging. *J Vasc Intervent Radiol* 1997; **8**: 9–18.

31 Smith TP, Cragg AH, Berbaum KS, Ryals TJ, Sato Y. Techniques for lower-limb angiography: a comparative study. *Radiology* 1990; **174**: 951–5.

32 Swanson DP, Thrall JH, Shelty PC. Evaluation of intravascular low-osmolality contrast agents. *Clin Pharmacy* 1986; **5**: 877–91.

33 Kozak BE, Bedell JE, Rosch J. Small vessel leg angiography for distal vessel bypass grafts. *J Vasc Surg* 1988; **8**: 711–5.

34 Morettin LB. 'Dry limb' femoral arteriography. *Radiology* 1974; **113**: 468–9.

35 Cardella JF, Smith TP, Darcy TP, Hunter DW, Castaneda'-Zuniga W, Amplatz K. Balloon occlusion femoral angiography prior to in-situ saphenons vein bypass. *Cardiovasc Intervent Radiol* 1987; **10**: 181–9.

36 Kahn PC, Boyer DN, Moran JM, Callow AD. Reactive hyperemia in lower extremity arteriography: An evaluation. *Radiology* 1968; **90**: 975–80.

37 Friedman J, Zeit RM, Cope C, Bernhard VM. Optimal use of tolazoline in arteriography. *Am J Radiol* 1984; **142**: 817–20.

38 Cohen MI, Vogelzang RL. A comparison of techniques for improved visualization of the arteries of the distal lower extremity. *Am J Radiol* 1986; **147**: 1021–4.

39 Rudnick MR, Berns JS, Cohen RM, Goldfarb S. Contrast media-associated nephrotoxicity. *Curr Opin Hypertens* 1996; **5**: 127–33.

40 Rudnick MR, Goldfarb S, Wexler L *et al*. Nephrotoxicity of ionic and nonionic contrast media in 1196 patients. *Kidney Int* 1995; **47**: 254–61.

41 Barrett BJ, Carlisle EJ. Metaanalysis of the relative nephrotoxicity of high and ion osmolality iodinated contrast media. *Radiology* 1993; **188**: 171–8.

42 Solomon R, Werner C, Mann D, D'Elia J, Silva P. Effects of saline, mannitol, and furosemide on acute decreases in renal function induced by radiocontrast agents. *N Engl J Med* 1994; **331**: 1416–20.

43 Rautenbery E. Roentgenphotographie der leber, der milz, und des zwerchfells. *Deutsch Med Wschr* 1994; **40**: 1205.

44 Seeger JM, Self S, Harwood TRS, Flynn TC, Hawkins IF. Carbon dioxide gas as an arterial contrast agent. *Ann Surg* 1993; **217**: 688–98.

45 Hawkins IF. Carbon dioxide digital subtraction angiography. *Am J Roentgenol* 1982; **139**: 19–24.

46 Kerns SR, Hawkins IF, JR. Carbon dioxide digital subtraction angiography: expanding applications and technical evolution. *Am J Radiol* 1995; **164**: 735–41.

47 Hawkins IF, Caridi JG, Kerns SR. Plastic bag delivery system for hand injection of carbon dioxide. *Am J Roentgenol* 1995; **165**: 1–3.

48 Caridi JG, Hawkins IF. CO2 digital subtraction angiography: potential complications and their prevention. *J Vasc Intervent Radiol* 1997; **8**: 383–91.

49 Rundback JH. Livedo reticularis, rhabdomyolysis, massive intestinal infarction, and death post carbon dioxide arteriography. *J Vasc Surg* 1997; **26**: 337–40.

50 Prince MR, Arnoldus C, Frisoli JK. Nephrotoxicity of high-dose gadolinium compared with iodinated contrast. *J Magn Reson Imaging* 1996; **1**: 162–6.

51 Spinosa DJ, Hartwell GD, Angle JF *et al*. Optimizing imaging technique for gadolinium contrast angiography. *J Vasc Intervent Radiol* 1998; **9** (suppl): 192.

52 Patel KR, Semel L, Clauss RH. Extended reconstruction rate for limb salvage with intraoperative prereconstruction angiography. *J Vasc Surg* 1988; **7**: 531–7.

53 Owen RS, Carpenter JP, Baum RA *et al*. Magnetic resonance imaging of angiographic occult run-off vessels in peripheral arterial occlusive disease. *N Engl J Med* 1992; **326**: 1577–81.

54 Owen RS, Baum RA, Carpenter JP *et al*. Symptomatic peripheral vascular disease: selection of imaging parameters and clinical evaluation with MR angiography. *Radiology* 1993; **187**: 627–35.

55 Yucel EK, Kaufman JA, Geller SC, Waltman AC. Atherosclerotic occlusive disease of the lower extremity: prospective evaluation with two-dimensional time-of-flight MR angiography. *Radiology* 1993; **187**: 637–41.

56 Laissy JP, Limot O, Henry-Feugas MC *et al*. Iliac artery patency before and immediately after percutaneous transluminal angioplasty: assessment with time-of-flight MR angiography. *Radiology* 1995; **197**: 455–9.

57 McCauley TR, Monib A, Dickey KW *et al*. Peripheral vascular occlusive disease: accuracy and reliability of time-of-flight MR angiography. *Radiology* 1994; **192**: 351–7.

58 Leyendecker JR, Elsass RD, Johnson SP *et al*. The role of infrapopiteal MR angiography in patients undergoing optimal contrast angiography for chronic limb-threatening ischemia. *J Vasc Intervent Radiol* 1998; **9**: 545–51.

59 Poon E, Yucel EK, Pagen-Marin H, Kayne H. Iliac artery stenosis measurements. Comparison of two-dimensional time-of-flight and three-dimensional dynamic gadolinium-enhanced MR angiography. *Am J Radiol* 1997; **169**: 1139–44.

60 Quinn SF, Sheley RC, Semonsen KG *et al*. Aortic and lower-extremity arterial disease: evaluation with MR angiography versus conventional angiography. *Radiology* 1998; **206**: 693–701.

61 Kaufman JA, McCarter D, Geller SC, Waltman AC. Two-dimensional time-of-flight MR angiography of the lower extremities: artifacts and pitfalls. *Am J Radiol* 1998; **171**: 129–35.

4

Risk factor assessment and indications for reconstruction

JOHN M MAREK AND JOSEPH L MILLS

INTRODUCTION

Few topics have generated as much controversy as the preoperative risk assessment of surgical patients. The vascular surgical patient undergoing an infrainguinal bypass represents one of the most challenging patient groups with respect to preoperative assessment. Atherosclerosis is a systemic process and patients with peripheral vascular disease (PVD) often have multiple medical problems including significant cardiopulmonary, renal and metabolic disorders. In addition, patients with severe lower extremity PVD frequently do not have symptoms of coronary ischemia because their limited exercise tolerance prevents them from attaining stress levels that induce cardiac symptoms.

Approximately 70 per cent of perioperative and late mortality following peripheral arterial reconstructions is due to coronary artery disease (CAD). To diminish such complications, some authors advocate aggressive preoperative cardiac evaluation of all patients. Others have devised elaborate cardiac risk indices to predict which patients are at higher risk for cardiac events and thereby select those requiring more intensive evaluation. Still others feel that excellent results can be obtained with careful intraoperative monitoring and medical therapy, and that the combined morbidity and mortality of coro-

nary revascularization in addition to the peripheral vascular procedure outweigh any potential benefit. A clear consensus is lacking. Although the focus of this chapter is the preoperative assessment of patients in whom a lower extremity revascularization is being considered, it is also applicable to the majority of vascular procedures. The indications for revascularization are also reviewed so that the physician advising the patient undergoing peripheral reconstruction can do so with a complete understanding of the present literature.

BACKGROUND

Perioperative cardiac morbidity is the primary cause of death following anesthesia and surgery. A total of 1 million patients per year will have perioperative cardiac complications (myocardial infarction, congestive heart failure, arrythmias or cardiac death) at an annual estimated cost of $20 billion for in-hospital costs and long-term care.[1] Of the 27 million patients who undergo surgery each year in the USA, approximately 8 million have coronary artery disease or associated risk factors. It has been estimated that over the next 30 years the number of noncardiac surgical procedures will increase by 50 per cent (to 38 million) and the percentage of surgical patients over age 65 will increase from 25 per cent to 35 per cent.[2]

Patients undergoing peripheral vascular reconstruction are at an increased risk for perioperative cardiac complications. The incidence of myocardial infarction (MI) following noncardiac surgery has been estimated at 0–0.7 per cent, but increases to 2–6.4 per cent in patients undergoing elective vascular reconstruction; nearly half of these are fatal.[3] Patients with vascular disease are at higher risk because of advanced age, associated medical conditions, such as diabetes, renal, cardiac or pulmonary disease, and the physiological stress of surgery. Routine preoperative cardiac catheterization performed in large series of peripheral vascular patients documented CAD in excess of 90 per cent of patients, with one-third having severe, potentially reconstructable disease.[4] Additionally, upwards of 50 per cent of vascular patients undergoing persantine thallium scanning show evidence of reversible ischemia.[5] The fact that the majority of vascular patients have coronary artery disease is undisputed. The difficulty remains in predicting which of these patients will have an untoward cardiac event.

Comparison of cardiac morbidity between different studies is often misleading because the frequency of cardiac complications is related to the diligence with which the diagnosis is pursued. For example, retrospective reviews generally report an incidence of perioperative MI approximating 3 per cent. More intensive prospective studies report rates of 10–15 per cent.[3] This disparity arises because the majority of perioperative MIs are silent and many are subendocardial, requiring more than daily history or electrocardiograms (ECGs) to detect. In addition, over 50 per cent of perioperative myocardial events occur after the third postoperative day and many studies do not rigorously follow patients after this period. Similarly, the detection of arrythmias requires the use of continuous ECG monitoring in the preoperative and postoperative period to distinguish acute from chronic conditions. The incidence of congestive heart failure (CHF) is problematic because the diagnosis of

CHF varies between studies, and postoperative pulmonary congestion may be precipitated by heart failure or may be due to pulmonary capillary leak associated with other factors. Furthermore, while included in many studies, the cardiac outcomes of arrhythmia, CHF and angina are usually transient, and respond to medical management without permanent sequelae. They indicate presence of CAD and the possible need for subsequent cardiac evaluation. Overall, it is not surprising to find widely disparate data on cardiac morbidity in different reports. For these reasons the most meaningful studies are prospective and focus primarily on the outcomes of MI and cardiac death.

PREVALENCE OF CORONARY ARTERY DISEASE IN VASCULAR PATIENTS

Several studies have examined the incidence of CAD in vascular surgical patients as determined by preoperative coronary angiography.[4,6–9] The collected results from 1545 patients in five studies indicates that the incidence of hemodynamically significant CAD (greater than 70 per cent stenosis) is 77 per cent for one-vessel disease and 44 per cent for three-vessel disease in patients with symptoms of CAD (Table 4.1). Also of significance was the observation that 40 per cent of patients with no history of CAD were found to have significant stenosis of at least one coronary vessel. The high incidence of occult CAD is important because the risk of a perioperative cardiac event has been shown to correlate with the severity of the disease and to be independent of the presence of symptoms. The largest of these series by Hertzer et al.[4] examined the distribution of CAD among patients with peripheral vascular disease at varying sites. They showed no significant difference in the distribution of CAD between patients undergoing abdominal aortic aneurysm (AAA) repair, lower extremity revascularization, or cerebrovascular procedures (Table 4.2).

Table 4.1 *Incidence of CAD in vascular surgical patients determined by preoperative coronary angiography. From Cutler BS. Assessment and importance of coronary artery disease in patients with aortoiliac occlusive and aneurysmal disease. In: Ernst CB, Stanley JC eds Current therapy in vascular surgery, 2nd edn. Philadelphia, BC Decker, 1991, by permission of Mosby-Year Book, Inc.*

Author	Number of patients	Asymptomatic CAD		Symptomatic CAD	
		1-vessel (%)	3-vessel (%)	1-vessel (%)	3-vessel (%)
Tomatis et al. (1972)[6]	100	28	16	—	—
Hertzer et al. (1984)[4]	1000	37	15	78	44
Young et al. (1986)[7]	302	46	20	85	52
Blombery et al. (1986)[a8]	84	48	9	44	22
Orecchia et al. (1988)[9]	59	64	29	84	36
Average	1545 (total)	40	16	77	44

[a] Critical stenosis defined as >50 per cent, all other studies >70 per cent.

Table 4.2 *Incidence of coronary artery disease by serial coronary angiography in 1000 elective vascular patients from the Cleveland Clinic series*

	Total (%)	Severe CAD (%)
Abdominal aortic aneurysm	94	36
Lower extremity ischemia	90	28
Cerebrovascular disease	91	32

In the latter series, severe CAD was present in 25 per cent of patients and was defined as greater than 70 per cent stenosis of one or more coronary arteries serving impaired myocardium and representing a potential risk for MI. Severe inoperable CAD was found in 6 per cent of all patients and was defined as greater than 70 per cent stenosis of multiple coronary arteries with inadequate targets for coronary artery bypass grafting (CABG) because of diffuse distal disease. While the primary vascular diagnosis did not affect the incidence of CAD, male sex and increasing age did correlate with the presence of CAD. In contrast, neither hypertension, severity of peripheral occlusive disease nor diabetes mellitus had a significant association with the incidence of severe correctable CAD. Diabetics did, however, have a statistically increased incidence of severe inoperable CAD when compared to nondiabetics (12 per cent vs 4.5 per cent). Impressively, 50 per cent of diabetics over age 70 had severe CAD and half of these had inoperable disease. Based on their findings, CABG was performed in 70/250 (28 per cent) patients with AAA, 63/295 (21 per cent) of patients with cerebrovascular disease and 70/381 (18 per cent) of patients with lower extremity vascular insufficiency prior to the planned vascular reconstruction. This approach was not without cost as the operative mortality for CABG alone was 5.2 per cent. The operative mortality for patients undergoing vascular procedures without CABG was 2.0 per cent overall (AAA 3.4 per cent; lower extremity revascularization 1.8 per cent; extracranial reconstruction 0.3 per cent).

CORRELATION OF CARDIAC COMPLICATIONS WITH CATEGORY OF VASCULAR RECONSTRUCTION

The majority of studies that have evaluated perioperative cardiac morbidity in vascular patients have focused on aortic procedures, or have combined patients undergoing carotid, aortic and infrainguinal operations. The occurrence of cardiac events after aortic surgery has been attributed to myocardial stress from anesthesia, aortic clamping, declamping hypotension, blood loss and metabolic abnormalities. The magnitude of such physiologic stress is significantly lower in the patient undergoing an infrainguinal bypass and therefore these operations

would be expected to produce fewer cardiac complications. Surprisingly, however, patients undergoing infrainguinal procedures have an equivalent incidence of cardiac morbidity as those having aortic reconstructions.

Krupski and colleagues prospectively compared the differences between perioperative cardiac ischemic events in 140 patients undergoing major abdominal and infrainguinal vascular operations.[10] In the infrainguinal group, more patients had diabetes (44 per cent vs 11 per cent), angina (36 per cent vs 15 per cent), heart failure (29 per cent vs 9 per cent), dysrhythmias (36 per cent vs 17 per cent) and used digitalis (23 per cent vs 6 per cent). During operation, more patients undergoing aortic procedures suffered ischemia determined by echocardiography (26 per cent vs 10 per cent). After operation, there were similar incidences of ischemic events in patients undergoing infrainguinal vs aortic reconstruction (24 per cent vs 28 per cent). Ischemia by Holter monitoring occurred after operation in 57 per cent of patients having infrainguinal bypass compared to 28 per cent of patients with aortic procedures. Cardiac causes resulted in all four deaths in this series for a mortality of 2.8 per cent (3.5 per cent infrainguinal, 2 per cent aortic). Adverse outcomes occurred in patients having aortic operations at a mean of 2 days postoperatively, compared with 10 days in patients having infrainguinal procedures. This study highlights several important distinctions between patients undergoing aortic and infrainguinal operations. Patients undergoing infrainguinal revascularization have a higher preoperative incidence of cardiac symptoms and risk factors. While there was less intraoperative ischemia in infrainguinal bypass patients, they had a two-fold increase in postoperative ischemia with the majority of cardiac events occurring after a longer postoperative interval. Bry *et al.* in a review of 237 patients undergoing aortic or infrainguinal procedures similarly found no significant difference in the incidence of MI (6 per cent infrainguinal, 5.8 per cent aortic), cardiac-related death (2.2 per cent infrainguinal, 0 per cent aortic) or selection of patients for myocardial revascularization (2.2 per cent infrainguinal, 5.8 per cent aortic).[11]

Patients undergoing carotid surgery have significantly less cardiac morbidity and mortality (Table 4.3). In the recent ACAS trial there was one fatal MI among 724 carotid endarterectomy patients during the 30-day peri-

Table 4.3 *Incidence of perioperative myocardial infarction (MI) with vascular surgery*[3]

Procedure	Overall MI incidence (%)	Fatal MI incidence (%)
Carotid endarterectomy	2.0	0.8
Abdominal aortic aneurysm repair	6.4	2.2
Lower extremity revascularization	6.0	2.3

operative period.[12] In the NASCET trial there was a 0.9 per cent MI rate in 328 surgical patients.[13] This should be noted when comparing trials of cardiac morbidity in peripheral vascular surgery that include cerebrovascular patients.

ASSESSMENT OF CARDIAC RISK

The goal of preoperative assessment is to identify a subset of patients with sufficient risk for a myocardial event that they would derive benefit from complete cardiac evaluation and intervention. Such intervention might consist of preoperative myocardial revascularization with CABG or percutaneous transluminal coronary angioplasty, more intensive optimization of medical therapy, or aggressive intraoperative and postoperative hemodynamic monitoring. In the high-risk cardiac patient the selection of alternative, less invasive peripheral vascular procedures (angioplasty or extraanatomic bypass) might be indicated. In the high-risk cardiac patient with only claudication, peripheral vascular surgery might best be deferred altogether.

In the 1960s, investigators began to identify predictors of cardiac morbidity obtainable from history and physical examination. In these studies, a history of a recent MI consistently had prognostic value resulting in the practice of delaying surgery 6 months following an MI. In 1977, Goldman published the first multifactorial risk index for predicting perioperative cardiac events.[14] Although the applicability of this index to vascular patients has been subsequently challenged, this was nevertheless an important study. Since that time other risk-factor indices have been described including the Dripps American Society of Anesthesiologists (ASA), Detsky modified cardiac risk index (CRI), Eagle criteria and Cooperman probability, the latter two of which are directed primarily at the vascular surgery population.[15–18] In the 1980s, studies began evaluating the utility of preoperative diagnostic testing in predicting perioperative cardiac events. These tests included exercise stress testing, dipyridamole thallium scanning (DTS) and radionuclide imaging. Studies have also evaluated the utility of intraoperative and postoperative tests, such as transesophageal echocardiography (TEE), Swan Ganz catheterization and Holter monitoring in decreasing perioperative morbidity.

RISK FACTORS BASED ON HISTORY AND PHYSICAL EXAMINATION

Preoperative assessment of cardiac risk should begin with a careful history and physical examination. Patients are questioned for specific risk factors associated with CAD including age, hyperlipidemia, diabetes, renal disease, smoking, and a history of angina or MI. The physical examination should concentrate on evidence of valvular disease, dysrhythmia or CHF. Features of the history and physical examination alone account for 35 of 53 points in the Goldman cardiac risk index. Simple laboratory screening tests should include a complete blood cell count and renal profile. In addition to a standard 12-lead ECG, a baseline chest x-ray should be obtained, which may show evidence of CHF or cardiomegaly.

Of these variables, recent MI, diabetes and active CHF have been consistently associated with an increased incidence of perioperative cardiac events. The remaining factors have either not been studied thoroughly or reported results have been inconclusive.

Recent MI

Patients with previous MI are at greater risk for perioperative reinfarction (5–8 per cent) than those without prior MI (0.1–0.7 per cent).[2] The more recent the MI, the greater the likelihood of reinfarction. Initial studies indicated that within 3 months the reinfarction rate is 30 per cent or more, at 3–6 months it drops to 15 per cent, and after 6 months is approximately 6 per cent.[19] Over the last decade, these figures have been challenged. Rao et al. found that reinfarction occurred in only 1.9 per cent of 733 noncardiac surgical patients with a prior MI. Perioperative reinfarction occurred in only 5.7 per cent of patients whose MI was less than 3 months old and 2.3 per cent of those whose MI was 4–6 months old.[20] Whether these reduced risks are due to the use of intraoperative pulmonary artery and arterial catheters, or prolonged intensive care unit (ICU) monitoring, is unclear. Several other studies have confirmed the reinfarction rate of 5 per cent in patients with an MI less than 3 months old.[21,22]

Congestive heart failure

Preoperative CHF is a predictor of cardiac morbidity but the value of specific signs is controversial. CHF is a constellation of findings and the criteria for diagnosis varies among reports. Goldman found that two signs of heart failure, a third heart sound and jugular venous distention, have predictive value. Other studies have used more objective testing of left ventricular (LV) dysfunction. Pasternack et al. showed that the degree of LV dysfunction measured by radionuclide angiography correlated highly with the risk of perioperative MI, with 70 per cent of patients undergoing infrainguinal operations having an adverse cardiac event when left ventricular ejection fraction (LVEF) was less than 30 per cent.[23]

Diabetes mellitus

Diabetes is clearly a risk factor for CAD, with nearly a three-fold increase in risk of atherosclerotic disease.[24]

Diabetics comprise a significant proportion of patients undergoing lower extremity revascularization, approaching 40–50 per cent in some series. While earlier reports found diabetes predictive only when associated with other factors, recent studies have shown an increased risk of perioperative cardiac morbidity in diabetics.[17,25]

CARDIAC RISK INDICES

In the last two decades, studies using logistic regression and multivariate analysis have attempted to identify the clinical risk factors most predictive of perioperative cardiac risk. Goldman and associates were among the first to quantify the relative risks of cardiac morbidity in patients undergoing noncardiac surgical procedures.[14] Multivariate analysis of 39 clinical variables in 1001 surgical patients identified nine factors that were predictive of perioperative cardiac morbidity (Table 4.4). Relatively few of the patients in Goldman's study (80/1001) underwent vascular reconstruction. Detsky et al. modified the original risk index by adding variables (angina and pulmonary edema) and altering the scoring scheme.[16]

Unfortunately, while these risk indices have been shown to provide estimates of risk for a broad population of surgical patients, they appear to be less effective in higher risk subgroups, such as patients undergoing vascular surgery.[26]

Eagle and colleagues attempted to improve the value of risk indices in vascular patients by evaluating 254 consecutive patients referred for DTS prior to major vascular surgery.[17] Fifty-four patients had surgery canceled based on DTS results. The remaining 200 patients formed the study population. There were 30 patients (15 per cent) with perioperative ischemic events including six patients (3 per cent) with cardiac death, nine (4.5 per cent) with nonfatal acute MI, nine (4.5 per cent) with pulmonary edema, and 19 (8.5 per cent) with unstable angina. Logistic regression analysis identified five clinical predictors of cardiac events: Q waves on preoperative ECG, history of ventricular ectopy requiring therapy, age > 70, diabetes and angina. Of 64 patients (32 per cent) with no clinical predictors, there was a 3.1 per cent incidence of events; in 116 patients (58 per cent) with one or two clinical predictors, there was a 15.5 per cent incidence of cardiac events; in 20 patients (10 per cent) with three or more predictors, there was a 50 per cent incidence of events. In the 116 patients with one or two

Table 4.4 *Comparison of clinical cardiac risk indexes: Goldman, Detsky, Eagle. CCS = Canadian Cardiovascular Society (anginal classification scores), Creat = creatinine, ECG = electrocardiogram, MI = myocardial infarction, PACs = premature atrial contractions, PVCs = premature ventricular contractions*

Factor	Goldman CRI Definition	Points	Detsky CRI Definition	Points	Eagle criteria Definition	Points
Ischemic heart disease	MI within 6 months	10	MI within 6 months	10	Q waves on ECG	1
			MI > 6 months earlier	5	History of angina	1
			CCS class III angina	10		
			CCS class IV angina	20		
			Unstable angina	10		
Congestive heart failure	S3, gallop or jugular venous distention	11	Pulmonary edema within 1 week	10		
			Ever	5		
Cardiac rhythm	Rhythm other than sinus or PACs	7	Rhythm other than sinus or PACs	5	History of ventricular ectopy requiring treatment	1
	>5 PVCs per minute at any time before surgery	7	>5 PVCs per minute at any time before surgery	5		
Valvular heart disease	Important aortic stenosis	3	Suspected critical aortic stenosis	20		
General medical status	PO_2<60mmHG, PCO_2>50 mmHG, Creat >3.0 mg/dl, Bicarbonate <20 mmol/dl	3	Same as original index	3	Diabetes requiring treatment	1
Age	>70 years	5	>70 years	5	>70 years	1
Type of surgery	Intraperitoneal, intrathoracic or aortic	3	Emergency operation	10		
	Emergency operation	4				
Cardiac risk			Total score			
Low		0–12	0–15			0
Intermediate		13–25	16–30			1–2
High		>25	>30			3 or more

clinical predictors, DTS correlated well with adverse events (3.2 per cent cardiac event without redistribution *vs* 29.6 per cent with redistribution). They concluded that: (1) patients with no predictors do not require preoperative testing; (2) patients with one or two predictors should have preoperative thallium testing; and (3) patients with three or more predictors do not benefit from thallium testing due to the extremely high incidence of events in this subgroup. In addition they found that the Goldman CRI, the Detsky modified CRI and the Dripps ASA index were not predictive of the outcomes of MI or cardiac death in this patient population.

Uniform agreement on the utility of predictive preoperative risk indices has not been reached. Lette and colleagues in a retrospective study of 125 patients undergoing vascular reconstructions evaluated cardiac risk indices and DTS.[5] They compared the Dripps ASA, Goldman CRI, Detsky CRI, Eagle criteria, Yeager criteria and Cooperman probability. All scoring indices failed to predict adverse perioperative cardiac outcome. Wong and Detsky re-examined Lette and colleagues' analysis and concluded that criteria were of use only in patients with intermediate clinical risk status.[27]

Overall, studies investigating the predictive value of risk indices in patients undergoing vascular surgery have reported variable results, perhaps due to differing patient populations or protocols for surgical, anesthetic and postoperative care between institutions. The high prevalence of occult coronary disease among vascular patients may decrease the utility of clinical criteria in the prediction of perioperative cardiac outcomes after vascular surgery. In general, however, data appear sufficient to justify the use of clinical risk indices, such as the Eagle criteria to stratify subgroups of vascular surgical patients for further cardiac testing.

DIAGNOSTIC TESTING PREDICTORS

Recent attention has focused on the development of adjunctive tests to enhance the sensitivity and specificity of preoperative risk assessment. Commonly employed tests include ECG, exercise ECG, ambulatory Holter monitoring, echocardiography, dipyridamole thallium scanning and coronary angiography. The implications of recommending additional testing are substantial. Testing procedures are expensive and increase the likelihood that further tests and treatments will be recommended. Such a course is justifiable only if the additional testing provides information that is unavailable by history and physical examination, and also improves patient management and outcome. Several investigators have suggested that special testing only be obtained in patients considered intermediate or high clinical risk. In these reports, 4 per cent of patients clinically identified as low risk suffered cardiac events, compared to 9–21 per cent identified as intermediate or high risk.[17,28,29]

PREOPERATIVE CARDIAC STUDIES

Resting 12-lead electrocardiogram

All patients should have a baseline preoperative ECG performed, which should be compared to prior tracings for interval changes. Preoperative ECG abnormalities commonly occur. The most frequent abnormalities are ST-T wave changes, left ventricular hypertrophy or strain, and Q-waves. Despite the widespread use of preoperative ECG, only a few studies have examined its predictive value. Carliner *et al.* studied 200 patients undergoing elective noncardiac surgery and found that an abnormal preoperative ECG was the only significant independent predictor of adverse cardiac outcome.[30] Von Knorring evaluated patients undergoing major noncardiac surgery with ECG patterns suggestive of previous MI, LV hypertrophy or strain, or myocardial ischemia, and noted that 17.7 per cent sustained a perioperative MI.[31] In contrast, Goldman noted that ECG abnormalities, including Q-waves, ST-T wave changes or bundle branch blocks, had no significant predictive value.[14] Overall, a resting ECG is useful as a baseline examination, to identify unsuspected changes from prior ECGs, or to indicate the need for further workup if ischemic changes are present. A normal tracing does not exclude significant CAD.

Stress electrocardiography

Stress ECG is a popular method of identifying myocardial ischemia in patients with chest pain. It is inexpensive, noninvasive and in patients with the ability to exercise has been shown to correlate with long-term prognosis.[32] There is less consensus on its ability to predict perioperative cardiac morbidity. Cutler *et al.* noted a 37 per cent incidence of perioperative MI in lower extremity occlusive disease patients with a positive stress ECG compared to 1.5 per cent in those with no ischemia on stress ECG.[33] McPhail and colleagues noted in 100 vascular patients that ST segment depression during exercise was not a predictor of perioperative cardiac morbidity. They did find, however, that the risk of a postoperative cardiac event correlated with ability to achieve 85 per cent of maximum predicted heart rate on exercise testing (7 per cent *vs* 24 per cent cardiac event rate) and suggested this was a valuable indicator. Unfortunately, 70 per cent of the patients in their study were unable to achieve this exercise level, calling into question its utility as a screening examination.[34]

Overall, stress ECG is frequently inapplicable in vascular patients, especially those with lower extremity occlusive disease. At least one-third of all vascular patients cannot complete the study because of claudication, orthopedic or pulmonary disease. Beta-blocking medications may limit heart rate response to exercise, and digitalis or electrolyte abnormalities may produce resting ST segment abnormalities. Stress ECG has been largely replaced in preoperative evaluation of peripheral vascular patients by tests not requiring exercise.

Ambulatory Holter monitoring

Holter monitoring has been shown to be a reliable method of detecting cardiac dysrhythmias and myocardial ischemia. Recently, it has been used in surgical patients during the preoperative, intraoperative and postoperative periods in an attempt to predict cardiac morbidity. During the preoperative period, 18–40 per cent of patients at risk for CAD demonstrate frequent ischemic episodes with more than 70 per cent of these episodes being clinically silent.[10,29,35] Holter monitoring has the advantage of not requiring exercise and is lower in cost than other methods such as DTS. Disadvantages are that 10 per cent of patients have baseline ECG abnormalities that limit or preclude interpretation, and ECG patterns such as left ventricular hypertrophy (LVH) may lead to false-positive results.

Raby and colleagues, in a prospective study of 176 vascular patients, identified preoperative ischemia detected by Holter as a significant predictor of cardiac events.[29] Eighteen per cent of patients had preoperative ST depression (97 per cent silent) and there was a 37 per cent incidence of cardiac events in this group. In contrast, less than 1 per cent of patients without detectable ischemia suffered perioperative cardiac morbidity. In a subsequent study, Raby et al. used Holter monitoring to evaluate the significance of intraoperative and postoperative ischemia in vascular patients.[36] Postoperative ischemia occurred in 30 per cent of the 115 patients studied and preceded nearly all cardiac events by a mean of 7 hours before the event. They concluded that Holter monitoring can identify perioperative ischemia that may be treatable with anti-ischemic therapy to prevent subsequent major events.

Similarly, Mangano and colleagues have reported an association between postoperative ischemia on Holter monitoring and subsequent major cardiac events.[35] In 100 patients with CAD or at risk for CAD, they demonstrated that 42 per cent of patients developed postoperative ischemia (94 per cent silent). Eighty per cent of all episodes occurred without acute change in heart rate and 77 per cent of intraoperative events occurred without acute change in blood pressure. Eleven of the 13 adverse cardiac outcomes were preceded by postoperative ischemia. Pasternack and colleagues studied 200 patients undergoing vascular procedures using pre-, intra- and postoperative monitoring, and found silent ischemia occurred in over 60 per cent of patients undergoing vascular procedures, especially in the postoperative period.[37] Duration and number of ischemic episodes correlated well with perioperative events. Patients who

suffered a perioperative MI had an increase in total duration (17.7 hours vs 5.5 hours) and number (42 vs 13 episodes) of ischemic events. There were nine postoperative MIs and two cardiac deaths in this study, all in patients exhibiting ischemia on monitoring.

Overall, these results suggest that perioperative cardiac morbidity is frequently preceded by silent myocardial ischemia detectable by Holter monitoring. Unfortunately, standard continuous two-lead ECG monitoring cannot provide the information needed to assess myocardial ischemia adequately. In the future, identification of ischemic episodes with newer, full-display, online monitoring using computerized analysis may allow immediate recognition of postoperative myocardial ischemia and direct prompt institution of appropriate medical therapy to prevent morbid events. This emerging technology offers exciting new potentials in identifying patients during the postoperative period who may benefit from more aggressive medical management.

Radionuclide ventriculography

Several studies have correlated preoperative ejection fraction determined by radionuclide ventriculography with the incidence of postoperative cardiac events. Data are inconclusive. Pasternack and colleagues evaluated 100 patients undergoing lower extremity revascularization with radionuclide angiography and demonstrated that, in 50 patients with a LVEF >55 per cent, there was no cardiac morbidity, in 42 patients with a LVEF of 36–55 per cent, there was a 19 per cent incidence of MI with one cardiac death, and in eight patients with LVEF<35 per cent, there was a 75 per cent incidence of MI with one cardiac death.[23] Subsequent studies have failed to confirm this relationship.[38,39] Baron and colleagues evaluated 457 patients undergoing aortic surgery and found that a LVEF of less than 50 per cent predicted postoperative CHF, but not MI or death.[40]

Echocardiography

Left ventricular dysfunction, valvular heart disease and prior MI can all be identified by echocardiography. There are, however, no data to suggest that preoperative resting echocardiography adds information that cannot be obtained from routine clinical and ECG data. The exception to this may be patients with a murmur or active CHF in whom echocardiography may be performed on the basis of these indications.

Recent studies do suggest an increase in cardiac complications in patients in whom wall-motion abnormalities can be induced by exercise or pharmacologic agents (dipyridamole, dobutamine or dobutamine with atropine). Poldermans et al. in a study of 300 patients undergoing major vascular surgery evaluated cardiac risk using echocardiography after the administration of dobutamine with supplemental atropine, if required, to reach the age-corrected target heart rate.[41] All 27 postoperative cardiac complications occurred in the 72 patients who had positive stress tests. While this approach holds promise, its utility will require further investigation.

Stress thallium imaging (dipyridamole thallium scintigraphy)

Dipyridamole thallium scintigraphy has emerged as a common method of preoperative cardiac screening for patients with peripheral vascular disease, in whom exercise induced physiologic cardiac stress testing is not possible. Thallium-201 is taken up by myocardial cells in proportion to blood flow. Coronary vasodilation with intravenous dipyridamole (persantine) is at least equal to that seen with exercise (albeit not the heart rate response) but with no significant increase in myocardial oxygen consumption. In effect, dipyridamole produces a steal phenomenon because stenotic vessels cannot dilate. Perfusion defects are classified as fixed or reversible on redistribution. Defects are evaluated for size and number either visually or using quantitative methods. Some institutions have replaced DTS with adenosine–thallium scans or dipyridamole–sestamibi scans. Adenosine is a short-acting coronary vasodilator that has fewer side effects than dipyridamole and technetium-99m sestamibi is a new myocardial perfusion agent that may offer some advantages over thallium.

Boucher and colleagues first reported DTS as an accurate, safe, noninvasive screening test for patients in whom claudication precluded exercise.[28] They evaluated DTS in 54 patients with suspected CAD undergoing elective vascular surgery. In their study, eight of 16 patients whose thallium scan showed redistribution had cardiac events, whereas there were no events in 32 patients with either normal or fixed defects. Since that time, DTS has been evaluated in multiple studies including more than 1500 patients.[1] In general, it has been shown to have an excellent negative predictive value for cardiac events (96–99 per cent). The low positive predictive value (10–20 per cent) of abnormal DTS, however, is a major shortcoming that can contribute to extensive unwarranted preoperative cardiac evaluation.

In earlier studies of DTS, physicians were not blinded to preoperative test results and studies included only those patients referred for DTS. Mangano and colleagues prospectively studied 60 patients undergoing elective vascular surgery and blinded physicians to DTS results.[42] Thirty-seven per cent of patients had reversible defects, 30 per cent had fixed defects and 33 per cent had no defects. Postoperative DTS redistribution defects did not correlate with either perioperative ischemia (by Holter and TEE monitoring) or adverse cardiac outcomes. In a larger study of 457 consecutive, unselected patients undergoing abdominal aortic surgery, Baron et al. confirmed that thallium redistribution was not significantly associated with adverse cardiac outcomes.[40] Reversible thallium defects were observed in 35 per cent of patients. Indications for coronary angiography were based only on clinical criteria of medically unstable angina, recent MI or persistent angina with prior MI. Thirty-seven patients underwent coronary angiography based on these clinical criteria alone. There was a 4.4 per cent mortality (2.2 per cent cardiac mortality) and 4.8 per cent incidence of MI. Neither MI nor cardiac death were associated with thallium redistribution.

Despite lack of proven efficacy, DTS is the most commonly used cardiac screening test prior to major vascular reconstruction. The studies cited above have shown no benefit in the routine use of DTS in screening vascular surgical patients. Studies by Eagle and colleagues showed that the specificity of the test could be improved by using it in certain subgroups of patients as indicated by clinical markers.[17] Eagle and colleagues concluded that patients with no clinical risk factors should proceed to surgery without screening, those with one or two risk factors should have DTS performed, and those with three or more risk factors should proceed to cardiac catheterization or have surgery canceled. Lette et al. tried to improve the specificity of DTS by quantifying the extent and severity of reversible defects.[5] The positive predictive value of DTS increased from 13 per cent when redistribution involved only one segment to 43 per cent when two or three segments were involved. While there are currently no large prospective trials reporting the selective use of DTS, based on the available data, a selective approach to screening seems reasonable with cardiac catheterization performed only in patients with severe symptoms or with multiple areas of redistribution on DTS.

INDICATIONS FOR PREOPERATIVE CARDIAC CATHETERIZATION AND MYOCARDIAL REVASCULARIZATION

Cardiac catheterization has been the 'gold standard' for quantifying ventricular function and assessing coronary circulation. The issue of which patients to subject to preoperative coronary angiography and possible subsequent myocardial revascularization is hotly debated. Clearly, the expense and morbidity of cardiac catheterization limits its application as a routine screening test. Most would also agree that patients with clinically unstable heart disease, those with severe or unstable angina or continued angina following MI, or those who show large or multiple areas of ischemia on noninvasive tests should have cardiac catheterization. The critical question then becomes which intermediate-risk group of patients would most likely benefit from selective coronary angiography and myocardial revascularization in an attempt to decrease the cardiac morbidity of the vascular surgical procedure as well as to improve long-term patient survival.

The reasoning behind consideration of myocardial revascularization prior to vascular reconstruction is based on studies which show a decreased cardiac morbidity in patients who undergo subsequent noncardiac operations. A total of 1600 patients enrolled in the Coronary Artery Surgery Study (CASS) registry, who subsequently required noncardiac surgery, were analysed. Patients without substantial CAD had an operative mortality of 0.5 per cent, patients with considerable CAD who had CABG before the noncardiac procedure had a operative mortality of 0.9 per cent, and those with CAD who received medical therapy had an operative mortality of 2.4 per cent.[25] A 1.6 per cent mortality was reported by Young and colleagues in patients with prior CABG undergoing abdominal aortic surgery compared to a 4.8 per cent mortality in those without prior CABG.[7] Other authors have reported no cardiac mortality in patients who had CABG prior to major vascular operations.[43] These results are often cited as arguments in favor of recommending CABG before major vascular operations to decrease perioperative cardiac complications. These studies, however, have an inherent selection bias because patients had already survived CABG before being considered candidates for a second major operation. If CABG is recommended specifically to improve perioperative cardiac morbidity in a prophylactic fashion, then the morbidity and mortality of the cardiac workup and CABG must be included in the analysis of overall morbidity and mortality.

Many reports concerning the benefit of prophylactic CABG may not be applicable to patients with symptomatic PVD who tend to be older, more often diabetic and with partially greater mortality risk for CABG. The mean age of patients undergoing peripheral vascular surgery is 65 years and the CASS data have shown CABG in this age group is clearly associated with increased complications. Mortality was 1.9 per cent after CABG in patients under 65 years of age compared to 5.2 per cent in those over age 65 and further increased to 9.5 per cent in patients older than age 75 years.[44] Mortality from CABG in patients older than age 80 years is 10 per cent and increases to 17 per cent in the presence of peripheral vascular disease.[46] In patients with peripheral vascular disease the mortality with CABG alone is approximately 6 per cent.[4,7,45] Rihal and colleagues conducted an analysis of patients from the CASS registry with combined coronary artery and peripheral vascular disease. Of these patients, 986 underwent CABG with a perioperative mortality of 4.2 per cent (2.9 per cent in those without PVD), a 7.4 per cent incidence of MI and a stroke rate of 1.6 per cent.[47] Overall, preoperative CABG in vascular patients is not without significant risk and may indeed increase overall mortality. It should be used selectively in patients at

high risk for cardiac complications or in patients who otherwise have clear indications for CABG.

Percutaneous transluminal coronary angioplasty (PTCA) has been advocated as an alternative to CABG as treatment for significant CAD prior to major surgery. There are, however, few data to support this practice. The Mayo Clinic reported a retrospective, uncontrolled series of 55 patients who had PTCA prior to a noncardiac operation.[48] The subsequent perioperative MI rate was 5.6 per cent, with a mortality rate of 1.9 per cent, which is not substantially different from the 2.4 per cent mortality rate of patients undergoing surgery without prior revascularization in the CASS study. In addition, PTCA is not without complications. In patients undergoing dilation of more than one coronary artery, success rates of 74–85 per cent are reported, with 4 per cent requiring emergency bypass, 3.5 per cent sustaining an MI and a 1 per cent mortality.[49] Recurrent stenosis continues to be a major problem with PTCA with 33 per cent of simple lesions and up to 66 per cent of complex lesions recurring within 6 months. Overall, it is untenable to support a role for prophylactic PTCA in decreasing postoperative complications or improving long-term outcome.

Mason and colleagues performed a decision analysis on vascular patients who had either no angina or mild angina with a positive DTS.[50] They evaluated three treatment strategies. The first was to proceed directly to vascular surgery. The second was to perform coronary angiography, followed by selective coronary revascularization prior to vascular surgery and to cancel vascular surgery in patients with severe inoperable CAD. The third strategy was to perform coronary angiography, followed by selective coronary revascularization prior to vascular surgery and to perform vascular surgery in patients with inoperable CAD. They excluded patients with acute limb-threatening ischemia and patients with severe angina (class 3 or 4, or unstable angina) in whom coronary angiography was felt to be mandatory. They concluded that proceeding directly to vascular surgery led to lower morbidity and cost. Preoperative coronary angiography reduced overall mortality only when the estimated operative mortality of the noncardiac surgery is substantially higher than 5 per cent and the estimated operative mortality of coronary revascularization is relatively low (2–3 per cent).

In patients with severe CAD myocardial revascularization improves long-term survival. In the Cleveland Clinic series, of 216 patients with surgically correctable CAD who underwent CABG, 72 per cent were alive at 5 years. In contrast, only 15 of 35 (43 per cent) of patients who were candidates but never received CABG, and 12 of 54 (22 per cent) with severe uncorrectable CAD remained alive at 5 years.[51] Rihal and colleagues studied patients with combined coronary artery and peripheral vascular disease.[47] Despite higher percentages of severe symptoms and coronary disease, the long-term outcome was improved in patients undergoing CABG (estimated survival at 8 and 16 years was 72 per cent and 41 per cent for the surgical group *vs* 57 per cent and 34 per cent for the medical group). Overall, while the morbidity and mortality of CABG is high in PVD patients, in small, select subgroups there may be a long-term benefit. Generally, however, prophylactic CABG prior to a vascular surgical procedure is unwarranted unless the patients meet criteria for myocardial revascularization based on their cardiac status alone.

ANESTHETIC TECHNIQUES AND UTILITY OF INVASIVE MONITORING

Several studies have attempted to identify the optimal anesthetic technique for patients undergoing infrainguinal reconstruction. Bode and colleagues recently reported a randomized, prospective study in which 423 patients undergoing infrainguinal reconstruction were randomized to general, epidural or spinal anesthetic.[52] All patients had radial artery and pulmonary artery catheter monitoring. There was no significant difference in mortality (epidural 3.4 per cent, spinal 2.9 per cent, general 2.9 per cent), nonfatal MI (epidural 4.7 per cent, spinal 5.2 per cent, general 3.6 per cent) or other complications.

Pulmonary artery pressure monitoring provides information useful in assessing volume status, ventricular function and measurement of pulmonary capillary wedge pressure (PCWP), and may serve as an indirect indicator of myocardial ischemia. Several authors, however, have questioned the sensitivity of changes in PCWP. Recent reports have even questioned the value of pulmonary artery catheters in the care of critically ill patients demonstrating increased mortality rates in those receiving pulmonary catheters despite adjustments for selection bias.[53,54] Haggmark *et al.* reported that in vascular surgery patients the sensitivity and specificity of PCWP abnormalities (>5 mmHg change from baseline or the development of abnormal waveforms) for ischemia ranged from 40 to 60 per cent.[55] Roizen *et al.* found that 11 out of 12 patients developed TEE wall-motion abnormalities when the aorta was cross-clamped above the celiac artery but the PCWP remained normal (<12 mmHg) in 10 out of 12 with only 2 out of 12 having transient increases.[56] The most sensitive detector of intraoperative ischemia appears to be TEE. London *et al.* reported a 33 per cent incidence of intraoperative TEE wall-motion abnormalities in 95 patients with CAD or at risk for CAD.[57] Eight of nine patients who developed adverse cardiac outcomes had preceding intraoperative wall-motion abnormalities. Few studies have evaluated other potential uses of TEE, such as assessment of volume status, valvular competence and overall left ventricular contractility. Overall, evidence suggests that the use of transesophageal echocardiography should be confined to patients with advanced heart failure, tight aortic stenosis or recent myocardial infarction.

NONCARDIAC RISK FACTOR ASSESSMENT

Coronary artery disease accounts for 70 per cent of the major morbidity for patients undergoing peripheral artery reconstructive surgery. Clearly, however, such patients have disease involving other organ systems, and careful attention must be paid to recognize and prevent complications. The high incidence of cerebrovascular disease present in patients with lower extremity occlusive disease is well documented. Approximately 25 per cent of claudicants without neurologic symptoms have hemodynamically significant (>50 per cent) carotid disease by duplex.[58] Nearly one-third of patients undergoing revascularization for limb salvage have greater than 50 per cent carotid stenosis despite the absence of neurologic symptoms.[59] The risk of neurologic events associated with noncardiac vascular surgery is, however, surprisingly low (0.4–0.9 per cent), and recognition of the high incidence of asymptomatic disease may benefit patients more in the long term than in the perioperative period.[60,61] The few strokes that occur are associated with intraabdominal procedures, perioperative hypotension and a greater than 50 per cent stenosis of the carotid ipsilateral to the neurologic event.

Despite the high prevalence of cigarette smoking and obstructive lung disease in this population, postoperative pulmonary complications, while not infrequent, are rarely the cause of perioperative mortality.[62] The increased use of aggressive pulmonary toilet and regional anesthesia for infrainguinal procedures may contribute to this. Patients undergoing abdominal procedures, those with recent bronchitis and longer duration of surgery are at increased risk of pulmonary complications.

Patients with chronic renal insufficiency constitute an important patient subgroup because significant renal impairment increases operative mortality. Renal function should be optimized before surgery, and patients with end-stage renal disease (ESRD) should be dialysed immediately preceding surgery and on the first postoperative day. Attention should be paid to avoid the dehydration and hypotension that is frequently associated with hemodialysis, especially after infrainguinal reconstruction. The long-term outlook for patients with ESRD who undergo infrainguinal bypass or amputation is poor, with less than 20 per cent of patients surviving 3 years after bypass.[63] Reconstruction may not be indicated in ESRD patients with claudication considering this poor prognosis.

INDICATIONS FOR ARTERIAL RECONSTRUCTION

The two primary indications for intervention in peripheral vascular disease are claudication and limb-threatening ischemia (Table 4.5). Claudication is a relative indication because the majority of such patients will remain stable throughout their lifetime, especially with the control of risk factors, such as smoking, and institution of an exercise program. The Framingham study demonstrated that patients with intermittent claudication had a 5 per cent risk of major amputation within 5 years of the onset of symptoms. Within the same time frame, 23 per cent developed symptoms of CAD, 13 per cent suffered cerebrovascular accidents and 20 per cent died.[64] Patient longevity, durability of the arterial reconstruction and improvement in quality of life must be weighed against the operative risk.

The degree of disability must be individualized for patients presenting with claudication. Symptoms that occur at one block may not interfere significantly with the elderly patient with a sedentary lifestyle, but to one who has retired with the expectation of an active life this may constitute a serious restriction. To the patient who is still working, short distance claudication is usually significantly limiting.

Ischemic rest pain is a disabling pain that often cannot be controlled with narcotics and is an indication for reconstruction. When disease has progressed to the point of ischemic rest pain or ulceration, the likelihood of eventual major amputation is substantial. In addition, the risks and costs of arterial reconstruction for limb salvage have been equivalent to those for major amputation in most reports. Furthermore, elderly patients are unlikely to be rehabilitated or use prostheses successfully after major amputation, and more often end up in a chronic nursing facility.

RECOMMENDED APPROACH

The vascular surgical patient undergoing an infrainguinal reconstruction represents a significant challenge with respect to proper preoperative assessment. These patients have a high incidence of both symptomatic and occult CAD. The goal of the preoperative assessment of these patients is to identify subsets that are at a high risk of a cardiac event who would benefit from some intervention to decrease their morbidity and mortality. The preoperative risk assessment should begin with a careful history and physical examination. Basic laboratory tests, resting ECG and chest x-ray are obtained. The control of hypertension is of importance because of its adverse effect on myocardial oxygen consumption. It is important to continue beta-antagonists and calcium channel blockers in the preoperative and postoperative period as their withdrawal is associated with rebound tachycardia and hypertension. There is evolving evidence that preoperative institution of beta-blocker therapy is cardioprotective.

Patients presenting with claudication deserve thorough evaluation as surgery may be canceled or postponed without serious consequences if cardiac risk is prohibitive. Patients without cardiac history or a low cardiac risk index can proceed to surgery with a risk of cardiac morbidity of less than 3 per cent. Patients with known symptomatic CAD or intermediate risk factors based on the Eagle criteria deserve noninvasive workup with DTS, stress echocardiography or ambulatory Holter monitoring. If negative, patients may proceed to surgery with little risk. Those with strongly positive tests should undergo cardiac catheterization, if they are reasonable candidates and willing to proceed with possible CABG. Those with high risk due to CHF, recent MI, or severe or unstable angina should have optimization of their medical condition before surgery is considered.

Table 4.5 *Clinical categories of chronic limb ischemia: AP = ankle pressure, BP = brachial pressure, PVR = pulse volume recording, TP = toe pressure, TM = transmetatarsal*

Grade	Category	Clinical description	Objective data
0	0	Asymptomatic – no hemodynamically significant occlusive disease	Normal treadmill/stress test
I	1	Mild claudication	Completes treadmill exercise,[a] AP after exercise <50 mmHg, but >25 mmHg less than BP
	2	Moderate claudication	Between categories 1 and 3
	3	Severe claudication	Cannot complete treadmill exercise and AP after exercise <50 mmHg
II	4	Ischemic rest pain	Resting AP <40 mm Hg, flat or barely pulsatile ankle or metatarsal PVR; TP <30 mm Hg
III	5	Minor tissue loss, nonhealing ulcer, focal gangrene with diffuse pedal ischemia	Resting AP <60 mmHg, ankle or metatarsal PVR flat or barely pulsatile; TP <40 mmHg
	6	Major tissue loss, extending above TM level, functional foot no longer salvageable	Same as category 5

[a] 5 minutes at 2 mph on a 12 per cent incline.

Patients who present with ischemic rest pain, ulceration or gangrene require lower extremity revascularization, or will otherwise require amputation. In this patient population, cancellation of surgery is not a good option and risks limb loss during a prolonged cardiac workup.[65] Patients at low or moderate cardiac risk should proceed directly to surgery. Patients at high risk due to recent MI, severe or unstable angina or CHF should undergo cardiac catheterization only if they are candidates for and willing to proceed with potential CABG. Patients requiring emergent revascularization for limb-threatening ischemia should proceed directly to the operating room. Intraoperative monitoring with pulmonary artery catheters or TEE should be reserved for selective patients with heart failure, aortic stenosis or recent MI.

Coronary angiography should be limited to patients who are suitable candidates and are willing to undergo CABG before their vascular procedure. This includes patients with unstable or severe symptomatic CAD or patients with multiple segments of thallium redistribution on DTS. If patients meet the standard criteria for myocardial revascularization (significant three-vessel or left main disease), they should have CABG performed preoperatively. While PTCA is appealing because of its lower risk, there are no data to support its use preoperatively in cardiac risk reduction.

Based on the available data, we developed an algorithm for the selective use of preoperative testing and cardiac catheterization with modification based on the patient's indication for revascularization (Fig. 4.1). There are few studies using a selective approach to preoperative risk assessment, however, results have been encouraging. Taylor and colleagues described their results after implementing a conservative preoperative screening program in 513 patients referred for vascular surgery.[66] Only in those patients with severe symptoms of CAD (5.8 per cent) (defined as unstable angina, uncontrolled arrhythmia, CHF or MI within 6 months) was further evaluation performed. Postoperative MI rate was 4.2 per cent with an overall death rate of 2.2 per cent (0.8 per cent cardiac).

Finally, patients considered at higher cardiac risk who undergo vascular surgery, especially infrainguinal reconstruction, should have close monitoring in the postoperative period as the majority of cardiac events occur during this time. Multiple-lead monitoring for silent ischemia offers an exciting potential for the detection and treatment of postoperative ischemic events to prevent subsequent morbid events. Beta-blocker therapy is also a promising adjunct.

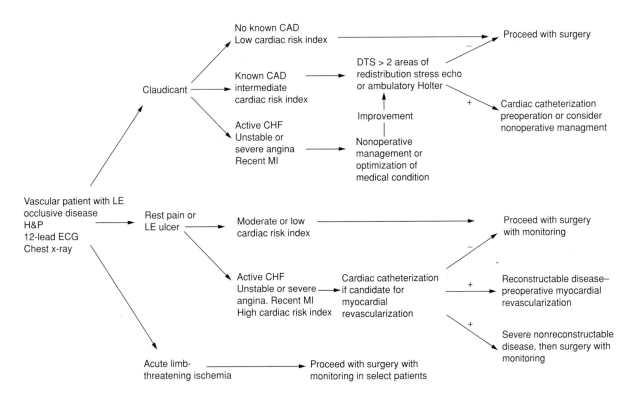

Figure 4.1 *Recommended approach in patients requiring lower extremity revascularization: CAD = coronary artery disease, CHF = congestive heart failure, DTS = dipyridamole thallium scanning, ECG = electrocardiogram, H&P = history and physical examination, LE = lower extremity, MI = myocardial infarction.*

REFERENCES

1 Mangano DT, Goldman L. Preoperative assessment of patients with known or suspected coronary disease. *N Engl J Med* 1995; **333**: 1750–6.

2 Mangano DT. Perioperative cardiac morbidity. *Anesthesiology* 1990; **72**: 153–84.

3 Yeager RA. Basic data related to cardiac testing and cardiac risk associated with vascular surgery. *Ann Vasc Surg* 1990; **4**: 193–7.

4 Hertzer NR, Beven KG, Young JR *et al*. Coronary artery disease in peripheral vascular patients: a classification of 1000 coronary angiograms and results of surgical management. *Ann Surg* 1984; **199**: 223–33.

5 Lette J. Waters D, Lassonde J. *et al*. Multivariate clinical models and quantitative dipyridamole–thallium imaging to predict cardiac morbidity and death after vascular reconstruction. *J Vasc Surg* 1991; **14**: 160.

6 Tomatis LA, Fierens EE, Verbrugge GP. Evaluation of surgical risk in peripheral vascular disease by coronary arteriography. A series of 100 cases. *Surgery* 1972; **71**: 429–35.

7 Young JR, Hertzer NR, Beven EG *et al*. Coronary artery disease in patients with aortic aneurysm: a classification of 302 coronary angiograms and results of surgical management. *Ann Vasc Surg* 1986; **1**: 36.

8 Blombery PA, Ferguson IA, Rosengarten DS *et al*. The role of coronary artery disease in complications of abdominal aortic aneurysm surgery. *Surgery* 1987; **101**: 150.

9 Orecchia PM, Berger PW, White CJ *et al*. Coronary artery disease in aortic surgery. *Ann Vasc Surg* 1988; **2**: 28.

10 Krupski WC, Layug EL, Reilly LM *et al*. Comparison of cardiac morbidity between aortic and infrainguinal operations. *J Vasc Surg* 1992; **15**: 354–65.

11 Bry JDL, Belkin M, O'Donnell TF *et al*. An assessment of the positive predictive value and cost-effectiveness of dipyridamole myocardial scintigraphy in patients undergoing vascular surgery. *J Vasc Surg* 1994; **19**: 112–24.

12 Executive Committee for the Asymptomatic Carotid Atherosclerosis Study. Endarterectomy for asymptomatic carotid artery stenosis. *JAMA* 1995; **273**: 1421–8.

13 North American Symptomatic Carotid Endarterectomy Trial Collaborators. Beneficial effect of carotid endarterectomy in symptomatic patients with high-grade carotid stenosis. *N Engl J Med* 1991; **325**: 445–53.

14 Goldman L, Caldera DL, Nessbaum SR, *et al*. Multifactorial index of cardiac risk in noncardiac surgical procedures. *N Engl J Med* 1977; **297**: 845.

15 Dripps RD, Lamont A, Eckenhoff JE. The role of anaesthesia in surgical mortality. *JAMA* 1961; **178**: 261.

16 Detsky AS, Abrams HB, Forbath N *et al*. Cardiac assessment for patients undergoing noncardiac surgery: a multifactorial clinical risk index. *Arch Intern Med* 1986; **146**: 2131–4.

17 Eagle KA, Coley CM, Newell JB *et al*. Combining clinical and thallium data optimizes preoperative assessment of cardiac risk before major vascular surgery. *Ann Intern Med* 1989; **110**: 859–66.

18 Cooperman M, Pflug B, Martin EW *et al*. Cardiovascular risk factors in patients with peripheral vascular disease. *Surgery* 1978; **84**: 505–9.

19 Steen PA, Tinker JH, Tarhan S. Myocardial reinfarction after anesthesia and surgery. *JAMA* 1978; **239**: 2566–70.

20 Rao TLK, Jacobs KH, El-Etr AA. Reinfarction following anesthesia in patients with myocardial infarction. *Anesthesiology* 1983; **59**: 499–505.

21 Rivers SP, Scher LA, Gupta SK *et al*. Safety of peripheral vascular surgery after a recent acute myocardial infarction. *J Vasc Surg* 1990; **11**: 70.

22 Shah KB, Kleinman BS, Sami H *et al*. Reevaluation of perioperative myocardial infarction in patients with prior myocardial infarction undergoing noncardiac operations. *Anesth Analg* 1990; **71**: 231.

23 Pasternack PF, Imparato AM, Riles TS, *et al*. The value of radionuclide angiogram in the prediction of perioperative myocardial infection in patients undergoing lower extremity revascularization procedures. *Circulation* 1985; **72** (suppl II): 2–13.

24 Kannel WB, McGee DL. Diabetes and cardiovascular risk factors: The Framingham Study. *Circulation* 1979; **59**: 8–13.

25 Foster ED, Davis KB, Carpenter JA *et al*. Risk of noncardiac operation in patients with defined coronary disease: the coronary artery surgery study (CASS) registry experience. *Ann Thorac Surg* 1986; **41**: 42–50.

26 Jeffrey CC, Kunsman J. Cullen DJ, Brewster DC. A prospective evaluation of cardiac risk index. *Anesthesiology* 1983; **58**: 462–4.

27 Wong T, Detsky AS. Preoperative cardiac risk assessment for patients having peripheral vascular surgery. *Ann Intern Med* 1992; **116**: 742.

28 Boucher CA, Brewster DC, Darling RC *et al*. Determination of cardiac risk by dipyridamole–thallium imaging before peripheral vascular surgery. *N Engl J Med* 1985; **312**: 389–94.

29 Raby KE, Goldman L, Creager MA *et al*. Correlation between preoperative ischemia and major cardiac events after peripheral vascular surgery. *N Engl J Med* 1989; **321**: 1296–1300.

30 Carliner NH, Fisher ML, Plotnick GD *et al*. Routine preoperative exercise testing in patients undergoing major noncardiac surgery. *Am J Cardiol* 1985; **56**: 51–7.

31 Von Knorring J. Postoperative myocardial infarction: A prospective study in a risk group of surgical patients. *Surgery* 1981; **90**: 55–60.

32 Bruce RA, Kasumi F. Hosmer J. Maximal oxygen uptake and normographic assessment of functional aerobic impairment in cardiovascular disease. *Am Heart J* 1973; **85**: 546–62.

33 Cutler BS, Wheeler HB, Paraskos JA *et al*. Applicability and interpretation of electrocardiographic stress testing in patients with peripheral vascular disease. *Am J Surg* 1981; **141**: 484–90.

34 McPhail N. Calvin JE, Shariatmadar A *et al*. The use of preoperative exercise testing to predict cardiac complications after arterial reconstruction. *J Vasc Surg* 1988; **7**: 6068.

35 Mangano DT, Hollenberg M, Fegert G *et al*. Perioperative myocardial ischemia in patients undergoing noncardiac surgery. I. Incidence and severy during the 4 day perioperative period. *J Am Coll Cardiol* 1991; **17**: 843.

36 Raby KE, Barry J. Creager MA *et al*. Detection and significance of intraoperative and postoperative myocardial ischemia in peripheral vascular surgery. *JAMA* 1992; **268**: 222–7.

37 Pasternack PF, Grossi EA, Baumann G *et al*. The value of silent myocardial ischemia monitoring in the prediction of perioperative myocardial infarction in patients undergoing peripheral vascular surgery. *J Vasc Surg* 1989; **10**: 617–25.

38 Kazmers A, Cequeira MD, Zierler RE. The role of preoperative radionuclide ejection fraction in direct abdominal aortic aneurysm repair. *J Vasc Surg* 1988; **8**: 128–36.

39 McCann RL, Wolfe RG. Resection of abdominal aortic aneurysm in patients with low ejection fractions. *J Vasc Surg* 1989; **10**: 240–4.

40 Baron J-F, Mundler O. Bertrand M *et al*. Dipyridamole–thallium scintigraphy and gated radionuclide angiography to assess cardiac risk before abdominal aortic surgery. *N Engl J Med* 1994; **330**: 663–9.

41 Poldermans D, Arnese M, Fioretti PM *et al*. Improved cardiac risk stratification in major vascular surgery with dobutamine-atropine stress echocardiography. *J Am Coll Cardiol* 1995; **26**: 648–53.

42 Mangano DT, London MJ, Tubau JF *et al*. Dipyridamole thallium-201 scintigraphy as a preoperative screening test. A reexamination of its predictive potential. *Circulation* 1991; **84**: 493–502.

43 Real GJ, Cooley DA, Duncan JM *et al*. The effect of coronary bypass on the outcome of peripheral vascular operations in 1093 patients. *J Vasc Surg* 1986; **3**: 788–98.

44 Gersh BJ, Kronmal RA, Frye RL *et al*. Coronary arteriography and coronary artery bypass surgery: morbidity and mortality in patients ages 65 or older. A report from the Coronary Artery Surgery Study. *Circulation* 1983; **67**: 483–91.

45 Mullany CJ, Darling GE, Pluth JR *et al*. Early and late results after isolated coronary artery bypass surgery in 159 patients aged 80 years or older. *Circulation* 1990; **82**(4): IV229–36.

46 Toal KW, Jacocks MA, Elkins RC. Preoperative coronary artery bypass grafting in patients undergoing abdominal aortic reconstruction. *Am J Surg* 1984; **148**: 825–9.

47 Rihal CS, Eagle KA, Mickel MC *et al*. Surgical therapy for coronary artery disease among patients with combined coronary artery and peripheral vascular disease. *Circulation* 1995; **91**: 46–53.

48 Huber KC, Evans MA, Bresnahan JF *et al*. Outcome of noncardiac operations in patients with severe coronary artery disease successfully treated preoperatively with coronary angioplasty. *Mayo Clin Proc* 1992; **67**: 15–21.

49 Illes RW, Levitsky S. Review of invasive treatments of coronary artery disease. *Surg Gynecol Obstet* 1989; **168**: 461–7.

50 Mason JL, Owens DK, Harris RA *et al*. The role of coronary angiography and coronary revascularization before noncardiac vascular surgery. *JAMA* 1995; **273**: 1919–25.

51 Hertzer NR. The natural history of peripheral vascular disease: implications for its management. *Circulation* 1991; **83**(suppl D): 1–12.

52 Bode RH, Lewis KP, Zarich SW *et al*. Cardiac outcome after peripheral vascular surgery: comparison of general and regional anesthesia. *Anesthesiology* 1996; **84**: 3–13.

53 Connors AF, Speroff T. Dawson NV *et al*. The effectiveness of right heart catheterization in the initial care of critically ill patients. *JAMA* 1996; **276**: 889–97.

54 Gore JM, Goldberg RJ, Spodick DH, Alpert JS, Dalen JE. A community-wide assessment of the use of pulmonary artery catheters in patients with acute myocardial infarction. *Chest* 1987; **92**: 721–7.

55 Haggmark S, Hohner P, Ostman M *et al*. Comparison of hemodynamic, electrocardiographic, mechanical, and metabolic indicators of intraoperative myocardial ischemia in vascular surgical patients with coronary artery disease. *Anesthesiology* 1989; **70**: 19–25.

56 Roizen MF, Beaupre PN, Alpert RA *et al*. Monitoring with two-dimensional transesophageal echocardiography: comparison of myocardial function in patients undergoing supraceliac, suprarenal-infraceliac, or infrarenal aortic occlusion. *J Vasc Surg* 1984; **1**: 300–5.

57 London MJ, Tubau JF, Wong MG *et al*. The natural history of segmental wall motion abnormalities in patients undergoing noncardiac surgery. *Anesthesiology* 1990; **73**: 644–55.

58 Marek JM, Mills JL, Harvich J *et al*. Utility of routine carotid duplex screening in patients presenting with claudication. *J Vasc Surg* 1996; **24**: 572–9.

59 Gentile AT, Taylor LM, Moneta GL, Porter JM. Prevalence of asymptomatic carotid stenosis in patients undergoing infrainguinal bypass surgery. *Arch Surg* 1995; **130**: 900–4.

60 Harris EJ, Moneta GL, Yeager RA *et al*. Neurologic deficits following noncarotid vascular surgery. *Am J Surg* 1992; **163**: 537.

61 Hertzer NR, Beven KG, Young JR *et al*. Incidental asymptomatic carotid bruits in patients scheduled for peripheral vascular reconstruction. *Surgery* 1984; **96**: 535–43.

62 Vodinh J, Bonnet F, Touboul C *et al*. Risk factors of postoperative pulmonary complications after vascular surgery. *Surgery* 1989; **105**: 360–5.

63 Whittemore AD, Donaldson MC, Mannick JA. Infrainguinal reconstruction for patients with chronic renal insufficiency. *J Vasc Surg* 1993; **17**: 32.

64 Peabody CN, Kannel WB, McNamara PM. Intermittent claudication: surgical significance. *Arch Surg* 1974; **109**: 693.

65 Krupski WC, Lawson RP, Whitehill TA *et al*. 'Cleared by Cardiology': The downside of routine preoperative cardiac evaluation before vascular surgery. Presented at the *11th Annual WVS*, Janiary 1996.

66 Taylor LM, Yeager RA, Moneta GL *et al*. The incidence of perioperative myocardial infarction in general vascular surgery. *J Vasc Surg* 1991; **15**: 52–61.

67 Rutherford RB, Flanigan DP, Gupta Sk *et al*. Suggested standards for reports dealing with lower extremity ischemia. *J Vasc Surg* 1986; **4**: 80.

5

Angioplasty, atherectomy and stenting of infrainguinal arteries

KLAUS SEE-THO AND E JOHN HARRIS

INTRODUCTION

The field of endovascular surgery is a relatively new area of medicine in which catheter-mediated intravascular manipulations are used for the diagnosis and treatment of vascular diseases. Endovascular surgical procedures are considered minimally invasive with vascular access usually obtained percutaneously at a site remotely located from the area of disease. Rapid advancement in technology and refinement in application have occurred since its introduction into clinical practice more than two decades ago. Although still in need of more rigorous clinical validation, prominent diagnostic and therapeutic roles have been accepted for several endovascular procedures. Moreover, continued development of new technology combined with new insights into the molecular mechanisms of vascular disease suggest increasing utilization of minimally invasive surgical techniques in the future treatment of diseased vascular tissue.

This chapter outlines the various facets of endovascular surgical applications in the diagnosis and treatment of lower extremity, arterial-occlusive disease. A brief historical overview is followed by a discussion of various diagnostic interventions and a detailed review of different therapeutic modalities. Indications for intervention, results of therapy, associated complications, a comparison with other medical or surgical treatment modalities, and current controversies in endovascular surgery are also discussed. Finally, future prospects in endovascular surgery with focus on developments in vascular biology and prevention of restenosis are outlined.

HISTORICAL PERSPECTIVE

The roots of endovascular therapies stretch back more than 100 years to the discovery of x-rays by Roentgen in 1895.[1] Several months thereafter, in 1896, Haschek and Lindenthal showed that x-rays could be used to visualize vessels from an amputated arm after injection with radio-opaque chalk.[2] Numerous pathologic animal and human studies of vascular anatomy followed but *in vivo* arteriograms were not made possible until the development of ionic contrast media in the 1920s.

At that time, catheter-mediated vascular access was also being developed. In 1928, Forssmann performed a right heart catheterization by passing a catheter from his own antecubital vein into his right atrium.[3] Vascular access was obtained by surgical cut-down until development of percutaneous methods in the 1950s. Seldinger's percutaneous wire-guided technique, introduced in 1953, quickly became a standard method for not only intravascular catheterization but most interventional procedures performed percutaneously to date.[4]

Arteriography became a powerful diagnostic tool for vascular surgeons, but therapeutic catheter-mediated intravascular interventions were largely undeveloped until the 1960s, when Fogarty developed his thrombo-embolectomy balloon catheter in 1963,[5] and Dotter attempted the first endoluminal angioplasty in 1964.[6] Using variably sized coaxial catheters placed over a guidewire, Dotter successfully dilated a series of stenotic femoropopliteal arteries. Dotter recognized the profound potential for endovascular treatment of vascular disease:

> Perhaps it is wishful thinking, but in any event, I am convinced that the relief of atheromatous obstruction in small arteries can best be accomplished by catheter technics. A flexible guide introduced percutaneously into an artery proximal to an area of atheromatous narrowing can be manipulated so as to traverse the obstruction. A mechanical attack upon the lesion would then become feasible, perhaps by gradual direct dilatation ...[7]

Dotter also pioneered efforts to dilate vessels using balloon-tipped catheters.[8] He attempted angioplasty with Fogarty thromboembolectomy catheters, but found the compliance of latex, even after reinforcement with fiberglass, did not allow for the generation of adequate radial dilating forces. Dotter also recognized the potential benefit of intravascular stenting to provide a rigid support within diseased vessels to counteract any tendency towards restenosis or occlusion, such as elastic recoil. In 1969, Dotter reported his experience with placement of spring-coil tube grafts in dog popliteal arteries.[9] Although he had only limited success with his procedures, Dotter nevertheless can be considered the father of endovascular surgery for developing the concept of intravascular catheter-mediated therapy.

Unfortunately, Dotter's pioneering work was largely ignored in the USA. However, in Europe, Porstmann, van Andel, Zeitler and their colleagues recognized the value of Dotter's work, and further refined his percutaneous angioplasty techniques.[7] In 1973, Porstmann developed a rigidly caged latex balloon to combat the problems of overcompliance.[10] However, this device was not favorably accepted because of concerns regarding excessive vascular wall trauma and predisposition to thrombosis.

Only after Gruentzig developed the first fixed-diameter, low-compliance, balloon catheter made from polyvinyl chloride in 1974 did the concept of catheter-mediated endoluminal dilatation gain recognition in the USA.[11] The low compliance of polyvinyl chloride allowed for generation of up to six atmospheres of radially exerted pressure within a fixed diameter. By using accurately sized catheters, risk for excessive vessel trauma, rupture or distal embolization was reduced. In 1976, Gruentzig created a double-lumen, single-end hole, balloon catheter, which subsequently has become the standard design for angioplasty catheters today.[12]

Since then, continued advances in guidewire, balloon, catheter, miniaturization, imaging and delivery system technology have enabled widespread application of balloon angioplasty throughout the human vascular tree. However, excitement with the new technique of balloon angioplasty has been tempered by disappointing success rates. Crossing longer complicated stenoses or occlusions, overcoming the residual stenosis of elastic recoil, developing luminal irregularity, acute thrombosis or dissection, and failing to maintain long-term patency due to the neointimal proliferative vascular injury response are significant problems limiting the widespread application of modern low-profile balloons and delivery systems.

With the never-ending search for improvement in the interventional arsenal against atherosclerotic disease and the desire to overcome many of the problems associated with balloon angioplasty, mechanical atherectomy and laser ablation devices have been developed. In parallel, diagnostic capabilities have improved, including the development of computer-assisted digital subtraction angiography with real-time road-mapping capabilities and the development of intravascular ultrasound imaging.

Laser technology, first developed in the late 1950s, was recognized for medical uses in the 1960s and 1970s for opthamologic, gynecologic, dermatologic, gastrointestinal and oncologic therapies. The therapeutic potential of photoablative therapy, combined with the development of percutaneous intravascular access, prompted intense interest in laser-assisted ablation of atheroma in the late 1970s and into the 1980s.[13–16] The concept was attractive, but significant complications and limitations of the technique have kept laser angioplasty interventions out of accepted medical practice. Nevertheless, interest in the development of 'high-tech' mechanisms for the dissolution of atheromatous disease remains enthusiastic.

The attractive concept of removal rather than rupture–dilatation of atheroma, led to the development of various mechanical atherectomy devices in the 1980s.[17–19] The underlying concept behind atherectomy was the hypothesis that removal, rather than stretching and fracturing, of atheromatous plaques would decrease the atherosclerotic burden and thus diminish the opportunity for restenosis or progression of disease.[20,21] In addition, removal of plaques without creation of intimal flaps or irregular luminal surfaces was also postulated to diminish the failure rate seen with conventional balloon angioplasty.

Finally, renewed interest in stent technology (fairly dormant since Dotter's work with coils in 1969) was brought on by the limitations associated with angioplasty, especially in overcoming postangioplasty restenosis from dissection or elastic recoil, and in attempts to improve long-term patency.[22] In the 1980s, Cragg, Dotter, Gianturco, Maas, Palmaz and others popularized stents with innovative designs, which were flexible or stiff, self-expanding or balloon expandable, and were made of advanced materials, such as shape-memory-retaining nitinol.[23–28] Additionally, stents were combined with graft materials to provide anchoring support for endoluminally placed 'stent-grafts'. Today, this stent-graft technology is rapidly evolving for the treatment of occlusive, aneurysmal and traumatic vascular diseases.[29–35]

DIAGNOSTIC PROCEDURES

The standard angiography of the late 1950s and early 1960s allowed excellent visualization of the aorta and its major branches, but required multiple plane-film projections and large amounts of potentially toxic contrast to view the entire lower extremity circulation. The 'cut-film' resolution of more peripheral vessels, especially those below the knee, was preferred by most surgeons, but required large volumes of contrast and multiple films at several stations. The development of computer-assisted angiography with digital subtraction to remove soft-tissue and bone artifacts and digital enhancement of contrast, allowed for decreased contrast volumes, while maintaining resolution of the distal vessels, albeit in a much smaller format than traditional cut films.[36] In addition, because the entire lower extremity could be visualized by following a single contrast bolus from the aorta to the foot in one sweep of the fluoroscope, real-time assessment of flow characteristics and a digitally subtracted 'road-mapping' capability became possible. Road-mapping allows one to maneuver guidewires and catheters in real time along a path marked by a contrast image retained by the computer. Refinement in angiographic techniques has also led to the development of less toxic, nonionic, contrast media and the use of non-toxic carbon dioxide gas as a contrast medium.[37] To date, angiography remains central to endovascular therapy, by providing accurate localization of disease and allowing near real-time maneuvering and placement of interventional catheters and devices. It also allows for direct assessment of technical success by completion angiography. At this time, angiography remains the 'gold standard' for preprocedural imaging of diseased arterial segments, although magnetic resonance and ultrasound imaging techniques are moving in a direction to supplant diagnostic arteriography.

Intravascular ultrasound (IVUS) devices were developed in the past decade to better visualize vascular wall morphology from within. External ultrasound devices have been used extensively to assist in the diagnosis and characterization of vascular disease.[38] Physiologic data was obtained with Doppler ultrasound, and morphologic characteristics of the arterial wall could be seen with B-mode and color Doppler technology. However, visualization of the vessel wall, especially in deep vessels like the iliac arteries, is often difficult due to overlying soft-tissue and gas interference. Thus, endovascular ultrasound devices were developed to circumvent these limitations. IVUS has been used to monitor the adequacy of various angioplasty and atherectomy procedures, as well as placement of endovascular stents.[39,40] Limitations include vessel size, interference from air bubbles, difficulty in differentiating fat, fresh thrombus and dissection planes that appear nonechoic, and interference from shadowing behind calcific lesions. IVUS has been shown to be an extremely accurate method for estimating luminal diameter and degree of stenosis. In addition, the ability to visualize images through blood without needing irrigation eliminates risks for systemic fluid overload. Therapeutically, ultrasound-guided angioplasty and atherectomy devices have been developed. Recent development of low-profile IVUS catheters, essentially the size of guidewires, allows real-time assessment of balloon angioplasty and stent deployment.[41]

BALLOON ANGIOPLASTY

As discussed above, balloon angioplasty was the first therapeutic endovascular technique conceived, dating back to the pioneering work of Dotter in the 1960s. Today, thousands of percutaneous transluminal angioplasties (PTA) of stenotic and occlusive lesions in the lower extremity are performed yearly. The basic technique involves antegrade percutaneous vascular access of the common femoral artery, and placement of guidewires and catheters under direct fluoroscopic or angiographic road-mapping guidance across the site of vessel stenosis or occlusion. Subsequently, low-profile balloon catheters are threaded over the wire down to the site of disease, and inflated rapidly to dilate and crack the atherosclerotic lesion, thereby re-establishing a functional lumen for arterial flow. These procedures are performed under systemic heparinization.

Adjunctive use of additional endovascular techniques and drug therapy to improve the technical success of angioplasty have been employed. Given the complexity of atherosclerotic lesions, not all lesions can be traversed and dilated. Thus mechanical atherectomy and laser ablation devices have been developed (see below). In addition, because many atherosclerotic lesions have adherent thrombi, adjunctive use of fibrinolytic therapy has been used to reduce the length of occlusive lesions and possibly convert total occlusions into stenoses, which are easier to traverse.[42,43] Occasionally, residual stenosis (defined as greater than 30 per cent diameter reduction) secondary to bulky complex lesions and elastic recoil of the dilated vessel occur and these lesions have been treated by placement of intravascular stents.[28] Following procedural heparinization to minimize thrombosis, long-term use of antiplatelet drugs (aspirin) before and after balloon angioplasty is recommended.[44]

Practically, multiple PTA procedures are often necessary and outcomes can be variable. Earlier case series from the 1980s reported results that appear comparable to surgical success rates but reporting standards were variable.[45] Patients selected for PTA had generally less severe disease (e.g. claudicants) than those undergoing surgical revascularization (i.e. for rest pain, gangrene or ulceration); primary and secondary patencies were ill-defined, specifically excluding initial failures; lesion characteristics were not uniformly recorded; follow-up intervals were frequently short; complications were inconsistently reported; and standard statistical methods with the use of life-table actuarial analyses were lacking. In the 1990s, guidelines for indications and reporting standards for endovascular therapy for lower extremity ischemia have been developed to resolve these deficiencies and allow more accurate comparisons.[46–49]

Acknowledging these shortcomings, trends for successful PTA have been identified.[50–52] In general, the best outcomes are from PTA of lesions in aortoiliac vessels in comparison to femoropopliteal or (even worse) infrapopliteal tibial arteries. Stenotic lesions fare better than occlusions, especially in regard to immediate technical success. Lesions that are more concentric than eccentric, and are less than 10–15 cm (and especially <3–5 cm) in length are more successfully dilated. Less diseased limbs as characterized by severity of symptoms (claudication vs rest pain, ulceration or gangrene), more focal disease (less than two segmental areas involved) and with good run-off (2–3 patent tibial vessels) fare much better than more diseased limbs. Other factors, such as the presence of comorbid cardiovascular or cerebrovascular disease, and diabetes, have been associated with poorer outcomes.[50]

The best results have been found in aortoiliac angioplasty of stenotic lesions in patients with claudication. In this group, greater than 90 per cent 1-year success and up to 70 per cent 5-year patency can be expected.[53–55] Results from iliac PTA series published over the past decade are summarized in Table 5.1. In addition, other more severe lesions in the aortoiliac vessels can be successfully dilated

with surprising long-term patencies from 50 to 70 per cent, especially when adjunctive use of stents and/or thrombolysis is employed.[56–58] Given this relatively good outcome, and a perceived low complication rate in comparison to surgical intervention, PTA and adjunctive use of stents and/or thrombolysis has been accepted by many as standard therapy for isolated aortoiliac occlusive disease.[59] In some situations, angioplasty may be used as an adjunct to infrainguinal bypass operations in order to provide adequate in-flow.[60,61]

Femoropopliteal or even more distal PTA, however, enjoys less initial success and disappointing long-term patencies and outcomes. Based on published series from the 1980s by Hunick, Gallino, Krepel, Hewes, Spence and Johnston and others, 1-year patency rates from 60 per cent to near 100 per cent and 5-year rates up to 70–80 per cent with lower extremity PTA are possible.[62–71] However, more recent studies using the more stringent, accepted reporting criteria indicate that 1-year patencies are closer to 50–75 per cent with 5-year rates as low as 30 per cent for infrainguinal PTAs.[52,72–80] By using a confidence profile metanalysis, Adar et al. reviewed 12 femoropopliteal PTA series totaling 1461 procedures, and reported 66 per cent 1-year and 60 per cent 5-year patencies.[77] When comparing indications, they found 62 per cent 3-year patency for angioplasty in claudicants compared to 43 per cent for limb salvage. In a separate review of 4304 femoropopliteal angioplasties, Becker et al. reported a 67 per cent 2-year patency rate.[44] In a large well-reported series from the University of Toronto, claudicants undergoing femoropopliteal PTA had a 1-year patency of 63 per cent and 5-year rate of 38 per cent.[78] Patency was judged by hemodynamic assessment as well as clinical outcome. Two factors were identified by multiple regression analyses as influencing patency: (1) stenoses vs occlusions; and (2) good vs poor distal run-off. It appeared that early procedural success was better in stenoses than occlusions and late patency was

Table 5.1 *Results of iliac artery angioplasty*

Author (year)	Procedures	Patency (years)					Comments
		1	2	3	4	5	
Spence (1981)[65]	148	93	87	79			
Gallino (1984)[63]	153	86	86	86	85	84	
Samson (1984)[83]	61	89	78	78			Excludes early failures
Van Andel (1985)[53]	194	100	98	95	94	90	Excludes early failures
Hewes (1986)[66]	141	91	89	89			
Henriksen (1988)[85]	55	85	80	80	75	75	
Wilson (1989)[81]	81	76	72	65	62	59	
Becker (1989)[44]	2697		81			72	Retrospective review
Clement (1990)[73]	61	93	88	69			Excludes early failures
Jeans (1990)[72]	180	69	62	60	59	57	
Harris (1991)[76]	148	88	88				
Johnston (1993)[55]	662	76	65	60	58	53	All iliac PTAs
Johnston (1993)[55]	580	77	67	61	58	54	Stenoses only
Johnston (1993)[55]	82	60	53	48			Occlusions only

determined by the presence of adequate distal outflow. These same factors were also influential in studies of patients with limb-threatening ischemia undergoing femoropopliteal PTA.[52] A summary of patency rates from PTA series published over the past decade is provided in Table 5.2.

Few reports document the results of infrapopliteal angioplasty.[88–92] While technically feasible with improved guidewire and balloon technology and improved angiographic resolution of distal vasculature, infrapopliteal PTA has been largely unsuccessful. Distal vessels are smaller and tend to be more diffusely diseased, thus making focal dilatations less successful and effective. In addition, since claudication usually results from occlusive disease above the tibial trifurcation, patients with distal disease tend to present with more significant ischemia and limb threat. Only 20–30 per cent of patients with distal PVD present with isolated tibial disease of which only lesions less than 5 cm long appear amenable to angioplasty.[90] Schwarten reports a 2-year limb salvage rate of 83 per cent in this small subset of patients,[90] but a more recent report by Treiman *et al.* suggests that infrageniculate PTA is not durable with hemodynamic success less than 20 per cent at 3 years.[92] It appears that distal lower extremity PTA should be reserved only for those patients with ideal, short, focal lesions (rare) or as a temporizing measure for patients with significantly limited life expectancy or severe contraindications to surgery.

LASER DEVICES

Since its invention in the late 1950s and its application to medical practice beginning in the late 1960s, the use of laser energy to treat atherosclerotic lesions has been attractive. Lasers emit electromagnetic energy of specific wavelengths based on electrical stimulation of a solid or gas medium in a mirrored chamber, which allows for amplified excitement of atoms. Photons of specific wavelengths (dependent upon the type of medium used) are emitted when the excited atoms return to baseline states. When delivered through fiber optics, this energy has been shown to be able to ablate atherosclerotic plaque precisely with limited injury to the underlying arterial wall.[15,16,93] Mechanisms for laser ablation include: thermal vaporization occurring when laser light is absorbed by tissues, converting the energy into heat; photochemical dissociation of molecular bonds without heat; electromechanical disruption of tissue where a free electron mass (plasma) creates a shock wave that disrupts tissue with minimal surrounding thermal injury; and by photochemical transformation of chromophobes resulting in local production of toxic intermediates causing tissue injury.[15,94]

Most medical lasers are continuous-wave type making use of argon ion, carbon dioxide (CO_2), or compounds with yttrium-aluminum-garnet (YAG) as the lasing medium. These lasers ablate tissue via thermal

Table 5.2 *Results of femoropopliteal artery angioplasty*

Author (year)	Procedures	Patency (years)					Comments
		1	2	3	4	5	
Gallino (1984)[63]	289	62	61	60	58	58	
Samson (1984)[83]	89	50	46	46			Excludes early failures
Krepel (1985)[64]	164	100	81	77	70	70	Excludes early failures
Hewes (1986)[66]	137	81	80	61	61		Stenoses only
Walden (1986)[84]	23	69	69				
Henriksen (1988)[85]	31	46	43	43	43	43	Claudicants only
Jorgenson (1988)[86]	58	40	33	25	25		
Milford (1988)[70]	27		47				Limb salvage rate
Adar (1989)[77]	1461	66	61	58		60	Confidence profile review
Becker (1989)[44]	4304		67		67	67	Review
Blair (1989)[82]	54		18				Limb salvage rate
Wilson (1989)[81]	49	62	59	59	59		
Clement (1990)[73]	85		58				Excludes early failures
Jeans (1990)[72]	190	48	43	42	41	41	
Stokes (1990)[54]	40	49	47	34	25	15	Diabetics only
Capek (1991)[50]	217	57	52	49	48	42	
Harris (1991)[76]	191	70					
Johnston (1992)[51]	254	63	53	51	44	38	
Hunink (1993)[52]	126	57	50	45	45	45	
Matsi (1994)[80]	208	47		42			Claudicants only
Stanley (1996)[87]	200		46				

vaporization. Around a central core of vaporization, concentric areas of cell necrosis/coagulation and acoustic (shock wave) injury occur. Remarkably, these lesions heal within 30 days and are associated with minimal inflammatory response and relatively normal re-endothelialization.[95] Studies in atherosclerotic monkeys demonstrate retardation of the neointimal hyperplastic response, which theoretically would slow the process of postprocedural restenosis.[95] Various absorption characteristics of different tissues results in variability in thermal ablation. For instance, argon lasers produce radiation at wavelengths of 488 and 514 nm, which are preferentially absorbed by fatty atherosclerotic plaque. However, white fibrous plaques are relatively insensitive and thus limit the ability for laser recanalization.[96] With the use of higher energies, the area of injury increases but depth remains a function of tissue absorption characteristics.

Pulsed-wave lasers, on the other hand, disrupt tissues by photochemical dissociation of molecular bonds with few thermal effects.[97] These 'cold lasers' are created by excitation and bonding of a noble gas/halogen medium producing excited dimers (eximer), which generate pulses of short-wavelength, high-energy ultraviolet light. The most common eximer laser is the xenon-chloride laser, which emits energy with a wavelength of 308 nm. Tissue is rapidly converted to vaporized fragments with minimal heat transfer to adjacent tissues, thus enabling disruption of thermally-resistant calcified lesions with little injury to the surrounding arterial wall. In contrast to continuous wave lasers, increasing energy of pulse-wave devices result in deeper penetration without change in width of tissue injury.

The first lasers approved for use in treatment of atherosclerosis used continuous-wave argon thermal ablation. Because vessel perforation was common with a bare optical fiber delivery system, a metal cap was added, resulting in the 'hot-tip' laser probe.[98] Another thermal contact probe was created by using a sapphire-tipped optical fiber.[99] A hybrid probe with a metal cap and recessed sapphire lens was also developed to deliver a fine beam directly and to heat through the metal cap diffusely.[93] Other laser devices make use of lens-tipped optical fibers to produce free beams, which are centered in the vessel via a balloon and use photochemical emulsions in a balloon to convert a linear laser beam into a diffuse cylindrical one.[93]

Clinical testing of all these laser devices has been uniformly disappointing, regardless of laser source, suggesting that, although theoretical use of laser energy to ablate atherosclerotic lesions is enticing, an effective device for delivery of this energy in a precise manner has yet to be developed. Most reports in the literature involve testing of continuous-wave 'hot-tip', sapphire or hybrid devices. Although initial success rates can be as high as 85 per cent for short (<3 cm) lesions, long-term patency has been disappointingly low with 1-year success rates rang-

ing from 11 to 57 per cent.[100–103] Eximer lasers appear to treat calcific lesions better than continuous-wave devices, but clinical success is less than 50 per cent before the first year of follow-up is over.[104,105] Interestingly, much of the initial successes have been attributed to the mechanical properties of the laser devices in enabling penetration through occlusive or tightly stenotic lesions, rather than to the ablative ability of laser energy. Indeed, the profile of the 'hot-tip' probe has been shown to enable crossing difficult lesions without turning on the laser device.[106]

Complications include perforation, hemorrhage, thrombosis, fistula formation, embolization, dissection and worsening of ischemia necessitating emergency operation. An increased complication rate has been attributed to a lack of a practical three-dimensional guidance system.[93] Subintimal deflection of laser probes due to bulky or calcific lesions, sets up the possibility for dissection and/or perforation. In addition, laser systems can only create small 2–3 mm channels, which then require subsequent balloon dilatation to enlarge the lumen. Thus, much of the theoretical and experimental benefit of laser therapy in limiting the proliferative response to injury is overshadowed by the significant vessel injury caused by balloon angioplasty. The theoretical decrease in restenosis with use of laser ablation without adjunctive balloon therapy remains clinically unproven.

Several newer devices have been developed to address some of these issues. Angioscopic guidance systems have been developed to enhance the ability to guide laser therapy and to inspect luminal effects of therapy directly.[107] However, perforation remains a problem because of the difficulty in differentiating plaque from arterial wall. Spectroscopic analysis of laser-induced tissue fluorescence to distinguish normal from diseased tissue has been used in the 'smart laser' systems where a diagnostic laser and detector for tissue photoexcitation are combined with a computer-controlled pulse-wave laser to attack only atherosclerotic lesions specifically.[108] Clinical failure to distinguish heterogeneous atheromatous lesions from normal vessel walls and a need to reposition the device continually until a lesion was identified, doomed this 'smart laser' device, and it is no longer manufactured. Finally, the use of intravascular ultrasound guidance promises accurate detailing of atherosclerotic lesions but trials with devices combining IVUS with laser angioplasty have yet to be reported.[93] Development of accurate guidance systems and utilization of new types of solid-state lasers, which selectively ablate atherosclerotic plaques with minimal surrounding effects (e.g. thulium-holmium-chromium:YAG) continue and may allow the future realization of the theoretic potential of laser ablative therapy.[109] For now, laser therapy has no advantage over angioplasty or surgery, and should only be used experimentally.

MECHANICAL ATHERECTOMY

Four types of atherectomy devices were approved by the Food and Drug Administration (FDA) for clinical trials: the Simpson Atherocath,[17] the Trac-Wright system (Kensey device),[19] the Auth Rotablator[18] and the Transluminal Extraction Catheter (TEC).[21] These devices were developed in an attempt to resolve some of the shortcomings of PTA. Postulated advantages included: better technical success with less subintimal dissection and avoidance of medial stretching resulting in diminished acute or intermediate restenosis; a reduction in atheromatous bulk thereby reducing longer term restenosis; and expanding therapeutic options to include treatment of diffuse disease and complete occlusions. Unfortunately, clinical results of the atherectomy devices have been extremely disappointing with no clear advantages over angioplasty alone, yet with higher rates of complications.

The Simpson directional atherectomy device has been the most widely tested device in the literature. The device makes use of a circular spinning blade inside a metal housing to cut atheromatous material, which has been forced through a window on the side of the housing by inflation of a balloon attached to the opposite side of the housing. Multiple passes and rotation of the device are required for complete circumferential atherectomy. The device is best suited for short, discrete, eccentrically placed stenoses, and has been able to remove ulcerative and intimal hyperplastic lesions, as well as debulk eccentric calcifications. Initial success rates are high, usually greater than 80 per cent, but restenosis is common with patency rates less than 50 per cent after 2 years.[17,110] Complication rates have been as high as 7 per cent and include dissections, embolization and catheter/guidewire-related problems.[111] Rupture of the vessel is rare. The device cannot be used to treat occlusive lesions unless the lesion can be penetrated by the device or converted to a stenosis with adjunctive therapy such as thrombolysis. Long, diffusely diseased vessels are also difficult to treat because of the multiple passages and piecemeal steps for removal that can take several hours to complete. If recanalization is successful, restenosis occurs at a very high rate.[21] Surgical bypass in this case takes less time to perform and has superior long-term patency. The device is also limited to use in fairly straight and large vessels due to its size and stiffness, such that tortuous iliac vessels and small tibial vessels cannot be effectively treated. However, as an adjunct to balloon angioplasty, the Simpson Atherocath has been successfully used to remove postangioplasty debris, residual stenotic lesions and hemodynamically significant intimal flaps.[20]

The Kensey device makes use of a rotating cam-tip attached to a central drive shaft that rotates at 100 000 rpm and seeks the path of least resistance.[19] There is no need to place a coaxial central guidewire, thus making treatment of total occlusions possible. Unfortunately, without a guidewire to keep the device on an intraluminal path, the device frequently deflects away from hard calcific or bulky atheromatous lesions, resulting in vessel perforation. Rates of perforation have been reported as high as 40 per cent, making use of this device prohibitive.[112]

The Auth Rotablator does use a central guidewire to direct it along an intraluminal path, and creates a smooth polished neolumen with its diamond-studded football-shaped tip, which rotates at a high frequency.[18] No flaps are created and atheromatous material, including hard calcifications are pulverized into microparticles that embolize distally. Usually, these particles pass harmlessly through the circulation, but cases of distal ischemia and transient hemoglobinuria have been reported.[21] This device requires use of multiple larger sized burrs or adjunctive angioplasty to enlarge the initial neolumen that was created. Also, the device does not burr effectively through chronic thrombus or soft rubbery intimal lesions. Patency rates have also been disappointingly low (less than 20 per cent at 2 years) despite leaving a smooth polished surface.[21]

The TEC catheter makes use of an irrigation/suction device to remove atheromatous particles from the circulation.[21] Using a coaxial guidewire for guidance, the atheromatous lesions are fed into a hollow conical tip where rotating blades cut up the lesion into small pieces, allowing them to be aspirated. Unfortunately, significant amounts of blood loss occurs with aspiration and instances of embolization have occurred from failure of effective aspiration. The device is capable of treating long lesions quickly, but restenosis rates have not been lower than treatment with standard angioplasty.[113]

Overall, mechanical atherectomy remains an experimental procedure with disappointing clinical success. It has failed to improve on the patency rates seen with standard angioplasty and is associated with significantly higher complication rates. Current indications for its use are limited to treatment of lesions where PTA is ineffective (e.g. long lesions) or relatively contraindicated (eccentric lesions). Indeed, given the success of surgical revascularization, one can question whether atherectomy has any significant role beyond adjunctive use to handle PTA complications, such as removal of intimal flaps.

STENTS

Some authors have estimated that the frequency of hemodynamically significant residual stenosis from elastic recoil or intimal dissection occurs in more than 5 per cent of attempted angioplasties.[114] Various intravascular stents have been developed since the mid-1980s to overcome these problems. Stents were intended to provide a relatively rigid frame to overcome elastic recoil mechanically, and to compress atheromatous plaques and intimal flaps against the vessel wall, such that a sufficient vascular channel for blood flow could be maintained. Stents have been made from various materials, including memory-retaining metals, such as nitinol, and in various designs to address problems with thrombogenicity, radial strength, flexibility, durability and ease of insertion and deployment.

In general, two major types of stents have been developed: the balloon expandable and the self-expanding. The most commonly used balloon-mounted stent, which is hydraulically dilated, is the Palmaz stent.[26] This stent has parallel slots that allow for low-profile compression over a balloon for insertion and very accurate intraluminal deployment upon balloon expansion. A frequent limitation is the lack of longitudinal flexibility making placement in tortuous vessels difficult. The Strecker stent[27] is a woven stent made of tantalum wire, which is also balloon expanded for accurate deployment, but also offers flexibility similar to the self-expanding Wallstent.[115] Wallstents are self-expanding stents with lower profiles, increased flexibility and are inserted into a sheath, which is withdrawn upon deployment. Their application is limited by small size (maximum 12 mm), decreased radial strength and diminished accuracy in deployment. For use in larger vessels, the self-expanding Gianturco Z stent[116] is capable of expanding to more than 35 mm in diameter but is less flexible than the Wallstent.

Clinical testing of stents in lower extremity PVD has mainly involved the use of Palmaz, Strecker or Wallstents in the iliac arteries. Patency rates from most recent reports are summarized in Table 5.3. In large multicenter trials with the Palmaz stent, technical success was greater than 90 per cent in treating iliac disease, with 2-year follow-up demonstrating secondary patencies close to 80 per cent.[117–119,120] The adjunctive use of stents with transluminal angioplasty has gained increasing acceptance, such that angioplasty and stent placement in iliac atherosclerotic disease has become standard therapy in some centers. In addition, angioplasty and stenting of iliac vessels is often used to provide adequate inflow to surgical femoropopliteal revascularization procedures.[60,61] Similar results have been obtained with the use of Strecker and Wallstents, which overcome many of the problems encountered with placement of stiff Palmaz stents in the tortuous pelvic vessels.[27,123,124]

Long-term results following stent deployment are only recently being reported, and a significant incidence of restenosis from neointimal hyperplasia persists.[115,125] Frequently, restenosis has been tempered with repeat angioplasty and stenting, resulting in higher secondary patency rates.[119,126,127,130] Complication rates for angioplasty and stenting have run as high as 10 per cent, with major complications, such as hematoma, hemorrhage, contrast extravasation, rupture, dissection, thrombosis and fistula formation being reported.[117,118] These complication rates have recently declined as improved delivery systems with smaller profiles have been developed.

Infrainguinal stent placement has not enjoyed the success of iliac stenting. Rates of thrombosis and reocclusion are significantly higher, especially when stents are placed in the region of the adductor canal.[124–126,129,130] Wallstents have been used more frequently than Palmaz stents in the femoropopliteal circulation. Because patency rates fall to below 60 per cent after 2 years and immediate thrombosis has been a problem due to the inherent thrombogenicity of stent materials, many centers testing infrainguinal stents are placing patients on heparin acutely and converting them to long-term anti-

Table 5.3 *Results of lower extremity stent placement*

Author (year)	Stent	Artery	Procedures	1	2	3	4	5	Comments
Palmaz (1990)[118]	Palmaz	Iliac	171	89					50% moderate claudicants
Zollikofer (1991)[124]	Wallstent	Iliac	26	96					Mean 16-month follow-up
		Femoralpopliteal	15	55					Mean 20-month follow-up
Sapoval (1992)[129]	Wallstent	Femoralpopliteal	22	49					Mostly occlusions
				67	56	43			Secondary patency
Cikrit (1995)[119]	Palmaz	Iliac	38	87	74	74	67	63	Stents for PTA failure
				91	91	91	91	86	Secondary patency
Henry (1995)[130]	Palmaz	Iliac	184	94	91	86	86		
				98	96	94	94		Secondary patency
		Femoral	116	81	73	72	65		
				96	95	95	95		Secondary patency
		Popliteal	10	50	50	50	50		
				90	80	80	69		Secondary patency
Vorwerk (1996)[127]	Wallstent	Iliac	118	95	88	86	82	72	Stenoses only
				96	93	91	91	83	Secondary patency

coagulation with warfarin.[129,130] Complication rates related to this anticoagulation are not well defined.

Overall, adjunctive stent deployment has only enjoyed short-term success in the iliac arteries, with long-term results still pending. The combination of vascular grafts with stents to form a covered stent has enabled the concept of endovascular bypass. Initially conceived for the treatment of aneurysmal disease, these stent grafts are now being applied to occlusive and traumatic arterial lesions. Several types of stent grafts have been developed for the treatment of patients with thoracic and abdominal aortic aneurysms, and, more recently, for treatment of iliac and popliteal aneurysms.[30,32–35,132] Preliminary experiences of stent grafting in femoral occlusive disease have been reported.[31] Finally, modifications of stent materials continue, with recent reports of hydrophilic coating, biologic stents and stents capable of delivering local drug therapy.[133–139] Clearly, the future of stents and stent-graft technology will rest in the development of novel stent materials, as well as in the ever-increasing knowledge of vascular wall biology and the response of the vascular wall to injury.

CURRENT INDICATIONS AND CONTROVERSIES

The driving force behind the development of endovascular technology is the hypothetical potential for improving cost effectiveness, decreasing critical complication rates, improving outcome, decreasing morbidity and mortality, and possibly extending applications to patients otherwise unfit or without clear indication for surgery. This potential, however, has yet to be realized for many reasons.

In the early 1980s, angioplasty was being touted as the ideal solution for treatment of lower extremity vascular disease. Initial reports with excellent technical success and good short-term patency, with acceptable complication rates, boosted enthusiasm for PTA. Indications for intervention broadened because of some technological improvements, which made PTA easier to perform, often despite sufficient symptoms or proven therapeutic benefit. Patients undergoing cardiac catheterizations for symptomatic cardiac disease, also underwent PTA of lower extremity lesions found incidentally.[140] Increasing numbers of angiograms and subsequent angioplasties were being performed on patients with mild to moderate intermittent claudication, despite evidence that mild disease is relatively benign with good prognosis if treated conservatively by exercise and reduction of risk factors.[141–143] Attitudes favoring treatment of technically easy and incidentally noted lesions without application of strict clinical selection criteria were viewed as harmful to the patient, and alarmed many leaders in the field of vascular disease.[140,144–152] Fortunately, the medical community has come together to reassess the status of lower extremity surgical and endovascular therapies, and to establish guidelines and standards for endovascular therapies.[46–49]

In several cost analyses reported in the 1980s, researchers found that initial hospital costs and lengths of stay were significantly lower in the group of patients undergoing angioplasty as compared to surgery.[153–156] However, these studies failed to consider the relative lack of durability of angioplasty and the costs of repeated interventions. Subsequently, others have shown that the potential cost savings and benefit to the patient have not been realized. In a study of amputation rates in Maryland hospitals over a 10-year span, comparing the impact of endovascular and surgical interventions for lower extremity occlusive disease, increased utilization of PTA failed to demonstrate cost savings or benefit to the patient.[157] Interestingly, when Doubilet and Abrams compared costs of angioplasty and surgery, they found that significant savings in millions of dollars and thousands of limbs could be realized with a strategy where angioplasty, as the first-line therapy, was combined with more durable surgical therapy as needed.[158] This strategy was superior to use of angioplasty alone (cheaper, with less morbidity but poorer long-term patency) or the use of surgery only (more expensive and with greater morbidity, but much more durable).

The concept that endovascular and surgical interventions are not competitive, but are instead complimentary, has been difficult to accept. Three major groups of practitioners have been involved with percutaneous therapy: vascular surgeons, radiologists and cardiologists. Controversy regarding which provider group should control this lucrative area of medical therapy has been escalating.[140,144,145,150,151] Surgeons argue that they are involved with the complete care of the vascular patient from the time of presentation through noninvasive conservative therapy, minimally invasive endovascular treatment and surgical intervention, and are thus best suited for decisions regarding management. Radiologists argue that they have the technology and skills required to perform endovascular procedures precisely; and cardiologists argue that they already have the patient base and also have the skills required for percutaneous access, and thus can best give complete care for the patient. The specter of self-referral and everyone wanting a 'piece of the pie' appears to be a significant problem in the application of endovascular technology.[140,144–151] Currently, several guidelines for a combined training program and a cooperative team approach to the vascular patient exist, but these ideals are not uniformly accepted.[46,49,140,145,159,160]

Arguments supporting the use of angioplasty are preservation of arterial flow in series, preservation of enlarged branch vessels and collaterals, saving the saphenous vein for future use (cardiac bypass or failed endovascular therapy), avoidance of operative morbidity or mortality, provision of temporarily increased distal perfusion to heal an ischemic lesion and a cheaper initial cost than surgery. Some authors argue that the low morbidity of PTA justifies more liberal criteria for intervention than surgical criteria.[44,151] Surgical techniques have been refined well enough to provide long-lasting graft patency, such that 10-year patencies of aortobifemoral grafts approach 90 per cent, and 5-year patencies of femoropopliteal bypasses are better than 70 per cent.[161–163] A randomized clinical trial comparing surgery to angioplasty in patients who are candidates for both therapies (i.e. mostly claudicants with short focal lesions) has shown that their results are comparable, especially if early angioplasty failure is excluded from analysis.[81] Most practitioners, however, consider surgical therapy much more durable than angioplasty, especially in regards to procedures for limb salvage.[82,140,161–163] However, the use of PTA in patients with a short life expectancy or who cannot tolerate surgery appears arguably justifiable. In addition, initial therapy with the less invasive endovascular procedures rather than surgery in those with clear indications for intervention (lifestyle-limiting severe claudication or limb threat) appears warranted, especially in younger patients.[164] Concerns that surgical options during rescue of failed or complicated PTAs would be compromised have not been confirmed. It appears that options for surgical intervention are not significantly affected by whether or not an endovascular procedure was previously performed.[81,83]

A more controversial indication for angioplasty has been in the treatment of those with mild to moderate intermittent claudication.[74] Immediate success and long-term patencies of PTA in this group are excellent, but a benefit above conservative management has not been shown. Only one small randomized trial comparing PTA to exercise therapy currently exists in the literature.[165] This study by Creasy et al. showed that patients undergoing exercise training had better symptomatic improvement compared to those undergoing PTA alone. However, this was confounded by two observations: (1) walking limitation in the PTA group was due to contralateral claudication; and (2) the exercise group decreased their smoking activities more than the PTA group. The authors conclude that a combined exercise training program and PTA program may be even better than either program alone, but this has yet to be proven. That an exercise program and risk modification plan were not applied to the PTA group speaks loudly to the fact that most interventionalists do not become involved in patient treatment.

Overall, the role of endovascular therapies in the treatment of lower extremity vascular disease remains to be completely defined. For now, a role for angioplasty as the initial line of therapy for treatment of short, discrete lesions in the iliac arteries in patients with severe limiting claudication or threat of limb loss appears justified. Additionally, angioplasty for patients with short life expectancies or severe contraindications to surgery appears reasonable. However, the increasing use of angioplasty, with or without stents, in patients with mild to moderate disease remains unjustified. Finally, realization of the cost savings to the patient and society from these endovascular therapies remains hypothetical and will require more thorough investigation.

PROSPECTS FOR THE FUTURE

The future for prevention and treatment of vascular disease lies in understanding the molecular mechanisms underlying the pathobiology of vascular disease. Despite refinement in techniques and instrumentation resulting in highly successful immediate revascularization, restenosis is the major factor limiting long-term success of surgical and endovascular procedures. Although advances in techniques and devices have made treatment of most peripheral atherosclerotic lesions possible, minimally invasive endovascular procedures will not become widely accepted as primary therapy until problems with restenosis can be minimized.

Insight into the pathobiology of restenosis has come from experiments with cultured cells, animal models of arterial injury and examination of pathologic human vessels. Two major hypotheses for development of restenosis can be found in the literature: (1) alterations in local hemodynamic physiology stimulate cellular responses that attempt to correct deviations in wall tension and shear stress, which under conditions of low flow results in development of restenosis;[166,167] and (2) as a result of vascular injury, a local inflammatory response follows, and a proliferative cascade of cellular and molecular interactions begins in an attempt to 'heal' the injury, which, if uncontrolled, eventually results in restenosis.[168–171] In the biology of restenosis, both processes are probably simultaneously at work.

The most commonly studied model of restenosis has involved studying effects of vascular injury occurring after angioplasty. Balloon angioplasty stretches and fractures atheromatous lesions leaving behind intimal flaps and dissection planes deep into the media.[44,168,171] A local inflammatory response as well as thrombus and platelet accumulation provides the stimulus for a fibroproliferative response to injury with intimal migration of smooth muscle cells and deposition of extracellular matrix. The molecular interactions between endothelial cells, macrophages, T lymphocytes, smooth muscle cells and a vast array of potent cytokines and growth regulatory molecules, including platelet-derived growth factors, basic fibroblast growth factors, transforming growth factors, interleukin, tumor necrosis factor and thrombin have been of intense interest.[169–177]

Various drug therapies, from antiplatelet agents to receptor antagonists and antiproliferative agents, have been employed in attempts to minimize the proliferative restenotic response.[170–177] Unfortunately, despite routine use of heparin, aspirin, dipyridamole and occasionally warfarin, and the experimental use of calcium channel blockers, ACE (angiotensin converting enzyme) inhibitors, chemotherapy drugs and other agents, success in preventing restenosis has been limited. In addition, concerns of potential side effects and toxicities have limited the use of pharmacologic agents systemically.

Physically, attempts to overcome restenosis have involved the design of less traumatic devices, thereby minimizing endovascular injury, as well as continuing to refine current methods of laser therapy, mechanical atherectomy and stent technology. To date success in preventing restenosis has been disappointing.

However, as the molecular events leading to restenosis are deciphered, new therapies, perhaps combining drugs with mechanical interventions, should be forthcoming. Technology is rapidly progressing such that endovascular devices with the ability to deliver pharmacologic agents locally will be developed. In addition, progress in the area of gene therapy may one day allow us to locally deliver antiatherosclerotic or antirestenotic agents, and allow for re-establishment of normal vascular function.[178–180]

Our experience with the development and use of endovascular devices to date, while disappointing with respect to long-term durability, has nevertheless taught us valuable lessons. As new technology is developed, we must continue to be cautious in its application to medical practice with emphasis on careful clinical testing, adherence to standards of reporting and continued cautious development of guidelines for application. With this approach, and continued cooperation between the various fields of vascular surgery, radiology and cardiology, the future of endovascular treatment of lower extremity vascular disease remains bright.

REFERENCES

1 Patton DD. Roentgen and the new light – Roentgen's moment of discovery. Part 2: The first glimmer of the New Light. *Invest Radiol* 1993; **28**: 51–8.

2 Haschek E, Lindenthal OT. A contribution to the practical use of the photography according to Roentgen. *Wien Klin Wochensch* 1896; **9**: 63.

3 Forssmann W. The catheterization of the right side of the heart. *Klin Wochensch* 1929; **8**: 2085–7.

4 Seldinger S. Catheter replacement of the needle in percutaneous arteriography. *Acta Radiol* 1953; **39**: 368–76.

5 Fogarty TJ, Cranley JJ *et al*. A method for extraction of arterial emboli and thrombi. *Surg Gynecol Obstet* 1963; **116**: 241.

6 Dotter CT, Judkins MP. Transluminal treatment of arteriosclerotic obstruction: description of a new technique and a preliminary report of its application. *Circulation* 1964; **30**: 654–70.

7 Dotter CT. Transluminal angioplasty: a long view. *Radiology* 1980; **135**: 561–4.

8 Dotter CT, Judkins MP, Frische LH. The nonsurgical treatment of iliofemoral arteriosclerotic obstruction. *Radiology* 1966; **86**: 871–5.

9 Dotter CT. Transluminally-placed coilspring endarterial tube grafts. Long-term patency in canine popliteal artery. *Invest Radiol* 1969; **4**: 329–32.

10 Portsmann W. Ein neuer Korseh-Balloon Katheter zur transluminalen Rekanalization nach Dotter unter Besonder Baruksichtigung von Obliterationen an den Beckenarterien. *Radiol Diagn (Berl)* 1973; **2**: 239.

11 Gruentzig A, Hopff H. Perkutane Rekanalisation chronischer arterieller Verschlusse mit einem neuen Dilatationskatheter. Modifikation der Dotter-Technik. *Deutsch Med Wochensch* 1974; **99**: 2502–10.

12 Gruentzig A. Die perkutane Rekanalization chronischer arterieller Verschusse (Dotter–Prinzip) mit einem neuen doppellumigen Dilatationskatheter. *ROFO* Fortschrite Auf Dem Gebiete Der Rontgonstrahlen und Der Nuklearmedicin. 1976; **124**: 80–6.

13 Choy DS, Stertzer SH, Rotterdam HZ. Transluminal laser catheter angioplasty. *Am J Cardiology* 1982; **50**(6): 1206–8.

14 Ginsberg R, Wexler L, Mitchell RS, Profitt D. Percutaneous transluminal laser angioplasty for treatment of peripheral vascular disease: clinical experience with sixteen patients. *Radiology* **156**: 619–24.

15 Geschwind HJ, Castaneda1985; -Zuniga WR, guest eds. Laser angioplasty. *Semin Intervent Radiol* 1986; **3**(1): 1–81.

16 Cragg AH, Gardiner GA Jr, Smith TP. Vascular applications of laser. *Radiology* 1989; **172**: 925–35.

17 Simpson JB, Selmon MR, Robertson LL, Lipriano PR, Hayden WG, Johnson DE, Fogarty TJ. Transluminal atherectomy for occlusive peripheral vascular disease. *Am J Cardiology* 1988; **61**: 96G–101G.

18 Ahn SS, Auth D, Marcus RR, Moore WS. Removal of focal atheromatous lesions by angioscopically guided high-speed rotary atherectomy. *J Vasc Surg* 1988; **7**: 292–300.

19 Kensey KR, Nash JE, Abrahams C, Zarins CK. Recanalization of obstructed arteries with a flexible rotating tip catheter. *Radiology* 1987; **165**: 387–9.

20 Maynar M, Reyes R, Cabrera V, Roman M, Palido JM, Castaneda F, Letourneau JG, Castaneda-Zuniga WR. Percutaneous atherectomy as an alternative treatment for postangioplasty obstructive intimal flaps. *Radiology* 1989; **170**: 1029–31.

21 Ahn SS. Status of peripheral atherectomy. *Surg Clin North Am* 1992; **72**(4): 869–78.

22 Sigwart U, Puel J, Mirkovitch V, Joffee F, Kappenberger L. Intravascular stents to prevent occlusion and restenosis after transluminal angioplasty. *N Engl J Med* 1987; **316**: 701–6.

23 Dotter CT, Buschmann RW, McKinney MK, Ronch J.

Transluminal expandable nitinol coil stent grafting: preliminary report. *Radiology* 1983; **147**: 259–60.

24 Cragg A, Lung G, Ryoavy J, Castaneda F, Castaneda-Zuniga WR, Amplate K. Nonsurgical placement of arterial endoprostheses: a new technique using nitinol wire. *Radiology* 1983; **147**: 261–3.

25 Maass D, Zollikofer CL, Larginder F, Senning A. Radiological follow up of transluminally inserted vascular endoprostheses: an experimental study using expanding spirals. *Radiology* 1984; **152**: 659–63.

26 Palmaz JC, Sibbitt RR, Rentor SR, Tio FO, Rica WJ. Expandable intraluminal graft: A preliminary study. *Radiology* 1985; **156**: 73–7.

27 Strecker EP, Liermann DD, Barth KH, Wolf WR, Freuchaborg W, Berg G, Westphal M, Tiskuras P, Savin M, Sohunder B. Expandable tubular stents for treatment of arterial occlusive disease: experimental and clinical results. Work in progress. *Radiology* 1990; **175**: 97–102.

28 Katzen BT, Becker GJ. Intravascular stents: status of development and clinical application. *Surg Clin North Am* 1992; **72**(4): 941–57.

29 Lawrence DD Jr, Charnsangavej C, Wright KC, Gianturco C, Wallace S. Percutaneous endovascular graft: experimental evaluation. *Radiology* 1987; **163**: 357–60.

30 Parodi JC, Palmaz JC, Barone HD. Transfemoral intraluminal graft implantation for abdominal aortic aneurysms. *Ann Vasc Surg* 1991; **5**: 491–9.

31 Diethrich EB, Papazoglou K. Endoluminal grafting for aneurysmal and occlusive disease in the superficial femoral artery: early experience. *J Endovasc Surg* 1995; **2**: 225–39.

32 Marin ML, Veith FJ, Garman J, Sanchez LR, Lyon RT. Initial experience with transluminally placed endovascular grafts for the treatment of complex vascular lesions. *Ann Surg* 1995; **222**: 449–69.

33 Lazarus HM. Endovascular grafting for the treatment of abdominal aortic aneurysms. *Surg Clin North Am* 1992; **72**(4): 959–68.

34 Blum U, Langer M, Spillner G, Mialbe C, Beyensdorf F *et al*. Abdominal aortic aneurysms: preliminary technical and clinical results with transfemoral placement of endovascular self-expanding stent-grafts. *Radiology* 1996; **198**: 25–31.

35 Razavi MK, Dake MD, Semba CP, Hyman UR, Liddell RP. Percutaneous endoluminal placement of stent-grafts for the treatment of isolated iliac aortic aneurysms. *Radiology* 1995; **197**: 801–4.

36 Murray KK, Hawkins IF Jr. Angiography of the lower extremity in atherosclerotic vascular disease. *Surg Clin North Am* 1992; **72**(4): 767–89.

37 Hawkins IF Jr, Caridi JG. CO_2 digital subtraction arteriography – advantages and current solutions for delivery and imaging. *Cardiovasc Intervent Radiol* 1995; **18**: 150–2.

38 Stewart JH, Grubb M. Understanding vascular ultrasonography. *Mayo Clin Proc* 1992; **67**: 1186–96.

39 Cavaye DM, White RA, Tabbara MR, Kopehok GE.

Intravascular ultrasonography. *Surg Clin North Am* 1992; **72**(4): 823–42.

40 Isner JM, Rosenfield K, Lasordo DW, Kelly S, Patatski P, Langevin RE. Percutaneous intravascular US as adjunct to catheter-based interventions: preliminary experience in patients with peripheral vascular disease. *Radiology* 1990; **175**: 61–70.

41 Liu JB, Goldberg BB. Endoluminal vascular and nonvascular sonography: past, present, and future. *Am J Roentgen* 1995; **165**: 765–74.

42 Jorgensen B, Tonnesen KH, Nielsen JD, Holstein P *et al*. Segmentally enclosed thrombolysis in percutaneous transluminal angioplasty for femoropopliteal occlusions: a report from a pilot study. *Cardiovasc Intervent Radiol* 1991; **14**: 293–8.

43 Hess H, Mietaschk A, Bruckl R. Peripheral arterial occlusions: a 6-year experience with local low-dose thrombolytic therapy. *Radiology* 1987; **163**: 753–8.

44 Becker GJ, Katzen BT, Dake MD. Noncoronary angioplasty. *Radiology* 1989; **170**: 921–40.

45 Wilson SE, Sheppard B. Results of percutaneous transluminal angioplasty for peripheral vascular occlusive disease. *Ann Vasc Surg* 1990; **4**: 94–7.

46 Guidelines for percutaneous transluminal angioplasty [from the Standards of Practice Committee of the Society of Cardiovascular and Interventional Radiology]. *Radiology* 1990; **177**: 619–26.

47 Rutherford RB, Becker GJ. Standards for evaluating and reporting the results of surgical and percutaneous therapy for peripheral arterial disease. *J Vasc Intervent Radiol* 1991; **2**: 169–74 [also published in: *Radiology* 1991; **181**: 277–81].

48 Ahn SS, Rutherford RB, Becker GJ, Comerota AJ *et al*. Reporting standards for lower extremity arterial endovascular procedures. *J Vasc Surg* 1993; **17**: 1103–7.

49 Pentecost MJ, Criqui MH, Derras G, Goldstone J *et al*. Guidelines for peripheral percutaneous transluminal angioplasty of the abdominal aorta and lower extremity vessels. *Circulation* 1994; **89**(1): 511–31.

50 Capek P, McLean GK, Berkowitz HD. Femoropopliteal angioplasty: factors influencing long-term success. *Circulation* 1991; **83**(2, suppl I): I70–I80.

51 Johnston KW. Factors that influence the outcome of aortoiliac and femoropopliteal percutaneous transluminal angioplasty. *Surg Clin North Am* 1992; **72**(4): 843–50.

52 Hunink MGM, Donaldson MC, Meyerowitz MF, Palak JF *et al*. Risks and benefits of femoropopliteal percutaneous balloon angioplasty. *J Vasc Surg* 1993; **17**: 183–94.

53 van Andel GJ, van Erp WFM, Krepel VM, Bresslau PJ. Percutaneous transluminal dilatation of the iliac artery: long-term results. *Radiology* 1985; **156**: 321–3.

54 Stokes KR, Strunk HM, Campbell DR, Gibbons GW *et al*. Five-year results of iliac and femoropopliteal angioplasty in diabetic patients. *Radiology* 1990; **174**: 977–82.

55 Johnston KW. Iliac arteries: reanalysis of results of balloon angioplasty. *Radiology* 1993; **186**: 207–12.

56 Wollenweber J, Henne W, Kiefer H, Meyes M, Schmerson Z. Early and late results after percutaneous transluminal angioplasty in peripheral arterial occlusive disease. *Vasa* 1986; **15**: 67–70.

57 Jorgensen B, Henriksen LO, Karle A, Sager P *et al*. Percutaneous transluminal angioplasty of iliac and femoral arteries in severe lower-limb ischaemia. *Acta Chir Scand* 1988; **154**: 647–52.

58 Gupta AK, Ravimandalam K, Rio VR, Joseph S *et al*. Total occlusion of iliac arteries: results of balloon angioplasty. CardioVascular and Interventional *Radiology* 1993; **16**: 165–77.

59 Rosenblum JD, Leef JA, Kostelier JR, Boyte CM. Angioplasty and intravascular stents in peripheral vascular disease. *Surg Clin North Am* 1995; **75**(4): 621–32.

60 Pfeiffer RB, String ST. Adjunctive use of the balloon dilatation catheter during vascular reconstructive procedures. *J Vasc Surg* 1986; **3**: 841–5.

61 Brewster DC, Cambria RP, Darling RC, Athanasoulis CA *et al*. Long-term results of combined iliac balloon angioplasty and distal surgical revascularization. *Ann Surg* 1989; **210**: 324–31.

62 Martin EC, Fankuchen EI, Karlson KB, Delgin C *et al*. Angioplasty for femoral artery occlusion: comparison with surgery. *Am J Roentgenol* 1981; **137**: 915–19.

63 Gallino A, Mahler F, Probst P, Nashbur B. Percutaneous transluminal angioplasty of the arteries of the lower limbs: a 5 year follow-up. *Circulation* 1984; **70**(4): 619–23.

64 Krepel VM, van Andel GJ, Van Erp WF, Breslane PS. Percutaneous transluminal angioplasty of the femoropopliteal artery: initial and long-term results. *Radiology* 1985; **156**: 325–8.

65 Spence RK, Freiman DB, Bretenby R, Hobbs CL *et al*. Long-term results of transluminal angioplasty of the iliac and femoral arteries. *Arch Surg* 1981; **116**: 1377–86.

66 Hewes RC, White RI, Murray RR, Kaufman SI *et al*. Long-term results of superficial femoral artery angioplasty. *Am J Roentgenol* 1986; **146**: 1025–9.

67 Rooke TW, Stanson AW, Johnson CM, Sheedy PF *et al*. Percutaneous transluminal angioplasty in the lower extremities: a 5-year experience. *Mayo Clin Proc* 1987; **62**: 85–91.

68 Murray RR Jr, Hewes RC, White RG Jr, Mitchell DE *et al*. Long-segment femoropopliteal stenoses: is angioplasty a boon or bust? *Radiology* 1987; **162**: 473–6.

69 Johnston KW, Rae M, Hogg-Johnston SA, Colapinto RF *et al*. 5-year results of a prospective study of percutaneous transluminal angioplasty. *Ann Surg* 1987; **206**: 403–13.

70 Milford MA, Weaver FA, Lundell CJ, Yellin AE. Femoropopliteal percutaneous transluminal angioplasty for limb salvage. *J Vasc Surg* 1988; **8**: 292–9.

71 Tonnesen KH, Sager P, Karle A, Henriksen L, Jorgensen B. Percutaneous transluminal angioplasty of the superficial femoral artery by retrograde catheterization via the popliteal artery. *Cardiovasc Intervent Radiol* 1988; **11**: 127–31.

72 Jeans WD, Armstrong S, Cole SE, Horrocks M, Baird RN. Fate of patients undergoing transluminal angioplasty for lower-limb ischemia. *Radiology* 1990; **177**: 559–64.

73 Clement C, Costa-Foru B, Vernon P, Nicaise H. Transluminal angioplasty performed by the surgeon in lower limb arterial occlusive disease: one hundred fifty cases. *Ann Vasc Surg* 1990; **4**: 519–27.

74 Whyman MR, Ruckley CV, Fowkes FGR. Angioplasty for mild intermittent claudication. *Br J Surg* 1991; **78**: 643–5.

75 Dacie JE, Daniell SJN. The value of percutaneous transluminal angioplasty of the profunda femoris artery in threatened limb loss and intermittent claudication. *Clin Radiol* 1991; **44**: 311–16.

76 Harris RW, Dulawa LB, Andres G, Oglath RW *et al*. Percutaneous transluminal angioplasty of the lower extremities by the vascular surgeon. *Ann Vasc Surg* 1991; **5**: 345–53.

77 Adar R, Critchfield GC, Eddy DM. A confidence profile analysis of the results of femoropopliteal percutaneous transluminal angioplasty in the treatment of lower-extremity ischemia. *J Vasc Surg* 1989; **10**: 57–67.

78 Johnston KW. Femoral and popliteal arteries: reanalysis of results of balloon angioplasty. *Radiology* 1992; **183**: 767–71.

79 Matsi PJ, Manninen HI, Suhonen MT, Pirinen AE, Soimakallio S. Chronic critical lower-limb ischemia: prospective trial of angioplasty with 1–36 months follow-up. *Radiology* 1993; **188**: 381–7.

80 Matsi PJ, Manninen HI, Yanninen ZL, Suhonen MT *et al*. Femoropopliteal angioplasty in patients with claudication: primary and secondary patency in 140 limbs with 1–3 year follow-up. *Radiology* 1994; **191**: 727–33.

81 Wilson SE, Wolf GL, Cross AP. Percutaneous transluminal angioplasty versus operation for peripheral arteriosclerosis. Report of a prospective randomized trial in a selected group of patients. *J Vasc Surg* 1989; **9**: 1–9.

82 Blair JM, Gewertz BL, Moosch H, Lu CT, Zarino CK. Percutaneous transluminal angioplasty versus surgery for limb-threatening ischemia. *J Vasc Surg* 1989; **9**: 698–703.

83 Samson RH, Sprayregen S, Veith FJ, Scher LA *et al*. Management of angioplasty complications, unsuccessful procedures and early and late failures. *Ann Surg* 1984; **199**: 234–40.

84 Walden R, Siegel Y, Rubinstein ZJ, Morag B *et al*. Percutaneous transluminal angioplasty. A suggested method for analysis of clinical, arteriographic, and hemodynamic factors affecting the results of treatment. *J Vasc Surg* 1986; **3**: 583–90.

85 Henriksen LO, Jorgensen B, Holstein PE, Tonnesen KH *et al*. Percutaneous transluminal angioplasty of infrarenal arteries in intermittent claudication. *Acta Chir Scand* 1988; **154**: 573–6.

86 Jorgensen B, Tonnesen KH, Holstein P. Late hemodynamic failure following percutaneous transluminal angioplasty for long and multifocal femoropopliteal stenoses. *Cardiovasc Intervent Radiol* 1991; **14**: 290–2.

87 Stanley B, Teague B, Raptis S, Taylor DJ, Berce M. Efficacy

of balloon angioplasty of the superficial femoral artery and popliteal artery in the relief of leg ischemia. *J Vasc Surg* 1996; **23**: 679–85.

88 Bakal CW, Sprayregen, Schienbaum K, Cynemon J, Veith FJ. Percutaneous transluminal angioplasty of the infrapopliteal arteries: results in 53 patients. *Am J Roentgenol* 1990; **154**: 171–4.

89 Horvath W, Oertl M, Haidinger D. Percutaneous transluminal angioplasty of crural arteries. *Radiology* 1990; **177**: 565–9.

90 Schwarten DE. Clinical and anatomical considerations for nonoperative therapy in tibial disease and the results of angioplasty. *Circulation* 1991; **83**(2, suppl I): I86–I90.

91 Durham JR, Horowitz JD, Wright JG, Smead WL. Percutaneous transluminal angioplasty of tibial arteries for limb salvage in the high-risk diabetic patient. *Ann Vasc Surg* **8**: 48–53, 1994;

92 Treiman GS, Treiman RL, Ichikawa L, Van Allan R. Should percutaneous transluminal angioplasty be recommended for treatment of infrageniculate popliteal artery or tibioperoneal trunk stenosis?' *J Vasc Surg* 1995; **22**: 457–65.

93 Self SB, Seeger JM. Laser angioplasty. *Surg Clin North Am* 1992; **72**(4): 851–68.

94 Cragg AH, guest ed. Update on laser angioplasty. *Semin Intervent Radiology* 1991; **8**(2): 89–159.

95 Abela GS, Crea F, Seeger JM, Franzini D *et al*. The healing process in normal canine arteries and in atherosclerotic monkey arteries after transluminal laser irradiation. *Am J Cardiol* **56**: 1985; 983–8.

96 Torres JH, Motamedi M. Disparate absorption of argon laser radiation by fibrous versus fatty plaque: implications for laser angioplasty. *Lasers Surg Med* 1990; **10**: 149–57.

97 Grundfest WS, Litvack IF, Goldenberg T, Sherman T *et al*. Pulsed ultraviolet lasers and the potential for safe laser angioplasty. *Am J Surg* 1985; **150**: 220–6.

98 Abela GS, Fenech A, Crea F, Conti CR. 'Hot-tip': another method of laser vascular recanalization. *Lasers Surg Med* 1985; **5**: 327–35.

99 Gerschwind HJ, Blair JD, Mongkolsmai D. Development and experimental application of contact catheter for laser angioplasty. *J Am Coll Cardiol* 1987; **9**: 101–7.

100 Perler BA, Osterman FA, White RI Jr, Williams GM. Percutaneous laser probe femoropopliteal laser angioplasty: a preliminary experience. *J Vasc Surg* 1989; **10**: 351–7.

101 Harrington ME, Schwartz ME, Sanborn TA, Mitty HA *et al*. Expanded indications for laser assisted balloon angioplasty in peripheral arterial disease. *J Vasc Surg* 1990; **11**: 146–55.

102 White RA, White GH, Mehringer MC, Chaing FL, Wilson SE. A clinical trial of laser thermal angioplasty in patients with advanced peripheral vascular disease. *Ann Surg* 1990; **212**: 257–65.

103 Blebea J, Ouriel K, Green RM, Fiore WM *et al*. Laser angioplasty in peripheral vascular disease: symptomatic versus hemodynamic results. *J Vasc Surg* 1991; **13**: 222–30.

104 Litvack F, Grundfest WS, Adler L, Hickey AE *et al*. Percutaneous excimer-laser and excimer-laser-assisted angioplasty of the lower extremities: results of initial clinical trial. *Radiology* 1989; **172**: 331–5.

105 McCarthy WJ, Vogelzang RL, Nemcek AR Jr, Joseph A *et al*. Excimer laser-assisted femoral angioplasty: early results. *J Vasc Surg* 1991; **13**: 607–14.

106 Ahn SS, Eton D, Moore WS. Endovascular surgery for peripheral arterial occlusive disease. *Ann Surg* 1992; **216**(1): 3–16.

107 Abela GS, Seeger JM, Barbieri E, Franzini D *et al*. Laser angioplasty with angioscopic guidance in humans. *J Am Coll Cardiol* 1986; **8**: 184–92.

108 Leon MB, Almagor Y, Bartorelli AL, Prevasti LG *et al*. Flourescence-guided laser-assisted balloon angioplasty in patients with femoropopliteal occlusions. *Circulation* 1990; **81**: 143–55.

109 Oz MC, Treat MR, Troker SL, Andrew JE, Nowgrod R. A fiberoptic compatible midinfrared laser with CO_2 laser-like effect: application to atherosclerosis. *J Surg Res* 1989; **47**: 493–501.

110 Polnitz A, Nerlich A, Berger H, Hofting B. Percutaneous peripheral atherectomy. *J Am Coll Cardiol* 1990; **15**: 682–8.

111 Graor RA, Whitlow PL. Transluminal atherectomy for occlusive peripheral vascular disease. *J Am Coll Cardiol* 1990; **15**(7): 1551–8.

112 Snyder SO, Wheeler JR, Gregory RT, Gayle RG, Mariner DR. Kensey catheter: early results with a transluminal endarterectomy tool. *J Vasc Surg* **8**1988;: 541–3.

113 Wholey MH, Jarmolowski CR. New reperfusion devices: the Kensey catheter, the atherolytic reperfusion wire device, and the transluminal extraction catheter. *Radiology* 1989; **172**: 947–52.

114 Becker GJ. Intravascular stents: general principles and status of lower-extremity arterial applications. *Circulation* 1991; **83**(suppl I): I122–I136.

115 Rousseau H, Puel J, Jeffre F, Sigwart U *et al*. Self-expanding endovascular prosthesis: an experimental study. *Radiology* 1987; **164**: 709–14.

116 Duprat G Jr, Wright KC, Charnsangavej C, Wallace S, Giantureu L. Self-expanding metallic stents for small vessels: an experimental evaluation. *Radiology* 1987; **162**: 469–72.

117 Palmaz JC, Garcia OJ, Schatz RA, Rees CR *et al*. Placement of balloon-expandable intraluminal stents in iliac arteries: first 171 procedures. *Radiology* 1990; **174**: 969–75.

118 Palmaz JC, Richter GM, Noeldge G, Schatz RA *et al*. Intraluminal stents in atherosclerotic iliac artery stenosis: preliminary report of a multicenter study. *Radiology* 1988; **168**: 727–31.

119 Cikrit DF, Gustafson PA, Dalaing MC, Harris VJ *et al*. Long-term follow-up of the Palmaz stent for iliac occlusive disease. *Surgery* 1995; **118**: 608–14.

120 Long AL, Sapoval MR, Beyessen BM, Auguste MC *et al*. Strecker stent implantation in iliac arteries: patency and

120 predictive factors for long-term success. *Radiology* 1995; **194**: 739–44.

121 Palmaz JC, Laborde JC, Rivera FJ, Encarnacion CE *et al*. Stenting of the iliac arteries with the Palmaz stent: experience from a multicenter trial. *Cardiovasc Intervent Radiol* 1992; **15**: 291–7.

122 Strecker EP, Hagen B, Liermann D, Boos I *et al*. Current status of the Strecker stent. *Cardiol Clin* 1994; **12**(4): 673–87.

123 Vorwerk D, Guenther RW. Stent placement in iliac arterial lesions: three years of clinical experience with the Wallstent. *Cardiovasc Intervent Radiol* 1992; **115**: 285–90.

124 Zollikofer CL, Antonucci F, Pfyffer M, Redha F *et al*. Arterial stent placement with use of the Wallstent: midterm results of clinical experience. *Radiology* 1991; **179**: 449–56.

125 Guenther RW, Vorwerk D, Bohndorf K, Peters I *et al*. Iliac and femoral artery stenosis and occlusions: treatment with intravascular stents. *Radiology* 1989; **172**: 725–30.

126 Vorwerk D, Guenther RW, Schurman K, Wendt G. Late reobstruction in iliac arterial stents: percutaneous treatment. *Radiology* 1995; **197**: 479–83.

127 Vorwerk D, Guenther RW, Schurman K, Wendt G. Aortic and iliac stenoses: Follow-up results of stent placement after insufficient balloon angioplasty in 118 cases. *Radiology* 1996; **198**: 45–8.

128 Rousseau HP, Raillat CR, Joffre FG, Knight CJ, Ginestet M. Treatment of femoropopliteal stenoses by means of self-expandable endoprostheses: midterm results. *Radiology* 1989; **172**: 961–4.

129 Sapoval MR, Long AL, Raynaud AC, Beyssen BM *et al*. Femoropopliteal stent placement: long-term results. *Radiology* 1992; **184**: 833–9.

130 Henry M, Amor M, Ethevenot G, Henry I *et al*. Palmaz stent placement in iliac and femoropopliteal arteries: primary and secondary patency in 310 patients with 2–4 year follow up. *Radiology* 1995; **197**: 167–74.

131 White GH, Liew SCC, Waugh RC, Stephen MS *et al*. Early outcome and intermediate follow-up of vascular stents in the femoral and popliteal arteries without long-term anticoagulation. *J Vasc Surg* 1995; **21**: 270–81.

132 Joyce WP, McGrath F, Leahy AL, Bonchier-Hayes D. A safe combined surgical/radiological approach to endoluminal graft stenting of a popliteal aneurysm. *Eur J Vasc Endovasc Surg* 1995; **10**: 489–91.

133 Slepian MJ, Schindler A. Polymeric endothelial paving/sealing: a biodegradable alternative to intracoronary stenting. *Circulation* 1988; **78**(suppl II): II409.

134 Tanguay JF, Zidar JP, Phillips HR 3rd, Stack RS. Current status of biodegradable stents. *Cardiol Clin* 1994; **12**: 699–713.

135 Murphy JG, Schwartz RS, Bailey KR *et al*. A new biocompatible polymeric coronary stent: Design and early results in the pig model (abstract). *J Am Coll Cardiol* 1990; **1S**: 10SA.

136 Slepian MJ. Polymeric endoluminal paving. *Cardiol Clin* 1994; **12**: 715–37.

137 Diethrich EB. Polymeric covers and coats for metallic stents: microporous PTFE and the inhibition of intimal hyperplasia. *J Endovasc Surg* 1995; **2**: 266–71.

138 Seeger JM, Ingegno MD, Bigaton E, Klingman N *et al*. Hydrophilic surface modification of metallic endoluminal stents. *J Vasc Surg* 1995; **22**: 327–36.

139 Fontaine AB, Dos Pasos S, Spigos D, Cearbek J, Urbaneja A. Use of polyetherurethane to improve the biocompatibility of vascular stents. *J Endovasc Surg* 1995; **2**: 255–65.

140 Veith FJ, Gupta SK, Wengerter KR, Rivers SP, Bahal CW. Impact of nonoperative therapy on the clinical management of peripheral arterial disease. *Circulation* 1991; **83**(2, suppl I): I137–I142.

141 McDaniel MD, Cronenwett JL. Basic data related to natural history of intermittent claudication. *Ann Vasc Surg* 1989; **3**(3): 273–7.

142 McDermott MM, McCarthy. Intermittent claudication: the natural history. *Surg Clin North Am* 1995; **75**(4): 581–91.

143 Cooke JP, Ma AO. Medical therapy of peripheral arterial occlusive disease. *Surg Clin North Am* 1995; **75**(4): 569–79.

144 Zarins CK. The vascular war of 1988: the enemy is met. *JAMA* 1989; **261**: 416–17.

145 Wexler L, Ginsburg R, Mitchell RS, Mehigan JT. The vascular war of 1988. *JAMA* 1989; **261**: 418–19.

146 Porter JM. Endovascular arterial intervention: expression of concern (editorial). *J Vasc Surg* 1995; **21**(6): 995–7.

147 Frisch R. Presidential address: endovascular techniques and the vascular surgeon. *Ann Vasc Surg* 1991; **5**(1): 1–3.

148 Diethrich EB. Deficiencies of the modern vascular surgeon: a dilemma, a solution (editorial). *Ann Vasc Surg* 1991; **5**(1): 99–100.

149 Porter JM. Interventional therapy: an alternative view'(editorial). *Ann Vasc Surg* 1991; **5**(1): 101–2.

150 Wholey MH. Controverisies in peripheral vascular intervention. *Radiology* 1990; **174**: 929–31.

151 Martin EC. The impact of angioplasty: a perspective. *J Vasc Intervent Radiology* 1992; **3**: 511–14.

152 Moore WS. Therapeutic options for femoropopliteal occlusive disease. *Circulation* 1991; **83**(suppl I): I91–I93.

153 Jeans WD, Danton RM, Baird RN, Horrocks M. The effects of introducing balloon dilatation into vascular surgical practice. *Br J Radiology* 1986; **59**: 457–9.

154 Jeans WD, Danton RM, Baird RN, Horrocks M. A comparison of the costs of vascular surgery and balloon dilatation in lower limb ischaemic disease. *Br J Radiology* 1986; **59**: 453–6.

155 Kinnison ML, White RI, Bowers WP, Dunlop ED. Cost incentives for peripheral angioplasty. *Am J Roentgenol* 1985; **145**: 1241–4.

156 Freiman DB, Freiman MP, Spencer RK, McLean GK, Berkowitz HD. Economic impact of transluminal angioplasty. *Angiology* 1985; **36**: 772–7.

157 Tunis SR, Bass EB, Steinberg EP. The use of angioplasty, bypass surgery, and amputation in the management of peripheral vascular disease. *N Engl J Med* 1991; **325**: 556–62.

158 Doubilet P, Abrams HL. The cost of underutilization: percutaneous transluminal angioplasty for peripheral vascular disease. *N Engl J Med* 1984; **310**(2): 95–102.

159 White RA, Fogarty TJ, Baker WH, Ahn SS, String ST. Endovascular surgery credentialing and training for vascular surgeons. *J Vasc Surg* 1993; **17**(6): 1095–1102.

160 Katzen BT. Optimal resources for peripheral vascular intervention. *Circulation* 1991; **83**(suppl I): I143–I145.

161 Shah DM, Darling RC III, Chang BB, Fitzgerald KM *et al.* Long-term results of in situ saphenous vein bypass. *Ann Surg* 1995; **222**: 438–48.

162 Taylor LM Jr, Porter JM. Clinical and anatomic considerations for surgery in femoropopliteal disease and the results of surgery. *Circulation* 1991; **83**(2, suppl I): I63–I69.

163 Dalman RL, Taylor LM Jr. Basic data related to infrainguinal revascularization procedures. *Ann Vasc Surg* 1990; **4**(3): 309–12.

164 Levy PJ, Close T, Tornung CA, Haynes JL, Rush DS. Percutaneous transluminal angioplasty in adults less than 45 years of age with premature lower extremity atherosclerosis. *Ann Vasc Surg* 1995; **9**: 471–9.

165 Creasy TS, McMillan PJ, Fletcher EW, Collin J, Morris PJ. Is percutaneous transluminal angioplasty better than exercise for claudication? Preliminary results from a prospective randomised trial. *Eur J Vasc Surg* 1990; **4**(2): 135–40.

166 Glagov S. Intimal hyperplasia, vascular modeling, and the restenosis problem. *Circulation* 1994; **89**: 2888–91.

167 Glagov S, Bassiouny HS, Giddens DP, Zarins CK. Pathobiology of plaque modeling and complication. *Surg Clin North Am* 1995; **75**(4): 545–56.

168 Waller BF, Orr CM, Pinkerton CA, Van Tassel JW, Pinto RP. Morphologic observations late after coronary balloon angioplasty: mechanisms of acute injury and relationship to restenosis. *Radiology* 1990; **174**: 961–7.

169 Ross R. The pathogenesis of atherosclerosis: a perspective for the 1990s. *Nature* 1993; **362**: 801–9.

170 Schwartz SM, deBlois D, O'Brien ERM. The intima: soil for atherosclerosis and restenosis. *Circ Res* 1995; **77**: 445–65.

171 Nicolini FA, Pepine CJ. Biology of restenosis and therapeutic approach. *Surg Clin North Am* 1992; **72**(4): 919–40.

172 Currier JW, Faxon DP. Restenosis after percutaneous transluminal coronary angioplasty: have we been aiming at the wrong target?' *J Am Coll Cardiol* 1995; **25**(2): 516–20.

173 Naftilan AJ. Chemical atherectomy: a novel approach to restenosis. *Circulation* 1991; **84**: 945–7.

174 Baykal D, Schmedtje JF, Runge MS. Role of the thrombin receptor in restenosis and atherosclerosis. *Am J Cardiology* 1995; **75**: 82B–87B.

175 Dzau VJ, Gibbons GH, Cooke JP, Ossoigui N. Vascular biology and medicine in the 1990s: scope, concepts, potentials, and perspectives. *Circulation* 1993; **87**(3): 705–19.

176 Kraiss LW and Johansen K. Pharmacologic intervention to prevent graft failure. *Surg Clin North Am* 1995; **75**(4): 761–72.

177 Pratt RE, Dzau VJ. Pharmocological strategies to prevent restenosis: lessons learned from blockade of the renin-angiotensin system. *Circulation* 1996; **93**: 848–52.

178 Finkel T, Epstein SE. Gene therapy for vascular disease. *FASEB* 1995; **9**(10): 843–51.

179 Carmeliet P, Collen D. Gene targeting and gene transfer studies of the plasminogen/plasmin system: implications in thrombosis, hemostasis, neointima formation, and atherosclerosis. *FASEB* 1995; **9**(10): 934–8.

180 McEwan J. Potential for antiviral therapy in the treatment of restenosis after angioplasty. *Br Heart J* 1995; **73**(6): 489.

6

The role of profundaplasty in lower extremity revascularization

SCOTT S BERMAN, ANDRES E TOVAR-PARDO AND VICTOR M BERNHARD

INTRODUCTION

The ability to improve blood flow to the lower leg in the setting of superficial femoral artery (SFA) occlusion through revascularization of a diseased profunda femoris artery (PFA) was first described in 1961 by Leeds and Gilfillan, and Morris et al.[1,2] Further support for the importance of the profunda as the main collateral pathway connecting the iliac artery in the pelvis with the popliteal and infrageniculate vessels in the leg was provided by Waibel and Wolf.[3] They demonstrated a significant fall in popliteal artery pressure when the profunda was clamped in patients with SFA occlusion. Direct measurements of profunda femoris blood flow by Bernhard and associates established the capacity of this artery to maintain adequate blood flow to sustain a functional extremity despite complete occlusion of the SFA.[4] They recorded blood flow volumes in the profunda which were twice that measured through femoropopliteal bypass grafts and equivalent to flow in the external iliac artery under normal anatomic circumstances. Despite this compelling physiologic evidence, the precise role that profunda revascularization plays in the treatment of lower extremity ischemia has remained somewhat controversial.

ANATOMY

The PFA is the main blood supply to the musculature of the thigh. It typically arises as a solitary trunk from the common femoral artery 2–4 cm below the inguinal ligament and courses posterolaterally under the sartorius and vastus lateralis muscles in Hunter's canal. A prominent surgical landmark is the lateral femoral circumflex vein, which passes deep to the SFA but courses anteriorly across the profunda femoris. This large venous structure, which often has multiple tributaries lateral to the profunda, must be carefully divided to gain exposure of the proximal portion of the artery (Fig. 6.1). The PFA can be divided into three anatomic segments that have surgical significance.[5] The proximal portion extends from the origin to the take-off of the medial and lateral circumflex femoral branches. This portion of the vessel lies within Scarpa's triangle and is easily exposed by division of the lateral circumflex vein. The medial and lateral circumflex artery branches originate from the PFA in 80 per cent of patients, whereas in the remaining 20 per cent, they derive their origin from either the common femoral or the superficial femoral arteries (Fig. 6.2). The circumflex femoral arterial branches and, in particular, the lateral circumflex, comprise a rich anastomotic network with the hypogastric artery in the pelvis through the inferior gluteal and perineal arteries. Designated as the cruciate anastomosis, this collateral complex effectively bypasses occlusions of the external iliac, common femoral and proximal profunda femoris vessels. The middle section of the profunda femoris extends from the circumflex branches to the take-off of the second perforating branch. This portion of the artery lies deep to the sartorius muscle. The distal portion of the profunda extends from the second perforating branch distally to

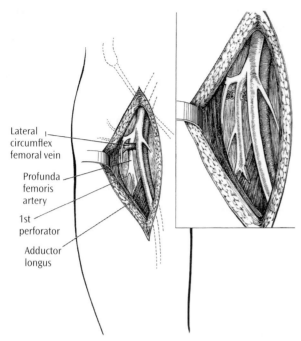

Lateral
circumflex
femoral vein

Profunda
femoris
artery

1st
perforator

Adductor
longus

Figure 6.1 *Exposure of the profunda femoris artery from an anterior approach. Reproduced with permission from Bernhard VM. The role of profundaplasty in revascularization of the lower extremities.* Surg Clin North Am *1979; 59: 681.*

the termination of the main trunk. The perforating branches of the distal PFA anastomose with the geniculate branches of the popliteal artery as well as with the recurrent tibial arteries to complete the collateral network, which extends from the pelvis to the lower leg.

PATHOPHYSIOLOGIC ASSESSMENT

Delineating the presence and significance of atherosclerotic occlusive disease involving the PFA requires diligence in the application of imaging modalities, and careful clinical assessment of the patient's historical and physical findings. Palpation of a profunda femoris pulse is often difficult due to its posterior position behind the SFA. Nonetheless, auscultation of a femoral bruit in a patient with a SFA occlusion provides indirect evidence of occlusive disease involving the profunda origin. Arteriography is the principal means of determining the existence of disease in the profunda femoris; however, multiple oblique views (Fig. 6.3) are usually necessary to visualize the proximal vessel and origin adequately without confounding overlap from the superficial femoral.[6]

The superficial location of the femoral vessels makes them amenable to interrogation with color-flow Doppler imaging, which provides both anatomic and physiologic data. Criteria have been established to define a greater

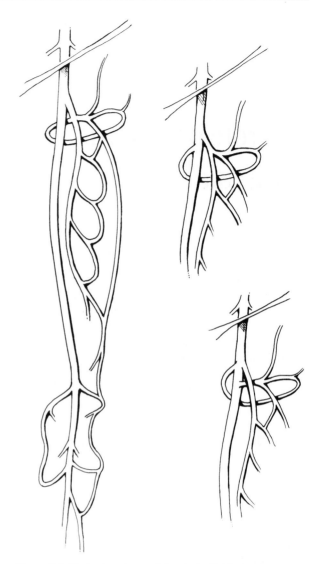

Figure 6.2 *Variant anatomy of the circumflex femoral artery branches and their contribution to collateral circulation of the thigh.*

than 50 per cent stenosis in the origin of the PFA.[7] A doubling of the peak systolic velocity in the narrowed area of the vessel coupled with the loss of flow reversal in diastole and the appearance of marked spectral broadening correlate well with greater than 50 per cent stenoses documented by arteriography.[8] These criteria assume that the normal velocity in the undiseased PFA approximates 65 cm/s. Color-flow Doppler imaging provides accurate noninvasive assessment of occlusive disease in the PFA as evidenced by sensitivity and specificity of 100 per cent and 86 per cent, respectively, achieved in numerous studies using this imaging modality.

Indirect measurements of profunda collateral adequacy using segmental Doppler pressures may be helpful in determining the physiologic significance of profunda occlusive disease. Well-developed collaterals between the profunda and infrageniculate branches of the popliteal

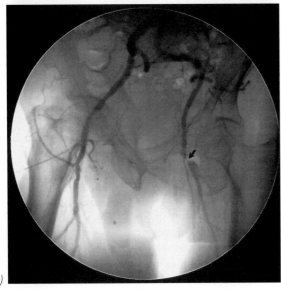

(a)

(b)

Figure 6.3 *Arteriogram of the femoral region. Adequate visualization of the profunda origin often requires oblique views (b) to unmask overlap from the superficial femoral seen in an anteroposterior view (a).*

and tibial vessels are crucial to the effectiveness of profunda revascularization. This collateral network can be assessed by calculating the profunda–popliteal collateral index (PPCI) as follows:

$$\text{PPCI} = \frac{\text{AKSP} - \text{BKSP}}{\text{AKSP}}$$

where the systolic pressure values above (AKSP) and below the knee (BKSP) are measured and compared.[9] A low index of less than 0.25 signifies a low pressure gradient across the knee joint and suggests that profunda revascularization may augment distal limb perfusion. By contrast, an index in excess of 0.25 indicates a large pressure gradient across the knee joint, poor collateral development and

predicts failure of profunda revascularization to improve limb ischemia.[10]

When discussing the options for revascularization of the PFA, three operative techniques and one nonoperative approach may be considered. The most common technique, whether as an isolated procedure or combined with an inflow or outflow bypass procedure, is that of endarterectomy with patch closure, termed profundaplasty. Bypass grafting of the profunda femoris is uncommonly utilized for isolated revascularization, and is usually combined with an inflow or outflow procedure when dealing with occlusive disease. Bypass grafting directly to the PFA beyond a proximal stenosis is, however, useful to revascularize the distal profunda when dealing with aneurysmal disease. This approach also finds applicability when scarring or infection in the groin preclude standard profundaplasty. Finally, percutaneous transluminal balloon angioplasty has been applied to lesions in the profunda femoris. Experience is limited and long-term follow-up is not yet available to draw reasonable conclusions as to the applicability of this technique on a wide scale.[11] The remainder of the chapter will be devoted to the selection of patients, techniques and results of profundaplasty for revascularization.

PATIENT SELECTION

In the presence of SFA occlusion, revascularization of the PFA using profundaplasty restores perfusion to the popliteal and crural arteries through the rich collateral network of the thigh. As such, profundaplasty is most frequently applied as an adjunctive procedure when treating inflow disease in the aortoiliac segments. Profundaplasty provides outflow in the presence of SFA occlusive disease for aortofemoral, iliofemoral, femorofemoral and axillofemoral bypass procedures. In these settings, profundaplasty reliably achieves limb salvage and improvement in claudication symptoms.[10] Pearce and Kempczinski reported a 5-year patency rate of 86 per cent and limb salvage rate of 72 per cent in 29 limbs undergoing extended profundaplasty in combination with aortofemoral bypass grafting.[12] Similarly good results were reported by McDonald and associates in their report of 21 patients undergoing femorofemoral bypass with concomitant profundaplasty with 100 per cent of patients attaining immediate relief of ischemia or improvement in claudication.[13] Even when direct bypass to the distal portion of the PFA is used as the outflow for aortofemoral and similar reconstructions, 5-year patency and limb salvage rates exceeding 90 per cent are achieved.[14]

When patients develop occlusion of a previously placed aortofemoral bypass graft limb, profundaplasty is often combined with graft thrombectomy to restore patency in a durable manner.[15,16] Profundaplasty, alone or occasionally in combination with an infrainguinal bypass, was required in 41 of 46 patients in our own series who presented with aortofemoral graft limb occlusion with limb salvage achieved in 95 per cent.[17]

In clinical situations in which a limited length of autogenous vein is available for infrageniculate bypass grafting, profundaplasty can establish the PFA as an adequate inflow source thereby limiting the length of vein required. Use of the PFA as an inflow source for distal bypass also permits avoidance of dissection through the scar of a previously operated groin incision if the proximal PFA is free of occlusive disease. Mills et al. have shown that the results for popliteal and tibial bypass grafts originating from the proximal or distal profunda were equivalent to those taking origin from the common femoral, superficial femoral or popliteal arteries.[18] Profundaplasty is often used as an adjunctive procedure at the time of infrainguinal bypass grafting, if the occlusive disease is limited to the PFA orifice and if profundaplasty can be accomplished without significantly complicating or prolonging the procedure. Although no data exist to justify this common practice, it is intuitive to believe that in this setting, profundaplasty may protect against limb-threatening ischemia if and when the infrainguinal bypass graft fails.

The principal controversy surrounding the use of profundaplasty is in the setting of critical limb ischemia when applied as the sole method of revascularization. At the center of this debate is the process of patient selection. A review of the reported series of isolated profundaplasty emphasizes the need to select appropriate patients carefully for a limited PFA procedure. Consistently good reports of the effectiveness of isolated profundaplasty for claudication have appeared in the literature. In one of the earliest compilations by Towne et al., 5-year patency in 83 patients operated upon for claudication was 77 per cent and exercise tolerance was invariably improved.[19] Similar results in patients with claudication were achieved by Liepe and associates.[20]

When the indications for profundaplasty are limb salvage, however, favorable results have been less consistently realized. For patients with ischemic rest pain, ulceration or gangrene, successful limb salvage in reported series of isolated profundaplasty has ranged from 14 per cent to 81 per cent.[21–23] Careful review of many of these reports identifies specific factors that may predict clinical success. The presence of a disease-free distal portion of the PFA combined with a well-developed collateral network between the PFA and crural vessels as evidenced by a low (<0.25) PPCI has been correlated with limb salvage in patients undergoing isolated profundaplasty.[9] Other factors that may correlate with favorable outcome include the presence of one or two patent tibial vessels, a low-thigh/ankle index of less than 0.55, an improvement in the postoperative ankle/brachial index of at least 0.10, and the absence of significant pedal gangrene.[24–26] When these selection criteria are applied, limb salvage comparable to distal

bypass procedures can be achieved using isolated profundaplasty alone.

Some important caveats must be considered before proceeding with profundaplasty as an isolated procedure. Compared with infrageniculate bypass, profundaplasty is a less stressful and time-consuming, procedure which can be performed under local anesthesia. This may be a substantial factor for the frail patient in whom a lesser procedure is warranted. Moreover, performance of profundaplasty does not preclude subsequent distal revascularization and might be contemplated as a less risky first step in a staged approach for higher risk patients. Finally, for the patient with distal gangrene facing limb loss, profundaplasty may improve perfusion through popliteal and geniculate collaterals sufficiently to permit healing of a below-the-knee, amputation and obviate the need for an above-the-knee amputation.[27] In some elderly and infirm patients with multiple co-morbid conditions, this simple benefit may make the difference between ambulation and relative independence versus being wheelchair bound or bedridden.

EXPOSURE OF THE PROFUNDA FEMORIS ARTERY

Direct exposure of the PFA from a standard groin incision requires only extension of the length of the incision to expose the artery distal to the endpoint of the obstructive plaque. Division of the lateral femoral circumflex vein is required to provide direct visualization of the proximal portion of the PFA to the level of the medial and lateral circumflex branches. Care should be exercised in dissecting and controlling the branches of the PFA, sparing them from damage or ligation as they may represent important collaterals between the profunda, the pelvic vasculature and the lower leg. The sartorius and vastus medialis muscles are retracted laterally, and the SFA is mobilized and retracted medially to provide exposure to the mid-portion of the PFA. Rather than initiating a long groin incision, extension of the incision continues as needed to expose as much PFA as necessary to reach beyond the occlusive disease. In most instances, the occlusive plaque is limited to the profunda orifice and the first portion of the vessel. Vascular control of the main trunk and multiple branches is obtained with soft silastic vessel loops to avoid damage to these delicate vessels. Since local groin wound complications are not infrequent and may be related to the extent of the incision and exposure, special attention to detail must be paid in ligating lymphatics, avoiding skin edge trauma, and undermining of groin skin flaps and meticulous multilayer closure techniques.[12]

When previous scarring in the groin or infection mandate avoidance of the standard approach to the PFA, it can be reached via a number of approaches in the upper thigh as classically described by Nunez *et al.*[28] and others (Fig. 6.4).[18,29] The three approaches are designated as the anterior, anteromedial and posteromedial. In the anterior approach, an incision is made in the upper thigh lateral to the sartorius. The muscle is retracted medially along with the superficial femoral vessels. The avascular raphé between the adductor longus and vastus medialis is incised providing exposure to the profunda vessels. This approach spares the blood supply to the sartorius, which enters segmentally on its inferomedial surface. By contrast, the anteromedial approach begins with an incision medial to the sartorius followed by retraction of the muscle laterally along with the superficial femoral vessels. Access to the PFA is again achieved by incision along the junction of the vastus medialis and adductor longus muscles. Finally, the posteromedial approach begins with a medial incision at the level of the mid-thigh, which is deepened in the plane between the sartorius and gracilis muscles. The sartorius and adductor longus muscles are retracted laterally, while the adductor brevis and magnus muscles are pulled medially. Access to the mid and distal PFA is provided in the plane lying deep to the adductor longus.

TECHNIQUE OF PROFUNDAPLASTY

Numerous technical approaches to profundaplasty have been described and are limited only by individual creativity. The specific configuration of the profundaplasty closure is usually dependent upon operative factors, such as the presence of an inflow or outflow graft, availability of the SFA for patch or flap closure, and the use of other options for patch closure, principally autogenous vein or prosthetic material. Some basic principles to be applied regardless of the method chosen for closure are worthy of emphasis. Arteriotomies on the PFA should be oriented longitudinally and traverse the vessel between the branches to avoid their orifices, which may be compromised during closure. Arteriotomies originating on the common femoral and extending through the profunda orifice should be placed laterally to avoid the angle between the PFA and SFA, which can add difficulty to the closure, often resulting in a narrowed area in the profundaplasty. Endarterectomy must be performed with the same care and diligence as in carotid surgery. The plane of dissection is defined between the inner and outer media to avoid excessive thinning of the endarterectomized wall. Careful completion of the distal endpoint to assure a smooth transition into the distal vessel may require fine cardiovascular tacking sutures to avoid raising an intimal flap upon restoration of flow. When extensive profundaplasty down into the mid and distal portion of the vessel is required, a completion arteriogram should be obtained to verify a techniquely adequate result.

When disease of the profunda is limited to the orifice and proximal portion of the artery, and the PFA will serve as the outflow for aortofemoral reconstruction, profundaplasty can be accomplished through an arteriotomy, which has its origin on the common femoral artery and extends through the PFA orifice just beyond the end of the obstructing plaque. Endarterectomy of the

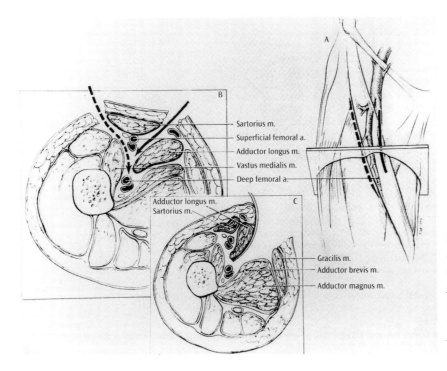

Figure 6.4 *Alternative approaches to exposure of the profunda femoris artery. Reproduced with permission from Veith FJ. Alternative approaches to the deep femoral, popliteal, and infrapopliteal arteries of the leg and foot, part 1. Ann Vasc Surg 1994; 8: 514–22.*

PFA is performed and closure completed by using the limb of the bypass graft as a patch over the limited arteriotomy (Fig. 6.5). When more extensive occlusive disease involves the PFA to the mid and distal portion the vessel, use of the graft limb as a patch is usually not adequate so other closure techniques must be considered. Alternatively, when the proximal PFA will serve as the inflow for an infrainguinal bypass, the proximal end of the bypass graft can be fashioned into a patch to achieve wide closure of a limited profundaplasty. Limited endarterectomy of the proximal PFA and SFA in combination with an inflow procedure can be closed by suturing the posterior and anterior walls of these vessels together, thereby repositioning the bifurcation at the distal junction of the endarterectomy endpoints. End-to-side anastomosis of the inflow graft is then performed on the common femoral artery.

If the SFA is patent but focally diseased proximally, femoral endarterectomy can be performed through an arteriotomy on the common femoral supplemented by division of the SFA (Fig. 6.6a). Endarterectomy of the SFA and common femoral are performed and the plaque is elevated completely from these vessels. Eversion technique can then be performed on the portion of the plaque extending down the PFA by prolapsing the artery toward the common femoral arteriotomy (Fig. 6.6b). Closure is obtained by end-to-end reanastomosis of the SFA and end-to-side anastomosis of the inflow bypass to the common femoral arteriotomy (Fig. 6.6c). This tech-

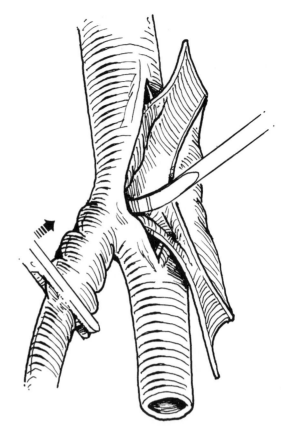

Figure 6.5 *A limited arteriotomy may be used for access to limited disease at the orifice of the profunda in aortofemoral reconstruction and closed with the limb of the aortofemoral graft as an overlying patch.*

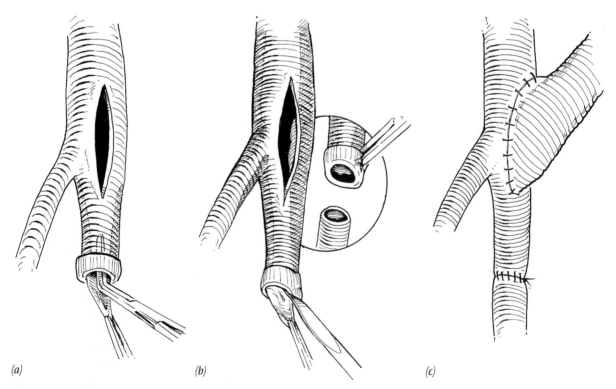

(a)   *(b)*   *(c)*

Figure 6.6 *Combined common femoral arteriotomy and transection of the superficial artery with eversion and patch angioplasty to accomplish profundaplasty as part of an inflow grafting.*

nique avoids the need for a patch closure specifically applied to the profundaplasty site.

When the SFA is completely occluded from its origin distally, patch closure of an extended profundaplasty can be completed using either a segment of endarterectomized SFA as a free patch after it is resected or by using a portion of the endarterectomized SFA as a flap closure of the profundaplasty (Fig. 6.7). These two techniques are applicable whether or not an inflow bypass graft is included in the revascularization. Similar patch closure can be obtained using either a proximal branch of the greater saphenous vein, a segment of upper extremity vein, or prosthetic patches made of Dacron® or polytetrafluoroethylene (Fig. 6.8).

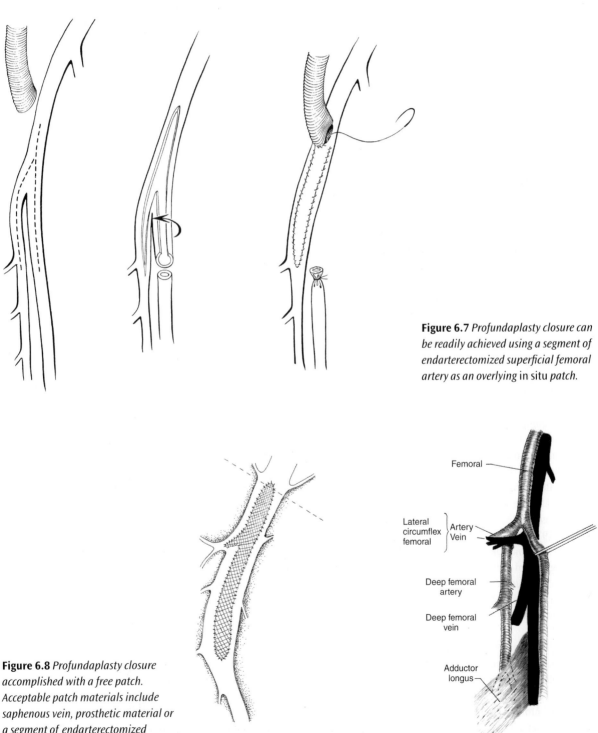

Figure 6.7 *Profundaplasty closure can be readily achieved using a segment of endarterectomized superficial femoral artery as an overlying* in situ *patch.*

Figure 6.8 *Profundaplasty closure accomplished with a free patch. Acceptable patch materials include saphenous vein, prosthetic material or a segment of endarterectomized superficial femoral artery.*

SUMMARY

Profunda femoris artery revascularization, executed using various profundaplasty techniques, can provide adequate outflow for managing aortoiliac occlusive disease with bypass procedures in the presence of SFA occlusion. Profundaplasty is also a useful and necessary adjunct in treating aortofemoral graft limb occlusions in this setting. Profundaplasty can create an adequate inflow source out of the PFA to reach distal vessels for infrainguinal bypass when autogenous conduit is limited. Combined with infrainguinal bypass procedures, profundaplasty may prevent limb threat if and when bypass patency is lost. In carefully selected patients, profundaplasty as an isolated procedure may be an effective treatment for claudication or severe ischemia manifested as rest pain or mild ulcerations, thereby avoiding extensive revascularization in poor-risk patients. When distal tissue loss is extensive, successful profundaplasty may limit amputations to the below-the-knee level in patients who are not candidates for other revascularization options.

REFERENCES

1 Leeds FH, Gilfillan RS. Revascularization of the ischemic limb. *Surgery* 1961; **82**: 25–32.

2 Morris GC, Edwards W, Cooley DA, *et al*. Surgical importance of the profunda femoris artery. *Arch Surg* 1961; **82**: 32–7.

3 Waibel PP, Wolf G. The collateral circulation in occlusions of the femoral artery: an experimental study. *Surgery* 1966; **60**: 912–16.

4 Bernhard VM, Ray LI, Militello JM. The role of angioplasty of the profunda femoris artery in revascularization of the ischemic limb. *Surg Gynecol Obstet* 1976; **142**: 840–4.

5 Lumsden AB, Colboon GL, Skandalakis G *et al*. Surgical anatomy of the deep femoral artery. In Merlini MP, Van Dongen RJAM, Dusmet M eds. *Surgery of the deep femoral artery*. Berlin: Springer-Verlag, 1994; 1–21.

6 Beals JSM, Adcock FA, Frawley JS *et al*. The radiologic assessment of disease of the profunda femoris artery. *Br J Radiol* 1971; **44**: 854–9.

7 Kohler RR, Nance DR, Strandness DE *et al*. Duplex scanning for diagnosis of aortoiliac and femoropopliteal disease: a prospective study. *Circulation* 1987; **76**: 1074–80.

8 Moneta GL, Yeager RA, Ruza A *et al*. Accuracy of lower extremity arterial duplex mapping. *J Vasc Surg* 1992; **15**: 275–84.

9 Boren CH, Towne JB, Bernhard VM *et al*. Profundapopliteal collateral index. A guide to successful profundaplasty. *Arch Surg* 1980; **115**: 1366–72.

10 Ouriel K, DeWeese JA, Ricotta JJ *et al*. Revascularization of the distal profunda femoris artery in the reconstructive treatment of aortoiliac occlusive disease. *J Vasc Surg* 1987; **6**: 217–22.

11 Varty K, London JM, Ratliff DA *et al*. Percutaneous angioplasty of the profunda femoris artery: a safe and effective endovascular technique. *Eur J Surg* 1993; **7**: 483–7.

12 Pearce WH, Kempczinski RF. Extended profundaplasty and aortofemoral grafting: an alternative to sychronous distal bypass. *J Vasc Surg* 1984; **3**: 455–8.

13 McDonald PT, Rich NM, Collins GJ Jr *et al*. Femorofemoral grafts: the role of concomitant extended profundaplasty. *Am J Surg* 1978; **136**: 622–8.

14 Prendiville EJ, Burke PE, Colgan MP *et al*. The profunda femoris: a durable outflow vessel in aortofemoral surgery. *J Vasc Surg* 1992; **16**: 23–9.

15 Bernhard VM, Ray LI, Towne JB. The reoperation of choice for aortofemoral graft occlusion. *Surgery* 1977; **82**: 867–74.

16 Goldstone J, Malone JM, Moore WS. Importance of the profunda femoris artery in primary and secondary arterial operations for lower extremity ischemia. *Am J Surg* 1978; **136**: 215.

17 Erdoes LS, Berman SS, Bernhard VM. Aortofemoral graft occlusion: strategy and timing of reoperation. *Cardiovasc Surg* 1995; **3**: 277–83.

18 Mills JL, Taylor SM, Fujitani R. The role of the deep femoral artery as an inflow site for infrainguinal revascularization. *J Vasc Surg* 1993; **18**: 416–23.

19 Towne JB, Bernhard VM, Rollins DL, Baum PL. Profundaplasty in perspective: limitations in the long-term management of limb ischemia. *Surgery* 1981; **90**: 1037–46.

20 Liepe B, Valesky A, Fritzenwanker B. Profundaplasty: a palliative operation in leg arterial occlusion of the aged? *Z Gerontol* 1985; **18**: 22–7.

21 Graham AM, Gewertz BL, Zarins CK. Efficacy of isolated profundaplasty. *Can J Surg* 1986; **29**: 330–2.

22 Harward TR, Bergan JJ, Yao JS *et al*. The demise of primary profundaplasty. *Am J Surg* 1988; **156**: 126–9.

23 van de Plas JP, van Dijk J, Tordoir JH *et al*. Isolated profundaplasty in citical limb ischemia: still of any use? *Eur J Vasc Surg* 1993; **7**: 54–8.

24 Kalman PG, Johnston KW, Walker PM. The current role of isolated profundaplasty. *J Cardiovasc Surg* 1990; **31**: 107–11.

25 McCoy DM, Sawchuck AP, Schuler JJ *et al*. The role of isolated profundaplasty for the treatment of rest pain. *Arch Surg* 1989; **124**: 441–4.

26 Fugger R, Kretschmer G, Schemper M *et al*. The place of profundaplasty in the surgical treatment of SFA occlusion. *Eur J Vasc Surg* 1987; **1**: 187–91.

27 Towne JB, Rollins DL. Profundaplasty: its role in limb salvage. *Surg Clin North Am* 1986; **66**: 403–14.

28 Nunez AA, Veith FJ, Collier P *et al*. Direct approaches to the distal portions of the deep femoral artery for limb salvage bypasses. *J Vasc Surg* 1988; **8**: 576–81.

29 Veith FJ. Alternative approaches to the deep femoral, popliteal, and infrapopliteal arteries in the leg and foot, part 1. *Ann Vasc Surg* 1994; **8**: 514–22.

30 Effney DJ, Stoney RJ. Profunda femoris reconstruction. In: Stoney RJ ed. *Wylie's atlas of vascular surgery. Disorders of the extremities*. Philadelphia: J.B. Lippincott Co., 1993; 30–41.

7

Interposition vein cuffs and collars for PTFE grafts

ANDREW W BRADBURY AND JOHN HN WOLFE

INTRODUCTION

In 1949, Kunlin first described the use of autogenous long saphenous vein (LSV) as an arterial conduit for bypass grafting to the leg.[1] Despite the subsequent introduction of alternatives, such as human umbilical vein (HUV), expanded polytetrafluoroethylene (ePTFE) and Dacron, there is a general consensus amongst vascular surgeons that vein offers the best prospect of long-term patency; especially when the distal anastomosis is placed below the knee. Unfortunately, even when imaginative use is made of alternative sources, such as arm and short saphenous vein, not all patients have vein of sufficient length or quality. The discussion then arises as to whether the use of prosthetic materials may be preferable to poor-quality vein or primary amputation. In other words, to what lengths should a surgeon go to splice short segments of small-caliber vein before using a prosthetic graft?

At the present time, the best prosthetic material for distal bypass appears to be externally reinforced PTFE. When the distal anastomosis is suprageniculate, patency rates for vein and PTFE are not significantly different, although no comparison has ever shown PTFE to be superior. Below the knee, the results of PTFE are clearly inferior, and the difference between PTFE and vein becomes greater the more distal the anastomosis is placed. For example, femorocrural grafting with vein produces 1- and 3-year patencies of 47–100 per cent and 47–71 per cent respectively. The same operation performed with PTFE produces patencies of 21–60 per cent and 14–38 per cent, respectively, at the same time intervals. Even enthusiasts find the latter figures demoralising. In the modern climate of dwindling healthcare resources, the reasons for not performing this sort of surgery at all may become overwhelming, despite evidence that primary amputation is no less expensive.[2]

Several pharmacological methods have been used in an attempt to improve prosthetic graft patency, including long-term aspirin, anticoagulation and prostacyclin infusions. However, at the present time, the best hope of improving PTFE graft performance lies in meticulous technique together with the construction of an arteriovenous fistula and/or venous interposition collar or cuff in certain circumstances. Although there are no controlled data to support the use of a fistula, there is increasing evidence, from both uncontrolled and randomized studies, that interposing a segment of vein between the PTFE graft and recipient artery increases patency.[3–5] The aim of the current paper is to examine the development of, as well as the evidence and current indications for, the use of venous interposition techniques in lower-limb arterial reconstruction.

DEVELOPMENT OF INTERPOSITION VEIN TECHNIQUES

Miller patch

This interposition technique involves suturing a piece of vein to one side of the distal arteriotomy, and then suturing PTFE to the rim of that vein on one side and to the opposite side of the arteriotomy on the other. Miller subsequently decided that a full cuff would be more effective.

Miller collar

A short segment of vein approximately 3–4 times the length of the distal arteriotomy is harvested from any available source, trimmed of valve cusps, if present, and opened longitudinally.[6] The vein is sutured to the margins of the arteriotomy with 7/0 Prolene and the PTFE graft is sutured to the rim of the collar with 6/0 Prolene (Fig. 7.1). Completion arteriography confirms wide patency of the distal anastomosis with good run-off (Fig. 7.2).

Taylor patch

The externally reinforcing rings or spiral are removed from the PTFE graft over a length of about 3 cm and a U-shaped slit of 1 cm or less made on the underside of the graft. The slit is minimally angled to ensure that the PTFE lies almost parallel to the recipient artery. The arteriotomy is made over 3–4 cm and should be 4–5 times longer than the diameter of the PTFE graft to be used (normally 6 mm). The PTFE graft is anastomosed to the proximal end of the arteriotomy using 6/0 Prolene

using a parachute technique or, if the artery is small (less than 2 mm), using four interrupted 6/0 Prolene sutures at the heel. The suture line is secured with a knot on each side and the PTFE graft incised longitudinally in the line of the arteriotomy to a point 2 cm proximal to the heel of the anastomosis. The limit of this incision is also fashioned into a U-shape and surplus graft material excised. A 5–6 cm length of vein is harvested, trimmed, opened longitudinally and fashioned into a diamond-shaped patch. The vein patch is sewn to fill the elliptical gap in the anastomosis. Placement of the patch is commenced distally using 6–8 interrupted 6/0 or 7/0 Prolene sutures, all inserted before tying. Several more interrupted sutures are inserted on each side and the anastomosis completed with a running suture. The widest part of the vein patch should overlie the most distal limit of the PTFE-arterial anastomosis. The vein patch lies thus: 2 cm along the PTFE graft, 1 cm overlying the PTFE-arterial anastomosis and 2–3 cm along the recipient vessel (Fig. 7.3). The vein patch should bulge gently and taper distally to enable a smooth transition from the 6 mm PTFE to the distal artery, which may be as small as 1.5 mm in diameter. The wider the available vein patch, the

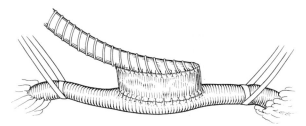

Figure 7.1 *The Miller collar.*

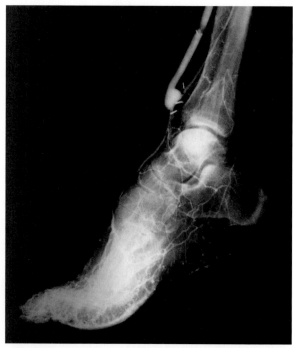

Figure 7.2 *Angiogram following femoral/dorsalis pedis graft using a Miller collar.*

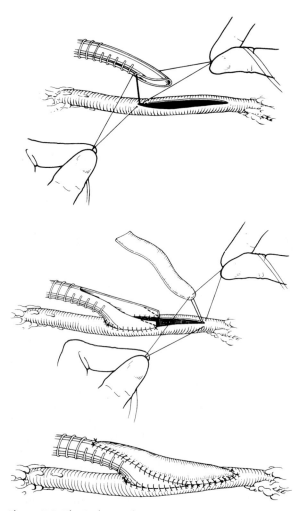

Figure 7.3 *The Taylor patch.*

more PTFE should be trimmed, so maximizing the amount of vein incorporated into the anastomosis. Because of limited access to the below-knee popliteal artery, there is merit in suturing the vein patch to the PTFE graft prior to tunneling. Taylor also advised suturing a 3 cm vein patch across the proximal anastomosis.[7,8]

St Mary's boot

Although both the 'Miller cuff' and the 'Taylor patch' have been associated with encouraging results, both have theoretical disadvantages. The cuff is associated with marked turbulence because of its shape and a high incidence angle of entry of the PTFE graft. The Taylor patch still necessitates suturing PTFE directly to the artery with the subsequent potential increase in myointimal hyperplasia at the heel of the anastomosis. Theoretically, the ideal patch would obviate direct PTFE-arterial anastomosis but maintain a smooth, streamlined angle of entry. The St Mary's boot attempts to combine these two favorable attributes.[4] A 6-cm length of vein is harvested and opened to form a rectangle. The corner of the venous sheet is then sutured to the apex of the arteriotomy using 7/0 Prolene to form the anastomotic toe. The remainder of the suture line is then fashioned in a

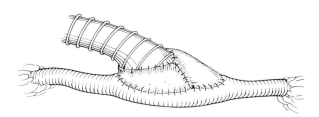

Figure 7.4 *The St Mary's boot.*

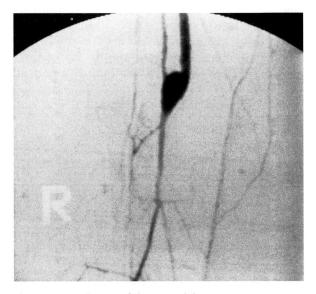

Figure 7.5 *Angiogram of the St Mary's boot.*

way similar to the Miller collar by draping the patch around the full circumference of the arteriotomy. The redundant length of vein is then excised obliquely and the suture line completed to form a 'boot-like' suture (Fig. 7.4). The heel of the boot is then tailored by incising it posteriorly. Lastly, the PTFE to vein anastomosis is completed. Although this modification possesses theoretical advantages, it remains to be seen whether it offers any clinically apparent advantages over the other venous interposition techniques already described. The anatomical difference with respect to the Miller collar is apparent in Fig. 7.5.

EVIDENCE FOR INTERPOSITION VEIN COLLARS AND GRAFTS

In 1992, Taylor reported his experience with 256 patients operated upon between 1982 and 1989 using the 'Taylor patch'.[8] Operations were performed under tourniquet control in order to avoid circumferential dissection, slinging and clamping of distal vessels. Externally reinforced PTFE was used once it became available. Aspirin was commenced preoperatively and continued postoperatively (300 mg daily). Heparin was given prior to proximal clamping: 5000 U for above-knee and 10 000 U for below-knee reconstructions. Prostaglandin infusions were also used for infrageniculate surgery and all patients underwent completion angiography. Graft patency was assessed at 3, 6, 9 and 12 months, and yearly thereafter. Recurrence of symptoms or a fall in ankle/brachial pressure indices were indications for angiography. The mean age of the patients was 72 years and, in 72 per cent of cases, operation was carried out for critical limb ischemia, including 100 per cent of infrageniculate reconstructions. The outflow was infrapopliteal in 32 per cent, to a single vessel or isolated popliteal segment in 53 per cent and 36 per cent of below-knee bypasses were secondary procedures. Data were evaluated by life-table analysis; the overall patency at 1 year was an excellent 85 per cent, at 3 years 74 per cent, at 5 years 65 per cent and at 8 years (17 grafts at risk) 51 per cent. There was no significant difference in patency between above- and below-knee popliteal reconstructions, although both were significantly better than bypasses to tibial vessels: 81 *vs* 58 per cent at 3 years, and 71 *vs* 54 per cent at 5 years. Although 26 occluded grafts were reopened, all but five failed within 2 years, making the difference between primary and secondary patencies small. During a mean follow-up period of 35 months, six grafts failed immediately (all bypasses to ankle level with poor run-off) and 65 grafts failed at a later date. Limb salvage was 96, 88 and 80 per cent at 1, 5 and 8 years, respectively. The authors attribute their excellent results to a reduction in perianastomotic neointimal hyperplasia, the shallow angle between graft and recipient artery reducing turbulence, the routine use of completion angiography and, of course, meticulous technique, particularly the use of interrupted sutures at the toe of the distal anastomosis. This allows placement of sutures under direct vision as well as arterial expansion in response to pulsatile inflow. On the basis of comparison with historical controls, the authors concluded that the vein patch was not of great value in the above-knee position, of some benefit in bypasses to the below-knee popliteal, and crucial to their improved results in crural bypass. The benefit of a patch at the proximal anastomosis remains unproven.

In 1995, the late J.H. Miller's unit reported retrospectively on all femoropopliteal bypass grafts performed with PTFE between 1978 and 1992.[9] Bypasses to the tibial vessels and secondary reconstructions were excluded. The majority of bypasses were performed for critical limb ischaemia or the acutely threatened ischaemic limb. This was not a randomized study and distal bypass technique (direct vs vein patch vs vein collar) was left to the discretion of the surgeon, although the authors point out that in difficult cases the surgeons usually chose to perform a venous interposition so potentially skewing the result against the cuff/collar technique. All patients underwent completion angiography and were followed up at 1, 3 and 6 months, and thereafter 6 monthly. The bypass was deemed patent if there was a pulse in the graft and/or a sustained rise in the ankle/brachial pressure index (ABPI). Cumulative patency at 12 and 36 months was presented in the form of actuarial life-table analysis. Overall, 559 grafts were performed in 506 patients. During the same time period, 768 primary femoropopliteal vein grafts were performed. There was no difference in risk factors between patients undergoing different PTFE techniques and patients undergoing vein grafts. At 30 days, 25 PTFE grafts had failed (4 per cent) and a further 25 patients had died (4 per cent) predominantly of myocardial infarction (MI). At 12 and 36 months, the overall patency of PTFE grafts was 82 and 62 per cent, respectively. For above-knee reconstruction, there was no significant difference in patency between cuffed and noncuffed grafts: cuff vs no cuff 85 vs 82 per cent at 12 months, and 69 vs 68 per cent at 36 months ($p = 0.89$). However, for below-knee reconstructions, there was a significant increase in patency for cuffed grafts: cuff vs no cuff 83 vs 66 per cent at 12 months, 57 vs 29 per cent at 36 months ($p = 0.01$). As might be expected, results were significantly better in patients undergoing operation for claudication rather than critical limb ischaemia. There was no significant difference in patency between cuffed PTFE grafts and vein grafts at 12 and 36 months. However, at 5 years the patency of cuffed PTFE grafts was significantly worse (47 vs 57 per cent), a difference that increased with time. Although 179 PTFE cuffed grafts occluded during the study, in 91 cases (51 per cent) the outflow vessel remained patent.

There are also data emerging from randomized stud-ies supporting the use of a venous interposition cuff in certain circumstances. In the UK, the Joint Vascular Research Group (JVRG) have conducted a multicenter randomized trial comparing the long-term patency of PTFE grafts performed with and without the addition of a Miller cuff.[5] The trial was instigated in 1991 and was closed in mid-1993, at which time 261 patients (133 cuff, 128 no cuff) had been randomized. The preliminary results were presented at the Vascular Surgical Society of Great Britain and Ireland, and published in abstract form in 1995. The patients had a mean age of 68 years and the male:female ratio was 2:1. There was no difference between the two groups with respect to age, sex, side, diabetes, patient reported smoking habits, previous graft failure, indication for operation, grade of surgeon, or site of distal anastomosis (150 above-knee popliteal, 96 below-knee popliteal and 15 tibial artery). There was a significant difference in operating time: 143 and 124 minutes for bypass with and without cuff, respectively. There was no difference in wound complications or length of postoperative stay (median 10 days). There was no difference in the use of aspirin or anticoagulation. At 30 days, five cuffed grafts had occluded necessitating two amputations, compared with 19 noncuffed grafts necessitating eight amputations. This difference was significant at the 5 per cent level. At a median follow-up of 16 months, life-table analysis of graft patency at 12 and 24 months showed no difference between cuffed and noncuffed grafts to the above-knee popliteal artery. However, there was a significant difference at the 1 per cent level between infrageniculate cuffed and noncuffed grafts with patencies of 78.7 vs 62.0 per cent at 12 months, and 49.4 vs 18.9 per cent at 24 months, respectively. There was a similar difference in limb salvage: 87.9 vs 67.4 per cent at 12 months, and 85.0 vs 54.3 per cent at 24 months.

At the present time, follow-up is being continued and the JVRG are recruiting patients to a follow-up study comparing the venous cuff with the Taylor patch for infrageniculate PTFE bypass. There are two current, randomized studies (in Sweden and Belgium) that will be reporting in a couple of years' time. In the USA, the Columbus Vascular Surgical Society initiated a randomized trial in 1994 comparing PTFE bypass performed with and without the Taylor patch.[10] At the time of writing, the data from these trials are not yet available.

WHY DO VEIN CUFFS WORK?

It is generally accepted that early graft failure (within 30 days) is due to surgical error: either there is a technical error, a defect in the graft itself or the run-off is inadequate. Approximately 10 per cent of distal grafts fail in this period. Failure occurring after 18 months is usually due to progression of disease either proximal or distal to the bypass, and accounts for 20 per cent of total failures. Between 30 days and 18 months PTFE graft failure is thought to be due predominantly to neointimal hyperplasia (NIH) at the distal anastomosis. There are three main theories as to how cuffs and collars might improve graft patency. They are not mutually exclusive and, to some extent, overlap each other.

Firstly, it is almost certain that the presence of an easily manipulated venous cuff allows the surgeon to construct a more perfect anastomosis than would be possible if a large diameter (6 mm) length of noncompliant PTFE were being anastomosed directly to a 2–3 mm crural vessel, especially where the latter is heavily diseased and/or calcified. After all, ease of reconstruction was the primary driving force behind the initial development of these interposition techniques. The subjective impression of numerous surgeons that this is so is supported by the 30-day failure rate in the JVRG venous collar trial described above. In addition, experimental work confirms the superiority of the cuffed anastomosis.[11] A perfect circle has the greatest cross-sectional area for any given circumference and anastomotic caste studies clearly indicated that direct PTFE anastomoses nearly always lead to oval narrowing of the recipient artery.[12] These studies also demonstrated that, even when the external appearance of the anastomosis is satisfactory, PTFE often protrudes into the lumen, so narrowing and creating turbulence at this critical site. These anatomical defects are found very much less frequently with cuffed anastomoses. The authors also found functional problems with direct PTFE–artery anastomoses in that the resistance to flow through the anastomosis did not relate directly to vessel and graft radius according to Poiseuille's law. By contrast, blood flow through a cuffed anastomosis correlated with radius of the outflow artery. This suggests that anatomical imperfections do give rise to additional and inherent functional resistance at direct PTFE–arterial anastomoses.

Secondly, it has been postulated that cuffed anastomoses improve prosthetic graft patency by increasing blood flow.[13] It is postulated that the cuff, by acting as an elastic venous reservoir, stores small volumes of blood and potential energy during systole, which is then converted to kinetic energy and subsequent onward flow down the recipient artery during diastole. However, this theory was not substantiated in the St Mary's experimental model.[12]

Thirdly, and probably most importantly, it has been observed that the presence of a cuff reduces and/or modifies the distribution of NIH at the anastomosis (Figs 7.6 and 7.7), which means that:

1 the anastomosis and run-off artery are not subject to the same degree of neointimal narrowing or distortion;
2 if the graft occludes, the run-off remains patent because NIH is confined to the cuff (Fig. 7.8).

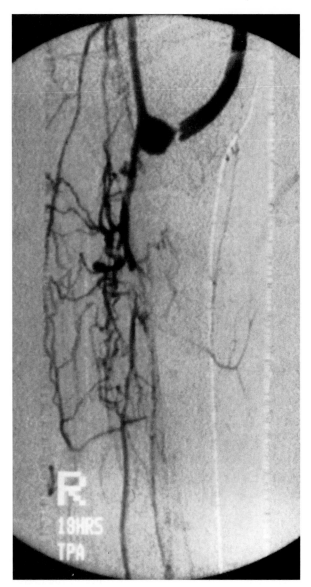

Figure 7.6 *Stenosis between PTFE and Miller collar.*

It is not yet understood how the interposition of a vein cuff reduces NIH and, indeed, the pathophysiology of NIH itself is far from completely defined. Nevertheless, the most popular theories are that the vein cuff acts by:

1 altering the haemodynamics of the anastomosis, such that the maximum stimulus to NIH is at the PTFE vein interface, where the conduit is a wide reservoir that can accommodate a degree of NIH without impairing flow;
2 reducing compliance mismatch between the PTFE and the recipient artery.

Understanding the mechanisms by which vein interposition cuffs 'protect' the artery from NIH may lead to further improvements in technique or cuff design with further graft–arterial anastomoses.[14] This has been attributed to reduction in compliance mismatch

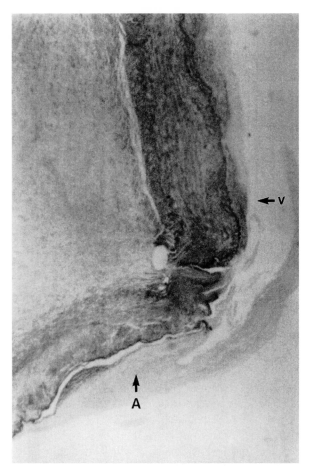

Figure 7.7 *Histology section showing sparing of the recipient artery from NIH (V = venous collar, A = artery).*

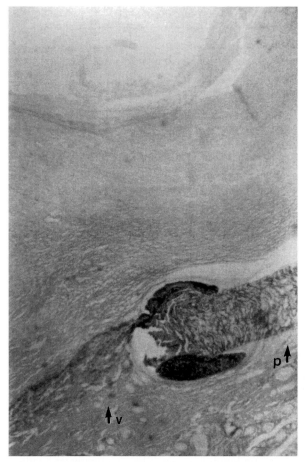

Figure 7.8 *Myointimal hyperplasia between PTFE and venous collar (P = PTFE, V = venous collar).*

between the stiff graft material and the relatively pliant artery. This is thought to diminish injury to the native vessel. However, in a recent study, where a PTFE jacket was placed around the vein cuff and incorporated into the anastomosis in order to render the cuff more like PTFE in terms of its distensibility, there was no difference in NIH between jacketed and nonjacketed cuffed anastomoses. This suggests that the protective effect of the vein cuff is not related to compliance. Instead, the authors suggest that the protective effect might relate to prolonged contact between the venous endothelium of the cuff and mitogenic substances within the plasma at areas of reduced flow.[15]

Although these studies have not yet provided a clear insight into the various factors that account for the beneficial effects of the vein cuff, they do indicate how mechanical and biological factors are inextricably linked. Mechanical stimulation of the endothelium through exposure to pressure, especially cyclical pressure, and shear forces does alter growth factor synthesis, collagen metabolism, smooth muscle cell activity, thrombosis and fibrinolysis, especially within a segment of vein that has been 'arterialized'.

CONCLUSION

There is good evidence from controlled and uncontrolled studies that vein cuffs significantly increase PTFE graft patency. The two most likely explanations for this phenomenon are that they improve technical accuracy and alter the amount or distribution of NIH.

Attempts have been made to increase prosthetic graft patency by trying to:

1 induce endothelium to line prosthetic graft materials;
2 manufacture compliant prosthetic grafts; and
3 understand and manipulate the complex molecular biology of NIH.

Ironically, perhaps the greatest single contribution to improving the patency of prosthetic grafts, namely the venous interposition cuff, was originally developed simply to make the process of attaching PTFE to recipient artery easier. The architects of these techniques appear to have unwittingly overcome fundamental problems related to the prosthetic anastomosis of which we were previously unaware. Many surgeons now feel it is obligatory to perform some form of interposition venous cuff or collar in infrageniculate PTFE bypasses. The next challenge is to perfect the anatomical form of this interposition and to use these data to try to understand the mechanisms underlying graft failure secondary to NIH.

REFERENCES

1 Kunlin J. Le traitement de l'arterite obliterante par la greffe veineuse. *Arch Mal Coeur* 1949; **42**: 371–3.

2 Cheshire NJW, Wolfe JHN, Noon MA, Davies L, Drummond M. The economics of femorocrural reconstruction for critical limb ischaemia with and without autologous vein. *J Vasc Surg* 1992; **15**: 167–75.

3 Harris PL, Bakran A, Enbi L, Nott D. ePTFE grafts for femoro-crural bypass – improved results with combined adjuvant venous cuff and arteriovenous fistula. *Eur J Vasc Surg* 1993; **7**: 528.

4 Tyrrell MR, Wolfe JHN. New prosthetic venous collar anastomotic technique: combining the best of other procedures. *Br J Surg* 1991; **78**: 1016–7.

5 Stonebridge PA, Howlett J. Prescott R. Ruckley CV. Randomised trial comparing polytetrafluoroethylene graft patency with and without a Miller cuff. *Br J Surg* 1995; **82**: 555–6 (abstract).

6 Miller JH; Foreman RK, Ferguson L, Aris I. Interposition vein cuff for anastomosis of prosthesis to small artery. *Austr NZ J Surg* 1984; 54: 283–5.

7 McFarland RJ, Taylor RS. Une amelioration technique d'anastomosis des prostheses arterielles femoro-distales. *Phlebologie* 1988; **41**: 229–34.

8 Taylor RS, Loh A, McFarland RJ, Cox M, Chester JF. Improved technique for polytetrafluoroethylene bypass grafting: long-term results using anastomotic vein patches. *Br J Surg* 1992; **79**: 348–54.

9 Raptis S, Miller JH. Influence of a vein cuff on polytetrafluoroethylene grafts for primary femoropopliteal bypass. *Br J Surg* 1995; **82**: 487–91.

10 Wright JG. A randomised prospective clinical trial of the Taylor patch. *J Vasc Surg* 1996; **23**: 376–7 (letter).

11 da Silva A, How TV, Harris PL. Imaging of local haemodynamics in interposition vein cuffs by dynamic duplex scanning and cine-DSA. In: Greenhalgh RM ed. *Vascular imaging for surgeons*. London: WB Saunders, 1995, 389–98.

12 Tyrrell MR, Chester JR, Vipond MN, Clarke GH, Taylor RS, Wolfe JHN. Experimental evidence to support the use of interposition vein collars/patches in distal PTFE anastomoses. *Eur J Vasc Surg* 1990; **4**: 95–101.

13 Harris PL, de Silva A, How T. Interposition vein cuffs. *Eur J Vasc Endovasc Surg* 1996; **11**: 257–9 (editorial).

14 Suggs WD, Henriques HE, De Palma RG. Vein cuff interposition prevents juxta-anastomotic neointimal hyperplasia. *Ann Surg* 1988; **2**: 207–717.

15 Norberto JJ, Sidawy AN, Trad KS *et al*. The protective effect of vein cuffed anastomoses is not mechanical in origin. *J Vasc Surg* 1995; **21**: 558–66.

8

Reversed vein bypass

JOSEPH L MILLS

INTRODUCTION

Autogenous vein, in the reversed configuration, remains the most applicable and durable conduit for infrainguinal revascularization.[1–2] Multiple authors have demonstrated that nearly all infrainguinal bypasses can be performed with autogenous vein if a diligent search for suitable vein is carried out.[3–6] While the conduit of choice is clearly greater saphenous vein (GSV), an increasingly large proportion of patients requiring infrainguinal bypass no longer have this option available, the vein having been previously utilized either for lower extremity or coronary revascularization. In such cases, our preference is to design the operation so as to utilize a single segment of vein whenever possible, but we do not hesitate to splice vein segments when necessary. In descending order of preference, we choose to harvest vein from the following sources: (1) ipsilateral GSV; (2) contralateral GSV; (3) ipsilateral lesser saphenous vein;[7,8] (4) upper extremity veins (cephalic and/or basilic, depending upon the length required);[9] and (5) contralateral lesser saphenous vein. When ipsilateral vein is unavailable, duplex scanning of alternative venous conduits is essential to identify the best available conduit. Duplex ultrasound vein mapping is helpful in measuring diameters of potential vein conduits, both by directing the surgeon to the selection of the optimal conduit available, and also by identifying calcified or sclerotic vein segments, which would not be usable if harvested, thus avoiding unnecessary incisions to harvest poor quality vein segments.

Some element of controversy remains over the superiority of the *in situ* versus the reversed vein configuration for infrainguinal bypass. In the 1970s and 1980s, the time period during which *in situ* bypass was resurrected, many authors claimed that results with *in situ* vein were superior.[10–20] Most of these studies were flawed by the use of historical controls. In addition to the problems inherent to the use of historical controls, many of these reports failed to distinguish between primary and secondary patency rates[21,22] (see Chapter 12 for a further discussion of these issues). Finally, *in situ* vein is only applicable to the best case scenario in which ipsilateral GSV of optimal diameter and adequate length is available. The historical 'control' groups frequently included reversed vein conduits consisting of veins other than GSV as well as patients undergoing reoperative leg bypass.[13,16,20,23] Alternate conduits and reoperative surgery result in patency and limb salvage results, which are distinctly inferior to those obtained when performing primary revascularizations using GSV. These reports were thus comparing apples and oranges. Fortunately, multiple prospective trials,[24–28] randomized to include patients undergoing first-time lower extremity bypass with GSV in whom either technique was potentially applicable, have demonstrated equivalent results with *in situ* and reversed vein (Table 8.1). In addition, in these randomized trials, vein quality was the most important factor with respect to long-term graft patency. Small-caliber veins (<3–3.5 mm) yielded inferior results regardless of graft configuration. For all these reasons, we continue to utilize reversed vein as our conduit of choice for infrainguinal bypass. It is applicable to nearly all patients requiring lower extremity reconstruction,[3,29–34] and is simpler and less tedious than techniques requiring valve lysis. Use of good-quality vein, meticulous operative judgment and technique, and vigilant postoperative duplex graft surveillance (see Chapter 13) are the most important factors in achieving long-term graft patency and limb salvage, not graft configuration.[2,35]

Since the first description of reversed vein bypass for revascularization of patients with chronic lower extremity arterial occlusive disease by Kunlin in 1949,[36] numer-

Table 8.1 *Randomized prospective trials of* in situ *versus reversed vein bypass*

| Type of grafts[a] | RVG | Patency (%) | |
		In situ	*p* value
Watelet *et al.* (1986)[26] (*n* = 100 grafts)			
AK/BK popliteal	88	71	NS
Harris *et al.* (1987)[25] (*n* = 215 grafts)			
AK/BK popliteal	77	68	NS
Veterans Administration Cooperative Study			
Group 141 (1988)[24] (*n* = 461 grafts)			
BK popliteal	75	78	NS
Infrapopliteal	67	76	NS
Wengerter *et al.* (1991)[28] (*n* = 125 grafts)			
Overall	67	69	NS
<3 mm veins	37	61	NS
Watelet *et al.* (1997)[27] (n = 91 grafts)	70.2	64.8	NS

NS = not significant, AK = above knee, BK = below knee, RVG = reversed vein grafts.

[a] Watelet *et al.* (1986) values at 36 months; Harris *et al.* values at 36 months; Veterans Administration Cooperative Study values at 24 months; Wengerter *et al.* values at 30 months; Watelet *et al.* (1997) – 10-year results.

ous techniques have been described to optimize vein conduit preparation and improve outcome. A common problem among busy surgeons is a failure to read the existing literature; many technical adjuncts have been rediscovered and reported by well-meaning surgeons who were unaware their inventive maneuvers to overcome technical obstacles had already been described.[37,38] In particular, Kunlin's 1951 article clearly and succinctly delineates essential techniques to aid infrainguinal bypass grafting when the native arteries are excessively thickened or the vein caliber is small relative to the native perianastomotic donor vessel.[39] In the space that follows, a practical approach to the technical conduct of lower extremity revascularization using reversed vein will be presented.

Prior to commencement of the operation, the operating surgeon should define the optimal inflow and outflow arteries. It is not obligatory to originate lower extremity bypasses from the common femoral artery. Shorter bypasses, originating from the deep femoral, superficial femoral and even the popliteal artery are frequently applicable, especially in diabetic patients requiring limb salvage bypasses.[40,41] A frequent pattern of arterial occlusive disease in diabetics involves severe obliterative atherosclerotic disease of the distal popliteal artery, and proximal trifurcation or infrapopliteal arteries in the calf, with reconstitution of the mid to distal peroneal, the posterior tibial or plantar arteries, or the dorsalis pedis artery. Many such patients have strongly palpable popliteal pulses, triphasic arterial Doppler waveforms at the popliteal level, and minimal disease in the common and superficial femoral arteries. Our preference is to perform short bypasses in such patients,[42] frequently using GSV from the thigh, especially if the thigh segment is of a better caliber as determined by pre-

operative vein mapping. The vein is then harvested from the thigh and tunneled subcutaneously from the popliteal artery to the appropriate outflow artery. This superficial tunnel is beneath intact skin, decreasing the chance that vein harvest incisional problems or infections will compromise the vein graft (Fig. 8.1). In addition, superficially tunneled vein grafts are easier to scan postoperatively and revision, if subsequently required, more readily carried out. If the superficial femoral artery is patent but harbors hemodynamically significant disease, it should be bypassed. Occasionally, if available vein conduit is severely limited, a focal superficial femoral artery lesion can be treated with percutaneous transluminal angioplasty, or if unsuccessful, endarterectomy and patch angioplasty to allow use of a more distal graft origin and shorten the length of vein required to perform the necessary bypass. If distal origin or 'short' bypass grafts are utilized, the native arterial tree proximal to the graft origin should be included in the postoperative duplex surveillance protocol to be certain that progressive or recurrent inflow disease does not compromise graft inflow.

Significant occlusive disease of the origin and proximal deep femoral artery should be addressed at the time of lower extremity bypass, especially if the bypass is to originate from the common femoral artery. The endarterectomy usually commences in the common femoral artery, although occasionally a portion of the inguinal ligament must be divided to allow access for clamp placement in a soft portion of the distal external iliac artery. Following division of crossing veins, the arteriotomy is then extended across the deep femoral artery orifice to allow complete removal of the posterior tongue of plaque, which invariably extends into the first or second portion of the deep femoral artery. Following com-

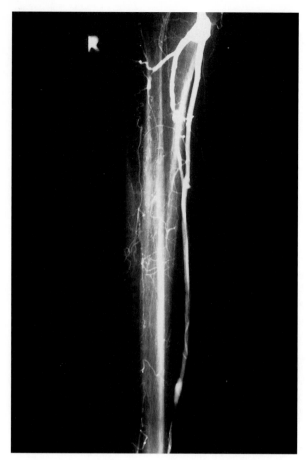

Figure 8.1 *Transfemoral arteriogram of a below-knee popliteal artery to distal peroneal reversed saphenous vein bypass graft, which was obtained 3 years postoperatively. This patient demonstrates the typical obliteration or 'wipe-out' of the proximal and mid-infrapopliteal vessels. The proximal anastomosis, vein conduit and distal anastomosis are all widely patent. The saphenous vein conduit had been harvested from the ipsilateral thigh and remains of adequate caliber, smooth and without intrinsic defects.*

infected or occluded prosthetic infrainguinal bypass is to repair previously unaddressed deep femoral artery obstruction. This maneuver may obviate the necessity to perform a redo leg bypass. The prudent surgeon, however, would always have corrected significant deep femoral disease at the primary bypass operation.

VEIN HARVESTING AND PREPARATION

The vein should be harvested carefully and expeditiously, and prepared by a senior member of the operating team. More junior members of the team can be kept occupied dissecting the donor and recipient arteries while the conduit is prepared. Greater saphenous vein harvest usually commences in the groin, two finger breadths lateral to the pubic tubercle. The saphenofemoral junction at the *fossa ovalis* should always be identified before the incision is extended distally to avoid the 'rookie' error of mobilizing the anterior branch or a large posteromedial collateral of the GSV, rather than the main trunk. Once the main trunk is identified, the incision should be extended with Cooley scissors or a 10 blade directly overlying the vein so as to avoid skin flaps in the thigh which might lead to significant postoperative wound complications. We frequently leave short skin bridges, especially in the thigh and about the knee, but if exposure or branch ligation is difficult, the skin directly overlying the vein should be divided. The periadventitial tissues, not the vein wall itself, are grasped with fine forceps. Side branches are meticulously identified, doubly ligated with 3-0 or 4-0 silk, and divided. It is preferable to leave a short stump of vein, rather than place a ligature too near the main trunk and compromise luminal integrity or to damage the vein at the origin of the branch. The vein should be soft and blue when the dissection originally begins. Sclerotic segments are whitish in hue and firm or rubbery in consistency, although vein spasm can sometimes blur the distinction. Spasm should be treated with direct irrigation of full-strength papaverine. Sufficient vein length should be harvested to allow performance of the optimum bypass length as defined by preoperative planning. If the vein quality or caliber is insufficient, and the operation cannot be reconfigured to permit use of a shorter conduit, then additional vein will need to be harvested. Since vein quality is of the utmost importance, marginal caliber (<3 mm) or sclerotic segments should not be used. Either shorten the length of the bypass by selecting an alternate inflow or recipient artery, or harvest additional good-quality vein and splice it to obtain a conduit of sufficient length. Once an adequate length has been obtained, the vein is carefully ligated proximally and distally and removed from its bed for preparation on a back table, while additional members of the team continue exposing the donor and recipient arteries.

pletion of the endarterectomy, the arteriotomy should be patched. If the vein to be used for the bypass is of good caliber (>4–4.5 mm), a long venotomy can be made and used both as the endarterectomy patch as well as the origin of the bypass. If the donor artery is excessively thick walled or if the vein bypass conduit is small, the endarterectomy site should be patched either with vein, or with a segment of endarterectomized superficial femoral artery used either as a free or rotated patch (see Chapter 4). The bypass graft is then sewn to a suitably sized opening in the patch, analogous to the Linton patch technique. Repair of correctable, hemodynamically significant, deep femoral artery occlusive disease is a fundamentally important surgical principle. Should the distal bypass subsequently fail, adequate deep femoral artery perfusion may prevent recurrent severe limb ischemia. In fact, one method of treatment for an

Preparing the vein on a back table allows the surgeon to be comfortably seated and work unhurriedly in a well-lighted environment using loupe magnification. The distal end of the vein is gently cannulated with a 3 mm olive or Marx tip needle and secured with a 3-0 silk tie. We prefer to distend the vein with autologous blood. Before the operation begins, we ask the anesthesiologist to withdraw 60 ml of blood from a peripheral vein or the arterial line, if present, into a syringe containing 1000 units of heparin. This blood is then labeled with the patient's name and hospital identification number, and placed in the refrigerator in the central operating room core. Once the vein is harvested, the circulating nurse retrieves the blood and places it into a small metal basin on the vein preparation table. A total of 30–60 mg of papaverine are placed into the metal basin before the blood is added. The mixture is then withdrawn into a 20 or 30 ml syringe, which is then connected to the olive tip needle. The vein is gently irrigated and flow assessed; blood should flow freely from the end. The vein is then sequentially compressed from distal to proximal between the thumb and forefinger of the surgeon's left hand while the vein is gently distended. Spasm should be overcome with time and papaverine, not overdistention and impatience. Overly forceful distention is unnecessary and should be avoided as it may generate pressures of up to 500 mmHg, potentially damaging the endothelium. Any branches which were missed are precisely grasped with a Jacobsen hemostat and carefully tied with 4-0 silk. Small defects are sutured in a longitudinal direction parallel to the long axis of the vein conduit with 7-0 prolene on a BV-1 needle. The entire length of the conduit is palpated and inspected to be sure there are no sclerotic segments and that no portions of the vein remain in spasm. Sites of branch ligation are doubly checked to be certain that the ligature does not narrow the lumen of the conduit. Blood should flow freely and easily from the end of the vein. When preparation is complete, the distal end of the vein is ligated with 3-0 silk, leaving the suture ends long, and the prepared conduit stored in the chilled blood until the graft is to be tunneled.

Although controversial, we believe that preparing the vein and storing it for the short time before its use in chilled, heparinized autologous blood optimizes endothelial preservation.[29,43–46] The addition of papaverine, a dilator acting directly on the smooth muscle in the vein wall, as well as deliberate avoidance of overdistention, ameliorates troublesome vasospasm. The amount of time the vein is left on the back table should be minimized by appropriate intraoperative planning with simultaneous dissection and exposure of the inflow and outflow arteries by other appropriately trained and experienced team members.

Arm veins, particularly the basilic vein, are more fragile and demanding to harvest.[9] Branches should be carefully identified and ligated a short distance away from their junctions with the main trunk, to avoid annoying bleeding from an injury at the crotch between the branch and its larger parent vein. The initial irrigation of arm veins is frequently performed with heparinized saline and papaverine. Defects in these thinner walled veins are more difficult to identify and repair if blood is used as the initial irrigant. Once major leaks are controlled, the remainder of the vein graft preparation is performed with chilled blood as outlined above. As emphasized by LoGerfo, Miller and others,[47] arm veins frequently harbor abnormal segments containing webs, synechiae and sclerotic valves. Angioscopy may be a useful adjunct in the preparation of such veins, identifying potentially significant intraluminal pathology in as many as 40 per cent of cases (see Chapter 11 for more details). If splicing is necessary, this is readily performed on the back table with running 7-0 suture after carefully spatulating the appropriate ends of the vein. The basilic vein is frequently of rather large caliber, and should be used as the proximal segment in a spliced graft to a small caliber tibial outflow artery.

TUNNELING

Proper tunneling is an important part of the procedure and should not be performed in a roughshod manner by an inexperienced member of the operative team. For primary leg bypasses with greater saphenous vein, we generally prefer tunneling in an anatomic plane, although, a subsartorial plane is frequently easier to utilize for bypasses to the above-knee popliteal artery segment.

When tunneling below-knee popliteal bypasses as well as those to proximal or mid tibial artery levels, the anatomic plane is usually chosen. A sturdy, large bore hollow tunneler with a handled and a bullet end is passed between the heads of the gastrocnemius muscles to the groin. The tunneler should pass easily without undue resistance if the proper plane has been entered. The bullet is then removed and the distal vein with silk ligature still attached is secured to the smaller bore obturator within the metal tunneler, and the vein gently drawn through the tunneler to the distal anastomotic site in a distended fashion to prevent twisting of the graft. The tunneler is then withdrawn over the vein and removed. Passing the vein in this manner avoids damaging the vein or tearing off branch ties, both of which can readily occur if a long tunneling clamp is used to pull the unprotected vein through the tissues. In addition, passing the vein through the tunneler in distended fashion minimizes the potential for graft twisting or kinking.

Grafts to the proximal or mid anterior tibial artery can either be tunneled through the interosseous membrane (Fig. 8.2) or via a lateral subcutaneous tunnel, usually with a single counter incision in the upper thigh (Fig. 8.3a. See p. 81).[33] The lateral tunnel is especially useful when performing a reversed vein bypass to the distal

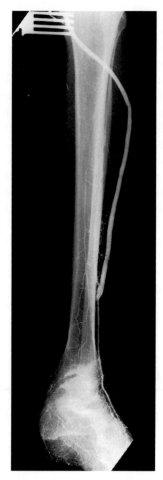

Figure 8.2 *Completion arteriogram of patient requiring femoral to distal anterior tibial artery bypass. In this instance, the graft was tunneled anatomically, through the interosseous membrane.*

anterior tibial artery or very distal peroneal artery (Fig. 8.3b and c). When bypassing to the paramalleolar or pedal arteries, the portion of the graft below the knee is usually tunneled subcutaneously. After tunneling, with the knee straight and the graft out to length, the graft should be irrigated and flow should be vigorous. If there is any question of graft twist or improper tunneling, the graft should be retunneled. When graft tunneling is completed, the patient can be systemically heparinized (75–100 units/kg).

ANASTOMOSES

The performance of venoarterial anastomoses is well illustrated in Chapter 9 for *in situ* bypass. However, there are certain anatomic factors that come into play with reversed vein grafts that are different, particularly with regard to size mismatch or disparity. This problem most frequently arises when attempting to create a successful proximal anastomosis between a small-caliber reversed vein and a larger caliber, often thicker-walled common or superficial femoral artery. Creating a standard posterior venotomy and direct anastomosis to the artery in such a case may lead to stricture of the heel of the vein at the proximal anastomosis (Fig. 8.4).This is avoidable by preserving a large side-branch near the distal end of the vein when performing the harvest. The venotomy is then carried out through the side branch (Fig. 8.5). This technique obviates the need to place a suture in the heel of the venotomy and also allows the heel of the anastomosis to sit up away from the artery, a factor of importance if the arterial wall is diseased or thickened (Fig. 8.6. See p. 82). This technique was originally described by Kunlin in 1951,[39] but has been forgotten, relearned and reported by subsequent generations of surgeons. If such a branch is not available, and the vein caliber is marginal or the arterial wall excessively thick, a Linton vein patch should be sewn to the donor artery first and the vein graft originated from the patch. If, despite all precautions, the proximal anastomosis looks tethered or has an hourglass deformity at the heel, and this defect is not alleviated by freeing up trapped adventitia, the heel should be patched with vein. The distal anastomosis is then carried out in routine fashion following verification of adequate flow through the graft and careful adjustment of graft length. If the distal vein diameter is excessively large, the edges can be trimmed after the heel is sutured. We prefer to make long distal arteriotomies, at least 10–15 times the diameter of the recipient artery, in order to flatten the angle of the distal anastomosis and create optimal hemodynamics. If the vein caliber is small, on occasion the side-branch technique can also be used for the distal anastomosis (Fig. 8.7. See p. 82). When the anastomoses are completed, flow is verified with continuous-wave Doppler and completion arteriography with inflow occlusion is performed to identify major defects in the conduit, its anastomoses, and the outflow vessels. We consider completion duplex scanning for all redo leg bypasses and when alternate vein conduits are required. The details of intraoperative duplex evaluation are addressed in a subsequent chapter.

Reversed vein remains the best all-purpose conduit for infrainguinal bypass. With thoughtfulness and care, it can be applied to the overwhelming majority of patients who require lower limb arterial reconstruction for chronic arterial obliterative disease. Vein caliber and quality are the most important determinants of outcome; therefore, these factors should be optimized at the first operation, since subsequent reoperative procedures are always more difficult. Performing leg bypass with marginal vein will produce marginal results. Thus the operation should be conducted so as to employ the best available vein; this may require tremendous ingenuity and perseverance on the part of the operating team, but optimal results are dependent upon the use of alternate inflow and outflow sites, adjunctive angioplasty or

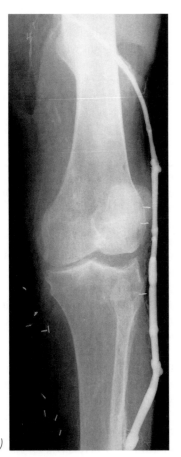
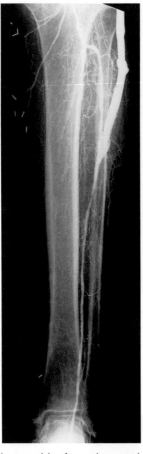
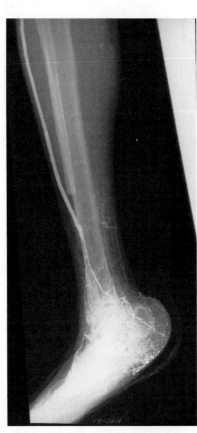

(a) (b) (c)

Figure 8.3 *(a) Intraoperative arteriogram of a patient requiring femoral to anterior tibial bypass. The patient had a previous bypass performed via a medial approach that had failed. In this situation, the graft was tunneled subcutaneously through a single lateral thigh counter-incision. (b) Shows the distal portion of the saphenous vein graft and its anastomosis to the proximal third of the anterior tibial artery. (c) Lateral subcutaneous tunneled grafts are also useful when the outflow artery is the distal peroneal. This artery segment is approached laterally via a segmental fibulectomy (arrow).*

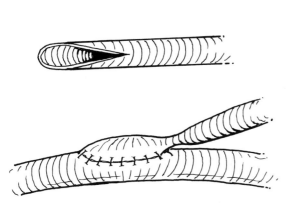

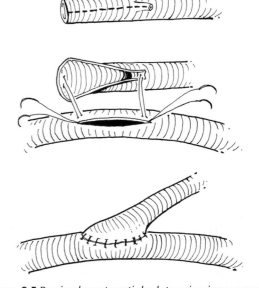

Figure 8.4 *Conventional longitudinal venotomy and end-to-side anastomosis may result in a napkin-ring or collar-like stricture at the heel of anastomosis. If such a defect is identified intra-operatively and is not alleviated by freeing up adventitial fibers, a patch angioplasty should be performed beginning on the hood of the graft and extending beyond the heel.*

Figure 8.5 *Proximal anastomotic heel stenosis using a reverse vein graft can be prevented by incorporating a side branch into the heel of the anastomosis thus elevating the anastomosis from the native thickened artery and preventing the necessity for placement of a heel stitch at the end of the venotomy.*

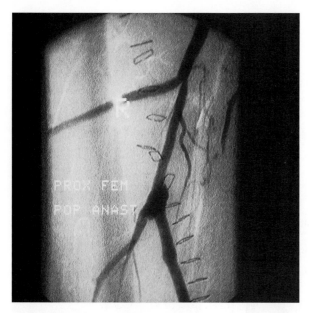

Figure 8.6 *Postoperative arteriogram obtained following bypass from the deep femoral artery to the posterior tibial artery. The proximal anastomosis, in which the heel branch technique was utilized is shown here. Note the elevation of the heel of the graft from the native profunda femoris artery.*

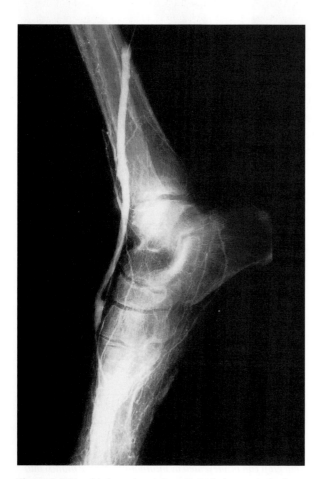

Figure 8.7 *The side branch anastomotic technique can also be used for distal anastomosis to small caliber arteries, such as a dorsalis pedis vessel shown here.*

endarterectomy, and harvesting of alternate conduits from any suitable extremity to create an appropriate conduit of sufficient length. Surgeons who compromise these principles at the primary operation may subsequently place themselves, and more unfortunately their patients, in an even more compromising position in the future.

REFERENCES

1 Porter J. In situ versus reversed vein graft: is one superior? *J Vasc Surg* 1987; **5**: 779–80.

2 Mills JL. In-situ versus reversed vein grafts: is there a difference? *Vasc Surg* 1999; **31**(6): 679–84.

3 Taylor LM, Phinney ES, Porter JM. Present status of reversed vein bypass for lower extremity revascularization. *J Vasc Surg* 1986; **3**: 288–97.

4 Bandyk DF, Kaebnick JW, Stewart GW, Towne JB. Durability of the in situ saphenous vein arterial bypass: a comparison of primary and secondary patency. *J Vasc Surg* 1987; **5**: 256–68.

5 Mannick JA, Whittemore AD, Donaldson MC. Clinical and anatomic considerations for surgery in tibial disease and the results of surgery. *Circulation* Suppl I 1991; **83**(2): I81–I90.

6 Green RM, Donayre C, DeWeese JM. Autogenous venous bypass grafts and limb salvage: 5-year results in 1971 and 1991. *Cardiovasc Surg* 1995; **3**(4): 425–30.

7 Chang BB, Paty PSK, Shah DM, Leather RP. The lesser saphenous vein: an underappreciated source of autogenous vein. *J Vasc Surg* 1992; **15**: 152–7.

8 Weaver FA, Barlow CR, Edwards WH, Mulherin JL, Jenkins JM. The lesser saphenous vein: autogenous tissue for lower extremity revascularization. *J Vasc Surg* 1987; **5**: 687–92.

9 Harris RW, Andros G, Dulawa LB *et al.* Successful long-term limb salvage using cephalic vein bypass grafts. *Ann Surg* 1984; **200**: 785–92.

10 Leather RP, Powers SR, Karmody AM. A reappraisal of the in situ saphenous vein artery bypass: its use in limb salvage. *Surgery* 1979; **86**: 453–61.

11 Bush HL Jr, Nabseth DC, Curl GR *et al.* In situ saphenous vein bypass grafts for limb salvage. A current fad or a viable alternative to reversed saphenous vein bypass grafts? *Am J Surg* 1985; **149**: 477–80.

12 Levine AW, Bandyk DF, Bonier PH *et al.* Lessons learned in adopting the in situ saphenous vein bypass. *J Vasc Surg* 1985; **2**: 145–53.

13 Fogle MA, Whittemore AD, Couch NP *et al.* A comparison of in situ and reversed saphenous vein grafts for infrainguinal reconstruction. *J Vasc Surg* 1987; **5**: 46–52.

14 Corson JD, Karmody AM, Shah DJ, Naraynsingh V, Young HL, Leather RL. In situ vein bypasses to distal tibial and limited outflow tracts for limb salvage. *Surgery* 1984; **96**: 756–62.

15 Leather RP, Shah DM, Chang BB, Kaufman JL. Resurrection of the in situ saphenous vein bypass 1000 cases later. *Ann Surg* 1988; **208**: 435–42.

16 Leather RP, Shah DM, Karmody AM. Infrapopliteal arterial bypass for limb salvage; increased patency and utilization of the saphenous vein used in situ. *Surgery* 1981; **90**: 1000–7.

17 Hallin RW. In situ saphenous vein bypass grafting. *Am J Surg* 1983; **145**: 626–9.

18 Harris RW, Andros G, Dulawa LB. The transition to 'in situ' vein bypass grafts. *Surg Gynceol Obstet* 1986; **163**: 21–8.

19 Leather RP, Shah DM, Buchbinder D. Further experience with the saphenous vein used in situ for arterial bypass. *Am J Surg* 1981; **142**: 506–10.

20 Bush HL Jr, Corey CA, Nabseth DC. Distal in situ saphenous vein grafts for limb salvage. Increased operative blood flow and postoperative patency. *Am J Surg* 1983; **145**: 542–8.

21 Rutherford R, Flanigan D, Gupta S *et al*. Suggested standards for reports dealing with lower extremity ischemia. *J Vasc Surg* 1986; **4**: 80–94.

22 Rutherford RB. Standards for evaluating results of interventional therapy for peripheral vascular disease. *Circulation* Suppl 1991; **83**: 6–19.

23 Gupta AK, Bandyk DF, Cheanvechai D. Natural history of infrainguinal vein graft stenosis, relative to bypass grafting technique. *J Vasc Surg* 1997; **25**: 211–25.

24 Veterans Administration Cooperative Study Group 141. Comparative evaluation of prosthetic, reversed, and in situ vein bypass grafts in distal popliteal and tibial-peroneal revascularization. *Arch Surg* 1988; **123**: 434–8.

25 Harris PL, How TV, Jones DR. Prospectively randomized clinical trial to compare in situ and reversed saphenous vein grafts. *Br J Surg* 1987; **74**: 252–5.

26 Watelet J, Cheysson E, Poels D. In situ versus reversed saphenous vein for femoropopliteal bypass: a prospective randomized study of 100 cases. *Ann Vasc Surg* 1986; **1**: 441–52.

27 Watelet J, Soury P, Menard JF *et al*. Femoropopliteal bypass: in situ or reversed vein grafts? Ten year results of a randomized prospective study. *Ann Vasc Surg* 1997; **11**: 510–19.

28 Wengerter KR, Veith FJ, Gupta SK. Prospective randomized multicenter comparison of in situ and reversed vein infrapopliteal bypasses. *J Vasc Surg* 1991; **13**: 189–99.

29 Mills JL, Taylor SM. Results of infrainguinal revascularization with reversed vein conduits: a modern control series. *Ann Vasc Surg* 1991; **5**: 156–62.

30 Imparato AM, Kim GE, Madayag M *et al*. The results of tibial artery reconstruction procedures. *Surg Gynecol Obstet* 1974; **138**: 33–8.

31 Szilagyi DE, Hageman JH, Smith RF *et al*. Autogenous vein grafting in femoropopliteal atherosclerosis: the limits of its effectiveness. *Surgery* 1979; **86**: 836–51.

32 Reichle FA, Martinson MW, Rankin KP. Infrapopliteal arterial reconstruction in the severely ischemic lower extremity. A comparison of long-term results of peroneal and tibial bypasses. *Ann Surg* 1980; **191**: 59–65.

33 Kacoyanis GP, Whittemore AD, Couch NP *et al*. Femoropopliteal and femoroperoneal bypass vein grafts. *Arch Surg* 1981; **116**: 1529–34.

34 Taylor LM Jr, Edwards JM, Phinney ES *et al*. Reversed saphenous vein bypass to infrapopliteal arteries. *Ann Surg* 1987; **205**: 90–7.

35 Mills JL, Harris EJ, Taylor LM Jr *et al*. The importance of routine surveillance of distal bypass grafts with duplex scanning: a study of 379 reversed vein grafts. *J Vasc Surg* 1990; **12**(4): 379–89.

36 Kunlin J. Le traitement de l'arterite obliterante par la greffe veineuse. *Arch Mal Coeur* 1949; **42**: 371–3.

37 Sharp WJ, Shamma AR, Kresowik TF, Gison JP. Use of terminal T junctions for in situ bypass in the lower extremity. *Surg Gynecol Obstet* 1991; **172**: 151–2.

38 Muller-Wiefel W. Femoropopliteal bypass. In: Bergan JJ, Yao JST eds. *Operative techniques in vascular surgery*. New York: Grune and Stratton. 1980: 131–40.

39 Kunlin J. Le traitement de l'ischemie arterique apres la greffe veineuse longue. *Rev Chir* 1951; **70**: 206–35.

40 Veith FS, Gupta SK, Samson RH *et al*. Superficial femoral and popliteal arteries as inflow sites for distal bypass. *Surgery* 1981; **90**: 980–90.

41 Mills JL, Taylor SM, Fujitani RM. The role of the deep femoral artery as an inflow site for infrainguinal revascularization. *J Vasc Surg* 1993; **18**: 416–23.

42 Mills JL, Gahtan V, Fujitani RM, Taylor SM. The utility and durability of vein bypass grafts originating from the popliteal artery for limb salvage. *Am J Surg* 1994; **168**: 646–51.

43 Cambria RP, Megerman J, Abbott W. Endothelial preservation in reversed and in situ autogenous vein grafts. *Ann Surg* 1985; **202**: 50–5.

44 Adcock OT Jr, Adcock GLD, Wheeler JR. Optimal techniques for harvesting and preparation of reversed autogenous vein grafts for use as arterial substitutes: a review. *Surgery* 1984; **96**: 886–93.

45 Gundry SR, Jones M, Ishihara T, Ferrans VJ. Optimal preparation techniques for human saphenous vein grafts. *Surgery* 1980; **88**: 785–94.

46 Cambria RP, Brewster DC, Hasson J. The evolution of morphologic and biomechanical changes in reversed and in situ vein grafts. *Ann Surg* 1987; **205**: 167–74.

47 Marcaccio EJ, Miller A, Tannenhaun GA *et al*. Angioscopically directed interventions improve arm vein bypass grafts. *J Vasc Surg* 1990; **17**: 994–1004.

9

In situ bypass

JAMES B KNOX AND MICHAEL BELKIN

HISTORICAL DEVELOPMENTS

In 1962, Karl Victor Hall from the University of Oslo, Norway, reported the first description of the *in situ* technique in an article entitled 'The greater saphenous vein used *in situ* as an arterial shunt after extirpation of the vein valves'.[1] Disappointed with the results of thromboendarterectomy and prosthetic bypasses for infrainguinal arterial occlusive disease, Hall preferred autogenous vein conduits. However, the reversed vein bypass described by Kunlin was frequently unsatisfactory for distal bypasses due to the narrow caliber of the distal saphenous vein.[2] The reversed technique also necessitated excessive handling of the vein with complete removal of the conduit from its native bed. Hall opted to perform arterial bypasses with the saphenous vein left *in situ*. Valve disruption was accomplished by palpating the distal extent of the arterialized pulsations and performing a transverse venotomy with direct valve excision.

The *in situ* technique was slow to gain popularity because of the tedious valve excision and uncertain efficacy of obtaining complete valve incompetence. Connolly in 1964, May in 1965 and Barner in 1969 reported small series of patients in whom blunt internal strippers were used to disrupt the valves, frequently tearing the leaflets and damaging the vein wall.[3–5] The resurgence in the use of the *in situ* technique was precipitated by a report by Mills in 1976.[6] Mills was concerned that even in the reversed position, the venous valves would create turbulence, collect thrombus and result in early failure in coronary artery bypass grafting. Mills therefore devised his technique for retrograde valve incision using an angled valvulotome.

In 1979, Leather reported 89 patients undergoing *in situ* bypass.[7] Eighty-two were performed for limb salvage

and the distal anastomoses were to tibial vessels in 38 patients. The saphenous vein was marked preoperatively with the patient in the standing position and the valves were lysed intraoperatively by passing microvascular scissors through branches into the vein in an antegrade fashion and cutting the valve leaflets. With this technique, veins as small as 2.5 mm were routinely utilized and even veins less than 2.0 mm were occasionally sufficient. Only 8 per cent of the patients evaluated had an inadequate vein for the intended procedure. The 30-day patency rate was 96 per cent and 30-month patency rate was 91 per cent.

Leather reported a larger series of *in situ* bypasses for limb salvage in 1981.[8] Scissors were still used for valve incision in the proximal vein; however, the Mills valvulotome was passed from below for the remainder of valve lysis. Mortality was low (3.2 per cent), 3-year patency was excellent (72 per cent), 8 per cent required subsequent procedures to ligate arterial-venous fistulas, and only 7 per cent of the ipsilateral saphenous veins could not be used for the procedure.

In addition to theoretical considerations regarding optimal handling of the saphenous vein and preservation of the *in situ* venous bed, Leather and others believed the 91–93 per cent vein utilization rate achieved by using smaller veins for *in situ* bypasses was a significant advantage over reversed vein bypasses in which greater than 25 per cent of patients were reported to have inadequate vein caliber for consideration of bypass.[8–10] In 1981, Buchbinder *et al.* reported a study comparing *in situ* and reversed vein bypass demonstrating improved patency with the *in situ* technique.[11] At 12 and 30 months, the *in situ* patency rates were 93 per cent and 91 per cent respectively, significantly better than the 68 per cent and 63 per cent patency rates with reversed bypass. Although controversy continues, the last 15 years have seen a vast increase in the number of *in situ* bypasses performed.

TECHNIQUE

Candidates for lower extremity revascularization with *in situ* saphenous vein are examined to determine the quality of the ipsilateral saphenous vein. Although historically this included venography, more recently the patient simply undergoes a clinical examination in the standing position taking care to note previous vein harvest or stripping, varicosities, leg edema, or signs of phlebitis, cellulitis or cutaneous lesions. Patients with a physical examination suggestive of inadequate vein, deep vein thrombosis or superficial varicosities undergo duplex venous mapping, which frequently reveals a surprisingly normal appearing saphenous vein. More recently, patients who undergo endovascular assisted *in situ* bypass (described below) obtain preoperative venous mapping. Patients with saphenous veins of questionable quality on the preoperative physical examination should have additional extremities prepared and draped for potential vein harvest.

The operation is performed by making a longitudinal incision in the femoral region centered about the inguinal ligament and slightly medial to the arterial pulse. The common, superficial and profunda femoral arteries are encircled with vascular tapes. The saphenous vein is identified and cleared of surrounding structures, and all branches are ligated and divided up to the saphenofemoral junction. Approximately 10 cm of proximal vein are mobilized.

The site for the distal anastomosis is chosen and a skin incision is performed taking care not to injure the saphenous vein. Once a suitable target vessel has been identified, the saphenous vein is mobilized distally to allow transposition of the vein to the deeper artery. If an 'open' technique is to be employed (as is typically our preference), the entire length of saphenous vein between the two existing incisions is exposed. The vein is left in its native bed and major branches are ligated. Lateral branches are collecting tributaries from the subcutaneous tissue and are less likely to result in significant arterial-venous fistulas. The posterior branches connect with the deep system and must be ligated. Care is taken not to constrict the lumen with branch ligation. At 20 cm intervals, a branch is ligated 1–2 cm from the vein to allow access for the valvulotome.

On initial inspection, the vein may appear inadequate. Occasionally, a minor branch of a duplicated saphenous system may have been exposed and a more suitable vein found with additional dissection. Twenty-six per cent of patients have duplicated saphenous systems in the upper leg and 46 per cent in the lower leg.[12] Veins with less than 2 mm outer diameter are generally not used, nor are thickened, grossly phlebitic segments. If the vein is of questionable quality, the distal vein may be transected and a silastic catheter introduced for gentle dilation with a heparinized saline with papaverine solution. A nicely dilated, thin-walled vein should be observed. If uncertainty still exists, the angioscope may be introduced. Although isolated synechia may be acceptable, dense synechia with partial obliteration of the lumen will result in early graft failure. Segmental vein defects may be excised and a composite bypass performed with the remaining saphenous vein or vein from other locations (Fig. 9.1).

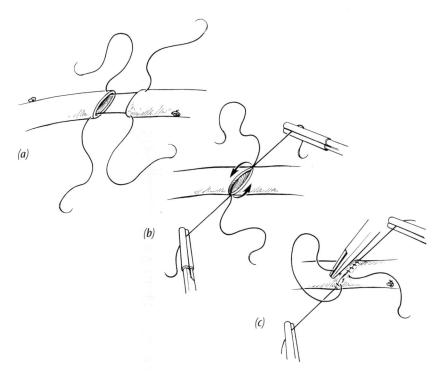

(a)

(b)

(c)

Figure 9.1 *The technique of venovenostomy is shown. (a) The two veins are cut at 45° angles and spatulated. The heels and toes are joined with simple 7-0 prolene sutures. (b) One tail of the suture from each end is gently distracted with a rubbershod clamp to maintain the length and orientation for the suture line. (c) The suture line is then completed and tied down as distraction is maintained on these two sutures. (Reproduced with permission from Belkin M, Donaldson MC, Whittemore AD. Composite autogenous vein grafts.* Semin Vasc Surg *1995; 8: 205.)*

Five thousand units of heparin are administered intravenously. A Satinsky clamp is placed at the saphenofemoral junction and the saphenous vein is transected sharply leaving a cuff of femoral vein for closure with a running 5-0 Prolene suture. Bleeding from the open saphenous vein is controlled with a soft 'bulldog' clamp. A valve is consistently found in the proximal saphenous vein and is excised under direct vision with Potts scissors. After placement of non-crushing vascular clamps, an arteriotomy is performed in the distal common femoral artery where the hood of the saphenous vein comfortably rests. A limited femoral endarterectomy may be required. If sufficient length of proximal vein is not available, the proximal anastomosis may be performed at the superficial femoral artery. The hood of the saphenous vein at the saphenofemoral junction is ideally suited for the proximal anastomosis. If the proximal saphenous vein is too narrow, it may be incised along its deep aspect creating a spatulated proximal end of comparable length to the arteriotomy. A standard Kunlin anastomosis is performed with 5-0 Prolene suture, whereby separate heel and toe sutures are placed as horizontal mattresses.[2] Carefully placed full-thickness bites are run towards each other and tied at the 'three o'clock' and 'nine o'clock' positions. Prior to completion, the arterial clamps are temporarily removed and the anastomosis is 'flushed'. After completion, the arterial clamps are removed and hemostasis is assessed (Fig. 9.2).

A careful valve incision is now performed using a device with a radial cutting blade such as the Mills valvulotome. This device fits comfortably into veins of all sizes in contrast to the fixed-diameter circumferential blade with the Hall or LeMaitre valvulotome. The occluding clamp is removed from the proximal arterialized vein and pulsations are noted to extend to the next competent valve. The vein is accessed by the valvulotome via previously designated branches. Valve leaflets are typically located immediately distal to branches and are oriented parallel to the skin.[13] As the valve sinus is distended from the arterial pressure, tension is distributed along the leading edge of the leaflet displacing the valve towards the center of the lumen, where it may be safely engaged by the valvulotome. The valvulotome is sharply retracted while angling the tip toward the center of the lumen, thereby minimizing the possibility of intimal tears. Direct visualization of the tip of the valvulotome will prevent inadvertent engagement and tearing of a vein branch site. Valves are predictably located at the saphenofemoral junction, 3–5 cm distal to the junction and 10 cm distal to the medial accessory branch of the saphenous vein[7] (Fig. 9.2).

The final passage of the valvulotome is via the distal open end of the saphenous vein. After complete valve lysis, vein quality and success of lysis are qualitatively assessed by documenting pulsatile flow from the end of the arterialized vein.

The distal anastomosis is performed by occluding the target artery with soft clamps, intraluminal occluders or a sterile tourniquet. The tourniquet is a particularly useful technique for obtaining vascular control in patients with troublesome companion venous branches, heavily calcified distal vessels and in secondary procedures. After controlling the vessels, an arteriotomy is performed, the vein cut to an appropriate length, and an anastomosis performed with 6-0 or 7-0 prolene (Fig. 9.2). For below-knee popliteal bypasses, we prefer to tunnel the graft through the anatomic popliteal space as this avoids the sharp angulation that occurs if the vein approaches the below-knee popliteal artery from a subcutaneous position.

A Doppler probe is placed over the vein graft with sequential distal occlusion to identify occult fistulas demonstrated by continuous outflow despite graft occlusion. Adequacy of revascularization is assessed by careful clinical assessment of pulses and tissue perfusion, continuous-wave Doppler, and completion arteriography, intraoperative duplex scan or angioscopy.

With both *in situ* and reversed vein bypass, careful handling of the venous conduit is mandatory. Gundry *et al.* notes that manipulation of the vein with forceps results in endothelial damage and destruction of the structural elements of the vein wall.[14] Trauma-induced vein wall edema and exposed extracellular matrix predispose the graft to thrombosis and early failure. Gundry emphasizes that blood is a superior preservative to saline and distention above physiologic pressures (200 mm Hg) should be avoided. LoGerfo encourages the use of papaverine (phosphodiesterase inhibitor) and an avoidance of cold solutions if flushing is to be employed.[15] Endothelial loss occurs with both the *in situ* and reversed vein techniques. Over a period of 1–2 weeks, re-endothelialization is achieved to a similar degree with both grafts and at 6 months there is little difference in intimal thickness or graft compliance.[16,17]

RESULTS

In situ bypass

Thirty day-operative mortality rates for the *in situ* bypass average 2 per cent, major morbidity 8 per cent, and early graft failures occur in approximately 5 per cent.[18–20] Five year primary patency rates range from 63 to 72 per cent and secondary rates from 81 to 83 per cent (Table 9.1). Belkin reported long-term (10 year) results with the *in situ* bypass[21] (Table 9.2). Primary patency rates are 60 per cent, secondary patency rates 76 per cent, and 90 per cent of survivors achieve limb salvage.

Most reports note little difference in patency rates between popliteal and infrapopliteal bypasses with no difference between anterior tibial, posterior tibial, or peroneal artery bypasses. Claudicants tend to fare

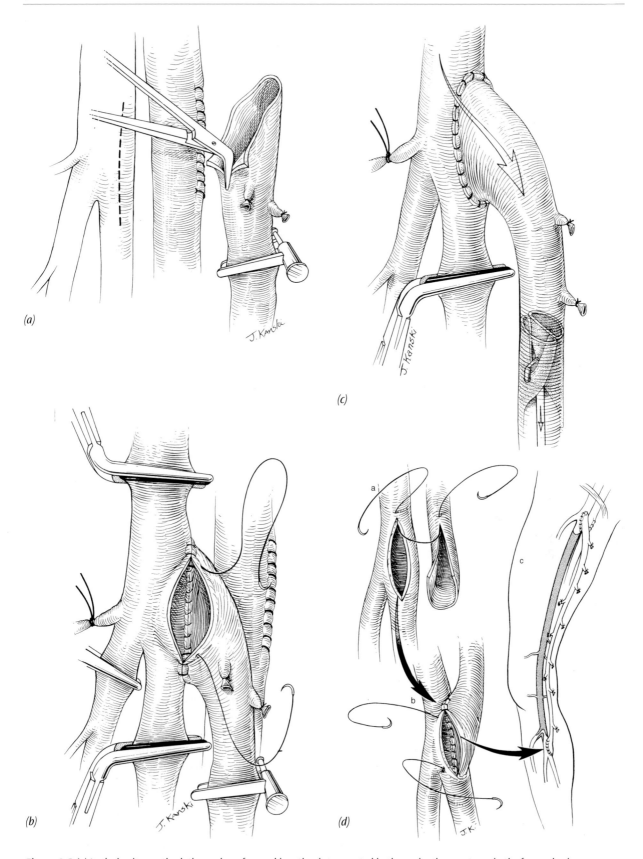

Figure 9.2 *(a) In the* in situ *method, the saphenofemoral junction is transected in the groin, the venotomy in the femoral vein overseen, and the proximal end of the saphenous vein prepared for anastomosis. (b) After the first venous valve is excised under direct vision, the graft is anastomosed end-to-side to the femoral artery. (c) Flow is then restored through the vein graft and the valvulotome inserted through side branches at appropriate intervals to lyse residual valve cusps. (d) The distal anastomosis is completed. (Reproduced with permission from Whittemore AD. Infrainguinal bypass. In: Rutherford RB ed. Vascular surgery. W.B. Saunders Co., Philadelphia, 1995.)*

Table 9.1 *Infrainguinal reconstruction with* in situ *saphenous vein*

Author	Number of limbs	Operative mortality (%)	5-year graft patency		5-year limb salvage (%)	5-year survival (%)
			Primary (%)	Secondary (%)		
Bergamini[18]	361	3	63	81	86	57
Donaldson[19]	440	2	72	83	84	66
Leather[8]	1688	3	70	81	92	58

Table 9.2 *Long-term (10-year) patency and limb salvage rates for* in situ *bypasses in men and women. No difference in patency or limb salvage between men and women was shown*

	Patients	10-year primary patency (%)	10-year secondary patency (%)	10-year limb salvage (%)
Men	338	58.2±7.7	77.2±4.6	92.0±1.8
Women	244	67.8±4.0	73.5±4.1	87.9±2.9
Total	582	59.8±5.4	75.5±3.5	90.4±1.6

slightly better than patients presenting with critical ischemia. Limb salvage rates approach 90 per cent, although 5-year survival in this population ranges from 28 to 66 per cent (Table 9.1).

Bypasses in patients with ischemic limb ulcerations may be performed to isolated tibial artery segments.[22] Although these patients do not achieve dramatic improvements in ankle pressures nor obtain the graft-flow velocities typically seen with standard *in situ* bypass, these grafts to disadvantaged outflow tracts do exhibit acceptable patency rates with excellent limb salvage.

In an examination of causes of failure of the *in situ* bypass, Donaldson *et al.* evaluated 455 *in situ* bypasses.[23] One hundred and four potential causes of failure were identified from a group of 85 graft failures. Twenty of the causes of failure were directly related to the *in situ* technique and included valvulotome injuries and consequent vein lesions (14), retained leaflets (4) and arterial-venous fistulas (2). These *in situ* errors accounted for 15 failures out of 455 grafts (3.3 per cent). Overall, the major causes of graft failure were compromised outflow (19), anastomotic (18), vein stricture (14), focal vein stenosis (10), hypercoagulability (9) valvulotome injury (9), and kinks (6).

In situ versus reversed vein bypass

Many authors preferentially perform an *in situ* bypass based upon several theoretical concerns: (1) with *in situ* bypass, the vein remains in its native bed with nutrient flow; (2) less manipulation is required than with the reversed technique; (3) size discrepancies at the proximal and distal anastomoses are minimized improving fluid flow hemodynamics and facilitating construction of the anastomosis; (4) smaller diameter veins may be utilized; (5) distal bypasses to the calf and ankle are more likely to be feasible; and (6) emerging endovascular techniques

are applicable to the *in situ* bypass. Greater vein utilization is achieved with the *in situ* bypass without incurring a greater rate of intrinsic vein lesions. On postoperative surveillance, 10–25 per cent of *in situ* bypasses demonstrate intrinsic lesions versus 6–29 per cent with reversed vein.[23]

Wengerter performed a prospective evaluation of 62 *in situ* and 63 reversed vein bypasses.[24] Demographics and indications were comparable between the groups. There was no difference in operative mortality (6 per cent *in situ* vs 6 per cent reversed), 30-month secondary patency (69 per cent *in situ* vs 67 per cent reversed) or limb salvage (76 per cent *in situ* vs 87 per cent reversed). Patency of vein grafts of less than 3 mm diameter differed between the *in situ* bypass (61 per cent) and the reversed (37 per cent), but this difference was not statistically significant. In a nonrandomized series reported by Fogle *et al.*, superior 3-year patency was achieved with the *in situ* bypass when the distal anastomosis was performed to infrapopliteal arteries (87 per cent patency with *in situ* vs 62 per cent patency with reversed vein).[25]

Nonreversed vein bypass

Once the optimal proximal and distal arterial vessels are identified for revascularization, the overlying saphenous vein may not be of adequate quality to complete the *in situ* bypass. If a sufficiently long segment of more distal or proximal vein is present, an appropriate length of this higher quality vein may be harvested, valves lysed and anastomoses performed with the translocated, nonreversed vein (Fig. 9.3). This preserves the improved fluid hemodynamics resulting from size matching between artery and conduit as in a standard *in situ* bypass and allows adaptation of the best available conduit to the patient's arterial anatomy.

Batson compared *in situ* and nonreversed grafting

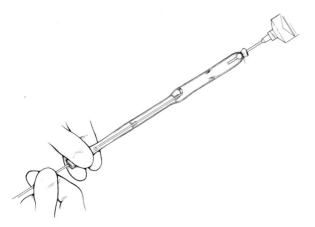

Figure 9.3 *The excised segment of ectopic vein may have its valves lysed* ex situ *by gently distending the vein graft with a syringe and a blunt needle as a Mills valvulotome is passed in the antegrade direction and the valves are lysed by withdrawing the valvulotome in a retrograde direction. (Reproduced with permission from Belkin M, Donaldson MC, Whittemore AD. Composite autogenous vein grafts.* Semin Vasc Surg *1995; 8: 205.)*

techniques and found no difference in early graft occlusion (6 per cent), limb salvage (94 per cent), or 13-month patency (88 per cent).[26] We have found the nonreversed translocated vein to be a useful modification of the *in situ* technique, particularly: (1) in secondary revascularizations; (2) when more distal sites are required for both inflow and outflow; and (3) when contralateral saphenous vein is required. Patency rates for the nonreversed bypass in our patients are similar to those obtained with *in situ* bypass.

FUTURE DIRECTIONS

Endovascular assisted *in situ* bypass

Patients undergoing conventional *in situ* bypass are subjected to incisions that frequently run the entire length of the leg. This may lead to considerable morbidity (15–44 per cent wound complication rates), long lengths of stay (average 12.8 days), and costly hospital admissions and outpatient services.[27] Several authors champion the use of endovascular techniques to occlude venous branches and lyse valves, thereby limiting the skin incision to the proximal and distal anastomotic sites.[27–29]

With endovascular-assisted *in situ* bypass, duplex mapping of the ipsilateral saphenous vein is performed preoperatively. Skin incisions are placed over the common femoral and distal target artery and the corresponding saphenous vein is mobilized. The vein is divided at the saphenofemoral junction, the most proximal venous valves excised and the proximal anastomosis

is performed. A long modified Mills' valvulotome is introduced through the distal vein, and the valves are lysed either blindly or under guidance from an angioscope placed via a proximal venous branch. The distal anastomosis is completed. Large venous tributaries may be identified angioscopically, using Doppler ultrasound, or arteriographically and ligated through a series of small incisions. Alternatively, trials have been performed in which a steerable catheter is introduced via the proximal venous branch and large tributaries are embolized with platinum coils, avoiding the additional incisions. Either angioscopy or fluoroscopy is used to direct the embolization. An average of 4–6 branches are embolized per limb. In veins less than 3 mm in diameter, the catheter may not be able to access the branches for embolization.

Completion angiography identifies missed branches or valves. Branches that are not successfully embolized are ligated through small separate incisions. In follow-up, 6–55 per cent of patients will require an additional procedure for arterial-venous fistula ligation.[27–29] The need to ligate these fistulas has been questioned by LeHeron who demonstrated that persistent fistulas are rarely of clinical significance.[30] Superficial arterial venous fistulas will frequently develop thrombophlebitis, which may be treated with heat and anti-inflammatories. Resolution of the symptoms signifies uncomplicated fistula thrombosis. Leather also noted that many persistent fistulas gradually close with time.[31]

In series comparing endovascular assisted with standard *in situ* bypass, wound complication rates range from 4 to 34 per cent with the endovascular procedure, significantly less than the 24–72 per cent rates with the open *in situ* bypass[27–29,32] (Table 9.3). Patency and limb salvage rates are similar between endovascular and open *in situ* bypass. Rosenthal and Cikrit noted significant reductions in length of stay, while Van Dijk and Clair showed no difference. Rosenthal believes the endovascular technique to be equivalent to the open technique in safety and efficacy, and with potential reductions in healthcare costs, the endovascular approach will become increasingly popular.

CONCLUSIONS

In situ bypass, once considered too tedious and technically demanding, has become a primary option in infrainguinal revascularization, particularly with small saphenous vein conduits and distal target arteries. Advances in valve lysis and microvascular surgical techniques coupled with an increasingly difficult limb-salvage patient population has resulted in an increase in popularity of the *in situ* bypass. Endovascular technologies promise exciting trends in limiting the morbidity and cost associated with infrainguinal bypass surgery.

Table 9.3 *Comparison of endovascular assisted* in situ *bypass (EAI) with conventional open* in situ *techniques (OPEN)*

Author	Patients EAI	OPEN	Wound infection (%) EAI	OPEN	Length of stay (days) EAI	OPEN	Patency rates (%)[a] EAI	OPEN
Clair[32]	32	27	9	4	8.0	8.6	79	91
Rosenthal[27]	53	41	4	24	4.2	11.6	88	83
Cikrit[29]	37	32	13	33	4.0	8.4[b]	83	79
					16.4	17.7[c]		
van Dijk[28]	47	50	15	36[d]	20	24	86	76
			13	30[e]				

[a] Patency rates: Clair (48 months – secondary), Rosenthal (15 months), Cikrit (18 months), van Dijk (12 months – secondary).
[b] Patients with uncomplicated postoperative course.
[c] Patients with complicated postoperative course.
[d] Superficial wound infection.
[e] Deep wound infection.

REFERENCES

1 Hall KV. The greater saphenous vein used in situ as an arterial shunt after extirpation of the vein valves. *Surgery* 1962; **51**: 492–5.

2 Kunlin JL. Le traitement di l'arterite obliterante par le greffe veineuse. *Arch Mal Coeur* 1949; **42**: 371–4.

3 Connolly JE, Harris EJ, Mills W Jr. Autogenous in situ saphenous vein for bypass of femoropopliteal obliterative disease. *Surgery* 1964; **55**: 144–53.

4 May AG, DeWeese JA, Rob CG. Arterialized in situ saphenous vein. *Arch Surg* 1965; **91**: 743–50.

5 Barner HB, Judd DR, Kaiser GC *et al.* Late failure of arterialized in situ saphenous vein. *Arch Surg* 1969; **99**: 781–6.

6 Mills NL, Ochsner JL. Valvulotomy of valves in the saphenous vein graft before coronary artery bypass. *J Thorac Cardiovasc Surg* 1976; **71**: 878–9.

7 Leather RP, Powers SR, Karmody AM. A reappraisal of the in situ saphenous vein arterial bypass: its use in limb salvage. *Surgery* 1979; **86**: 453–61.

8 Leather RP, Shah DM, Karmody AM. Infrapopliteal arterial bypass for limb salvage: increased patency and utilization of the saphenous vein used 'in situ'. *Surgery* 1981; **90**: 1000–7.

9 Levine AW, Bandyk DF, Bonier PH, Towne JB. Lessons learned in adopting the in situ saphenous vein bypass. *J Vasc Surg* 1985; **2**: 145–53.

10 Corson JD, Karmody AM, Shah DM *et al.* In situ vein bypasses to distal tibial and limited outflow tracts for limb salvage. *Surgery* 1984; **96**: 756–63.

11 Buchbinder D, Singh JK, Karmody AM, Leather RP, Shah DM. Comparison of patency rate and structural change of 'in situ' and reversed vein arterial bypass. *J Surg Res* 1981; **30**: 213.

12 Shah DM, Chang BB, Leopold PW *et al.* The anatomy of the greater saphenous venous system. *J Vasc Surg* 1986; **3**: 273–83.

13 Samuels PG, Plested WG, Cincotti JJ *et al.* 'In-situ' saphenous vein arterial bypass. *Am Surg* 1968; **34**: 122.

14 Gundry SR, Jones M, Ishihara T. Ferrans VJ. Optimal preparation techniques for human saphenous vein grafts. *Surgery* 1980; **88**: 785–94.

15 LoGerfo FW, Quist WC, Crawshaw HM, Haudenschild C. An improved technique for preservation of endothelial morphology in vein grafts. *Surgery* 1981; **90**: 1015–24.

16 Cambria RP, Megerman J, Abbott WM. Endothelial preservation in reversed and in situ autogenous vein grafts. *Ann Surg* 1985; **202**: 50–5.

17 Cambria RP, Brewster DC, Hasson J *et al.* The evolution of morphologic and biomechanical changes in reversed and in situ vein grafts. *Ann Surg* 1987; **205**: 167–74.

18 Bergamini TM, Towne JM, Bandyk DF *et al.* Experience with in situ saphenous vein bypasses during 1981 to 1989: Determinant factors of long term patency. *J Vasc Surg* 1991; **13**: 137.

19 Donaldson MC, Mannick JA, Whittemore AD. Femoral–distal bypass with in situ greater saphenous vein: long term results using the Mills valvulotome. *Ann Surg* 1991; **213**: 457.

20 Whittemore AD. Infrainguinal bypass. In: Rutherford RB ed. *Vascular surgery*. Philadelphia: W.B. Saunders Co., 1995; 794–814. (Personal communication from Leather RP, Fitzgerald K. Albany Medical College, 1992.)

21 Belkin M, Conte MS, Donaldson MC, Mannick JM, Whittemore AD. The impact of gender on the results of arterial bypass with in situ greater saphenous vein. *Am J Surg* 1995; **170**: 97–102.

22 Belkin M, Welch H. Mackey WC, O'Donnell TF. Clinical and hemodynamic results of bypass to isolated tibial artery segments for ischemic ulceration of the foot. *Am J Surg* 1992; **164**: 281–5.

23 Donaldson MC, Mannick JM, Whittemore AD. Causes of primary graft failure after in situ saphenous vein bypass grafting. *J Vasc Surg* 1992; **15**: 113–20.

24 Wengerter KR, Veith FJ, Gupta SK, Goldsmith J, Farrell E, Harris PL, Moore D, Shanik G. Prospective randomized

multicenter comparison of in situ and reversed vein infrapopliteal bypasses. *J Vasc Surg* 1991; **13**: 189–99.

25 Fogle MA, Whittemore AD, Couch NP, Mannick JA. A comparison of in situ and reversed saphenous vein grafts for infrainguinal reconstruction. *J Vasc Surg* 1987; **5**: 46–52.

26 Batson RC, Sottiurai VS. Nonreversed and in situ vein grafts. *Ann Surg* 1985; **201**: 771–9.

27 Rosenthal D. Endoscopic in situ bypass. *Surg Clin North Amer* 1995; **75**: 703–13.

28 van Dijk LC, van Urk H. du Bois JJ *et al*. A new 'closed' in situ vein bypass technique results in reduced wound complication rate. *Eur J Vasc Endovasc Surg* 1995; **10**: 162–7.

29 Cikrit DF, Fiore NF, Dalsing MC *et al*. A comparison of

endovascular assisted and conventional in situ bypass grafts. *Ann Vasc Surg* 1995; **9**: 37–43.

30 Le Heron D, Serise JM, Tingaud R. et al. Postoperative evaluation of in situ saphenous vein bypass with technetium-labeled albumin microspheres. *Texas Heart Inst J* 1982; **9**: 27–32.

31 Leather RP, Chang BB, Darling RC *et al*. In situ vein bypasses then and now: a story of New York neighbors. *Cardiovasc Surg* 1994; **2**: 146–53.

32 Clair DG, Golden MA, Mannick JA, Whittemore AD, Donaldson MC. Randomized prospective study of angioscopically assisted in situ saphenous vein grafting. *J Vasc Surg* 1994; **19**: 992–1000.

10

Complex reconstruction

JOSEPH L MILLS

INTRODUCTION

Certain clinical situations in which lower extremity revascularization is required may tax even the most ingenious and experienced of vascular surgeons. In the preceding seventh chapter, Andrew Bradbury and John Wolfe outlined intriguing techniques to improve outcome when adequate vein is unavailable and prosthetic must be utilized. Nevertheless, we remain firmly committed to the use of autogenous vein conduits whenever possible. Dogged persistence and extreme dedication are required to apply such a philosophy, however, and the purpose of the present chapter is to present the reader with additional useful techniques and tools of the trade to employ when standard procedures are not applicable. Such situations include reoperative lower extremity bypass, the performance of sequential or composite venous bypass grafts, the use of alternative conduits such as upper extremity veins, and the use of alternate inflow and outflow arteries with unusual operative exposures in order to avoid scarring from previous operations or to minimize the length of the bypass because of limited conduit availability.

Prevention of lower extremity arterial bypass failure is of paramount importance. There is no question that vein graft surveillance with appropriate intervention for graft-threatening lesions is well worth the effort. Techniques for repair of patent but hemodynamically failing grafts are presented in Chapter 13. Nonetheless, despite our best efforts, we continue to see patients who present with recurrent limb-threatening ischemia in whom a previously placed bypass has failed. If the initial operation was performed with prosthetic, the best course of action is to construct a new bypass with autogenous vein.[1-3] In this scenario, the patient may have available greater saphenous vein in the ipsilateral leg, which can be verified and mapped by preoperative duplex vein mapping. If the initial distal anastomosis was to the above-knee popliteal artery, the redo leg bypass should generally be anastomosed to the below-knee popliteal artery if this vessel reconstitutes and is continuous with at least one infrageniculate run-off artery. This approach avoids exposing a scarred and often diseased above-knee popliteal artery. The origin of the bypass will usually be the common femoral artery. At this level, the previous prosthetic anastomosis can be taken down and patched with vein, or if the venous conduit is of sufficient diameter, the anastomosis can be created at the same site after removing the prosthetic and trimming the arterial edges. If the common femoral and deep femoral arteries are widely patent, the mid-portion of the deep femoral artery can be used as a graft origin site after exposure is obtained via an approach lateral to the sartorius muscle (see Chapter 6, Fig. 6.4), thus obviating the need for repeat dissection in a scarred femoral triangle and shortening the length of conduit required.

Not infrequently, significant profunda femoral artery disease was left unaddressed at the initial operation or has progressed significantly since the primary operation. In such cases, particularly if the patient suffers only from severe claudication or rest pain without ulceration or tissue loss, a profundaplasty alone may suffice and obviate the need for a more difficult redo distal bypass. This consideration may be especially applicable to patients with prosthetic graft infections. Graft removal with autogenous deep femoral artery reconstruction may be sufficient to tide the patient's limb over until wounds have healed completely and infection has been eliminated.

If the initial bypass was constructed with ipsilateral greater saphenous vein, then the stakes are raised considerably. If the occlusion is recent, and particularly if the graft was known to harbor a stenosis by duplex surveillance, which was not addressed due to reluctance on the part of the patient or surgeon, we would consider lysis of the graft with urokinase or tissue plasminogen activator, followed by correction of the underlying responsible defect. If this approach succeeds, the patient should be anticoagulated chronically with sodium warfarin, maintaining an international normalized ratio (INR) between 2.5 and 3.0. However, this approach likely yields 1–2-year patency rates of only 40–50 per cent at best.[4–6]

If thrombolytic therapy fails, or if the graft is not freshly occluded, a new bypass with alternative vein conduit should be constructed. There are several maneuvers to obtain a conduit of sufficient length: (1) use of contralateral saphenous vein; (2) splicing of two or more segments of alternative (arm or lesser saphenous) vein conduit; (3) shortening the bypass length by using more distal inflow or graft origin sites such as the deep femoral artery, the superficial femoral artery, or the popliteal artery; (4) shortening the bypass length by using a more proximal insertion site or outflow artery (i.e. the per-

oneal artery after a failed pedal bypass); or (5) performing an endarterectomy of a diseased or occluded proximal artery to allow use of a shorter vein segment. In the latter situation, up to 10–20 cm of superficial femoral artery can be endarterectomized, frequently using eversion technique (Fig. 10.1) to serve as the proximal conduit.

CONDUIT SELECTION AND USE OF ALTERNATIVE ARTERIAL EXPOSURES

If the contralateral limb is not ischemic, and especially if the ankle–brachial index (ABI) is normal, we would not hesitate to harvest contralateral saphenous vein. Contralateral greater saphenous vein (GSV) seems to perform as well as ipsilateral GSV, with nearly equivalent patency results. We do not believe in saving this vein for later. Numerous reports testify that the contralateral GSV is only needed for subsequent use in 20–25 per cent of patients.[3,7] We therefore advocate using it when necessary, thus saving a more difficult alternate vein graft reconstruction for later. If the contralateral limb is already ischemic, as manifested by severe claudication, rest pain or ulceration, then we would not harvest vein from that extremity. If the contralateral limb is clinically asymptomatic, but the ABI is less than 0.6 or the foot is pulseless, we would harvest vein to the level of the knee or proximal calf if this would allow a single segment bypass to be performed.

If the length of conduit requires splicing, we look to alternate vein sources. Duplex vein mapping is very helpful in directing the surgeon to the most suitable caliber veins. If the ipsilateral lesser saphenous vein is of good quality and of sufficient length to perform a redo bypass without splicing, it would be our second choice. The lesser saphenous vein will reach from the deep femoral or proximal third of the superficial femoral artery to the below-knee popliteal artery. The lesser saphenous vein is also useful for popliteal distal bypasses. If the inflow source is the below-knee popliteal artery and the target is the distal peroneal artery, the entire operation can be conducted using a posterior approach with the patient in the prone position. Figures 10.2–10.4 illustrate the use of this technique in a diabetic patient with forefoot necrosis in whom the ipsilateral GSV had been previously expended for coronary revascularization. She had a palpable popliteal pulse with trifurcation wipe-out. The only distal vessel that reconstituted was the most distal portion of the peroneal artery. The lesser saphenous vein and popliteal artery were both exposed via a posterior approach with the patient in the prone position and the knee slightly flexed. The distal peroneal artery was also exposed deep to the lesser saphenous harvest incision between the tibia and the fibula just proximal to the ankle joint. This

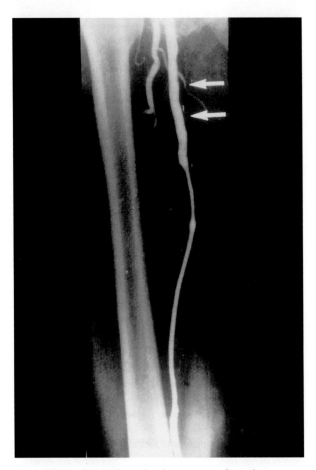

Figure 10.1 *Vein length was inadequate to perform the necessary bypass, therefore, an eversion endarterectomy (double arrow) was performed of the proximal superficial femoral artery, which was then anastomosed end-to-end to the available venous conduit, allowing a completely autogenous bypass without the need to harvest and splice additional saphenous vein.*

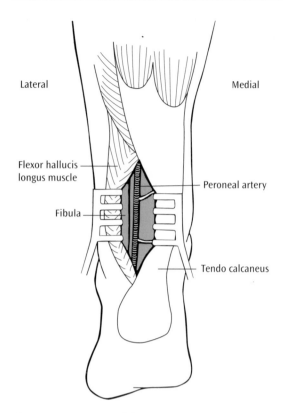

Lateral

Medial

Flexor hallucis
longus muscle

Fibula

Peroneal artery

Tendo calcaneus

Figure 10.2 *Exposure of the peroneal artery through the posterior approach. The tendon of the calcaneus is retracted medially and the flexor hallucis longus muscle is reflected laterally to expose the artery in the groove next to the fibula. The same incision is extended proximally to the popliteal fossa to mobilize the lesser saphenous vein. Reproduced with permission from Ouriel K. The posterior approach to popliteal–crural bypass. J Vasc Surg 1994; 19: 74–80.*

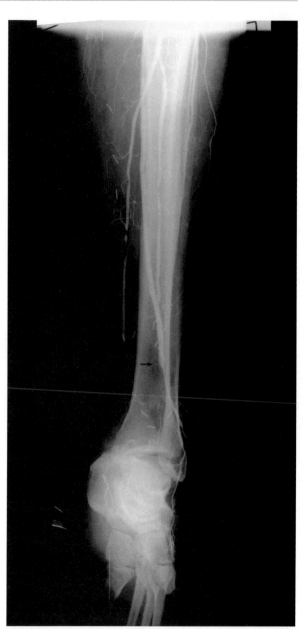

Figure 10.3 *Arteriogram obtained 3 years postoperatively in a patient with a lesser saphenous vein bypass from the below knee popliteal artery to the distal peroneal artery. The distal anastomosis is clearly visualized here.*

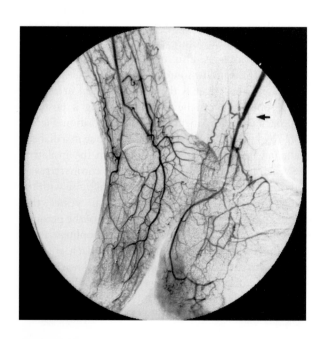

Figure 10.4 *Selective pedal and digital arteriography (same patient as Fig. 10.3) shows the distal anastomosis of the lesser saphenous to the peroneal artery (black arrow) and abundant collateralization from the distal peroneal artery to the foot. This patient's transmetatarsal amputation remained healed for 3 years after the initial bypass procedure. This arteriogram was obtained to evaluate right foot ischemia and resulted in the performance of a right femoral to posterior tibial bypass.*

approach has been well described by Ouriel and associates,[8] and is readily applicable to patients with the appropriate anatomy (Fig. 10.5). The posterior tibial artery may also be exposed via a posterior approach (Fig. 10.6). Such alternative surgical approaches should be considered not only in reoperative situations, but also in primary operations and in any situation in which available conduit length is limited.

Alternate distal exposures, both lateral and medial, of the deep femoral artery are important and should become familiar to the surgeon performing infrainguinal bypass (Chapter 4, Fig. 4.1). These techniques are useful to avoid dissection in the femoral triangle if previous operations or infection have occurred at this level.[9,10] In addition, if the common and deep femoral arteries are free of significant disease, origination of the bypass from a more distal site on the deep femoral artery shortens the length of the conduit required.[11,12] The origin of such a bypass from the mid-profunda femoris artery is demonstrated in Fig. 8.6 (Chapter 8).

USE OF ARM VEINS

When using arm veins, the surgeon should be aware that veins that appear outwardly normal during harvesting may contain intraluminal synechiae, webs, or sclerotic segments, presumably at the site of previous venipuncture. The median cubital vein at the elbow frequently harbors such culprits. For this reason, we advocate either intraoperative angioscopy prior to bypass or completion duplex scanning after bypass construction to be sure there are not significant intraluminal lesions within arm vein conduits. We also do not hesitate to harvest both the cephalic and basilic veins from the same upper extremity, if required, to provide a conduit of sufficient length. Such extensive harvests seem to result in minimal upper extremity swelling or morbidity. If both the upper arm basilic and cephalic veins are harvested, they can be anastomosed end-to-end. This may be necessary if the median cubital vein is sclerotic from previous venipuncture or intravenous access. Alternatively, the entire

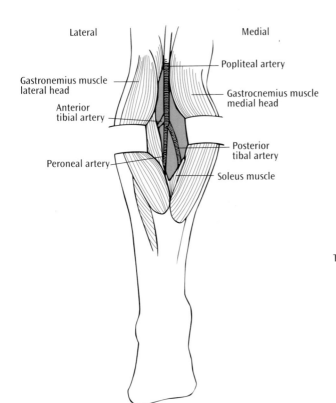

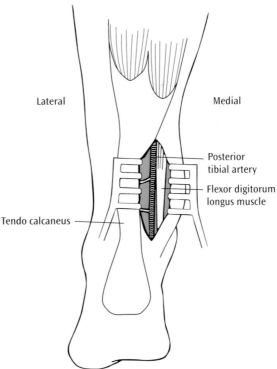

Figure 10.5 *Exposure of the popliteal and proximal crural arteries can be performed via a posterior approach between the heads of the gastronemius muscles. The origin of the soleus muscle can by lysed from the tibia to expose the proximal crural vessels if necessary. Reproduced with permission from Ouriel K. The posterior approach to popliteal–crural bypass. J Vasc Surg 1994; 19: 74–80.*

Figure 10.6 *Exposure of the posterior tibial artery can also be readily performed via a posterior approach. The tendo calcaneus is retracted laterally. The flexor digitorum longus muscle is reflected medially in the lower portion of the leg. The artery lies posterior to the lateral border of this muscle near the level of the malleolus. Reproduced with permission from Ouriel K. The posterior approach to popliteal–crural bypass. J Vasc Surg 1994; 19: 74–80.*

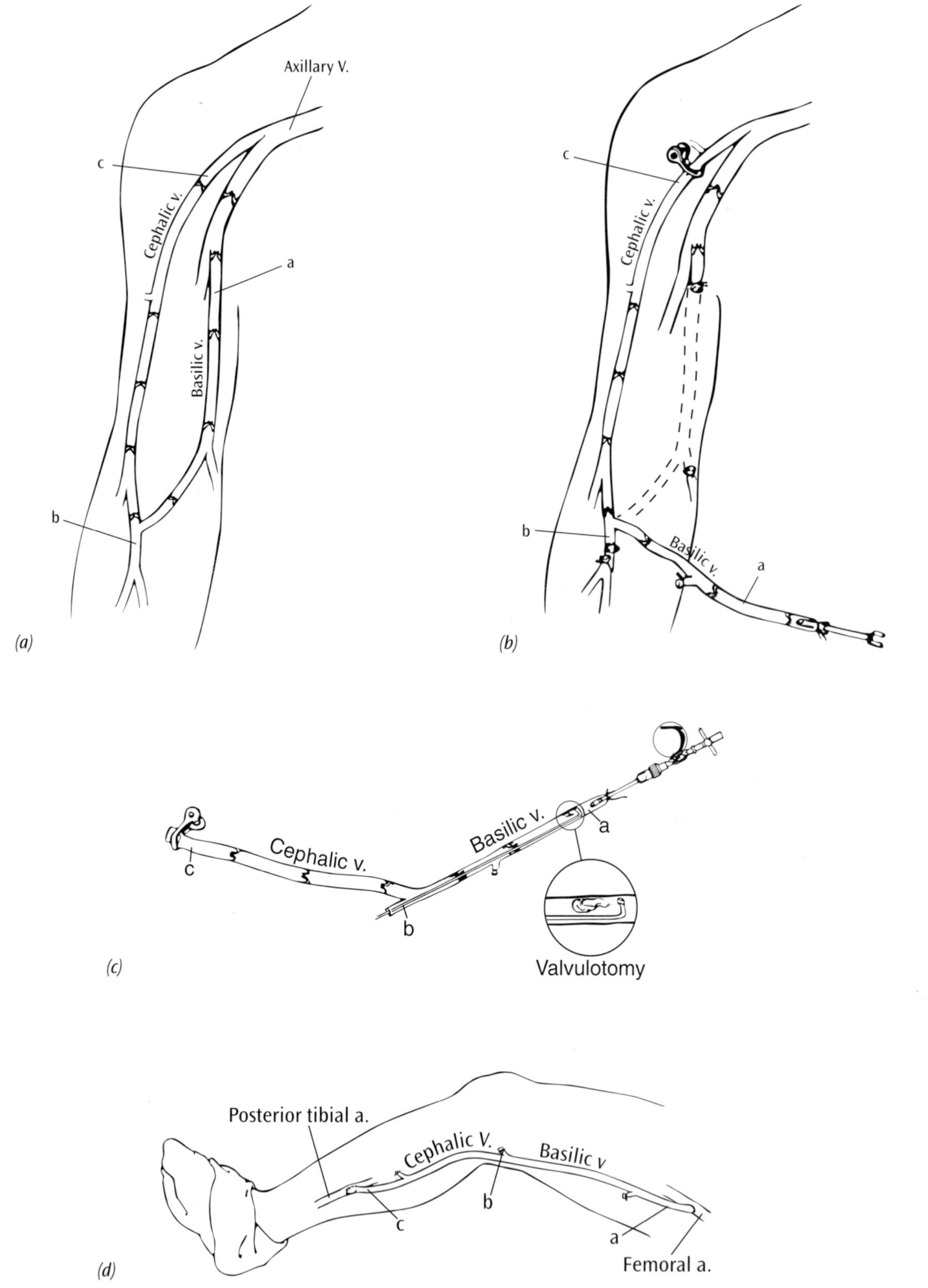

Figure 10.7 *(a) Both the cephalic and basilic veins can be harvested through separate incisions directly overlying the veins. (b) A cannula is then placed in the basilic vein for irrigation and gentle vein distention. (c) A valvulotome is then placed through a side branch to lyse the valves in the basilic portion of the conduit. (d) Such a combined cephalic and basilic conduit can be readily used to perform a bypass from the superficial femoral or deep femoral artery to the level of the mid-posterior tibial artery in the calf. Reproduced with permission from LoGerfo F. et al. A new arm vein graft for distal bypass. J Vasc Surg 1989; 5(6): 889–91.*

complex can be harvested intact and valve lysis of the basilic component performed, allowing this segment to be used proximally as a nonreversed conduit, continuous with the cephalic component in reversed configuration, obviating the need for splicing (Fig. 10.7a–d). Such a conduit will easily reach from the proximal superficial femoral artery (SFA) or mid-profunda femoral artery (PFA) to a mid-tibial artery. This ingenious technique is occasionally quite useful when longer arm vein grafts are necessary.

SEQUENTIAL BYPASS

Sequential bypasses are another useful alternative. If there is a patent popliteal island, this approach may obviate the need for splicing multiple venous segments to perform a long redo leg bypass to a distal tibial artery. For example, a sequential bypass can be constructed to a blind popliteal segment, using the proximal portion of this segment as outflow for a proximal bypass and the distal portion of the segment as the origin for a more distal bypass. Figures 10.8–10.11 illustrate the use of such a popliteal island to treat a diabetic patient with great toe gangrene 18 months following occlusion of a femoroperoneal saphenous vein graft. In this case, left cephalic vein was used to perform a common femoral to above-knee popliteal artery bypass: left basilic and available ipsilateral lesser saphenous vein were then spliced to construct a bypass from the below-knee popliteal artery to the paramalleolar posterior tibial artery. The patient's contralateral greater saphenous vein and right basilic vein had previously been utilized to reconstruct the left lower extremity.

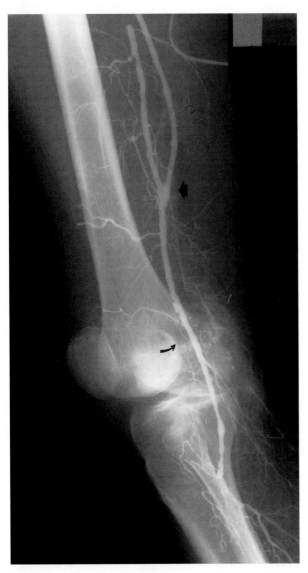

Figure 10.8 *Large arrow demonstrates anastomosis of cephalic vein conduit to above-knee popliteal artery. The small arrow identifies the native blind popliteal artery segment.*

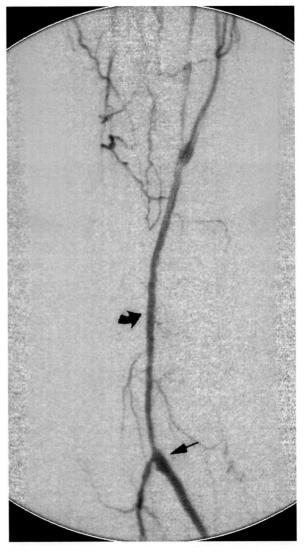

Figure 10.9 *Large arrow demonstrates a blind popliteal segment. Small arrow demonstrates the origin of a more distal bypass based on the distal portion of the blind popliteal segment.*

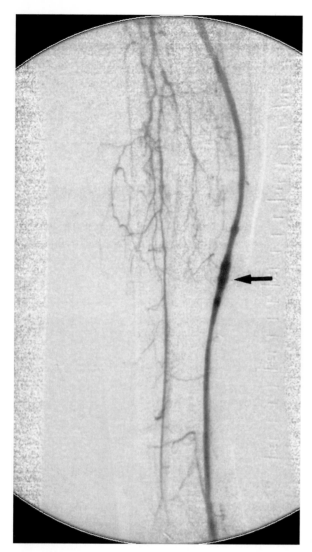

Figure 10.10 *Arteriogram from proximal calf to ankle level demonstrating a venovenous anastomosis (arrow) between the basilic and lesser saphenous veins used to perform a below-knee popliteal to posterior tibial artery sequential bypass.*

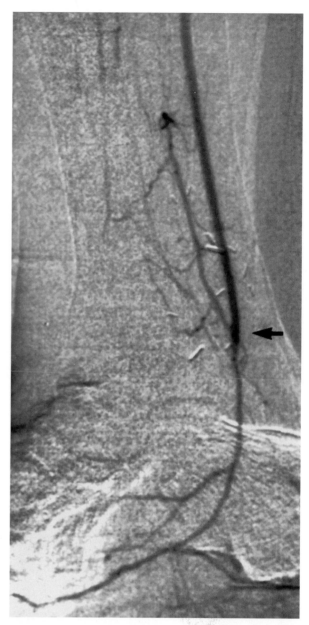

Figure 10.11 *Arrow demonstrates distal anastomosis of the spliced vein conduit to the paramalleolar posterior tibial artery. This patient's sequential bypass has remained patent with functional limb salvage 2 years after the procedure was performed.*

FREE TISSUE TRANSFER

An additional scenario, in which complex reconstructions may be required, occurs in patients with extensive gangrene of the distal lower extremity, frequently involving the heel.[13] In many such patients, particularly those with renal failure and exposed calcaneus, a bypass alone is insufficient to result in healing and subsequent independent ambulation. We have developed extensive experience with free tissue transfer combined with lower extremity arterial bypass.[14,15] In select ambulatory patients with large soft-tissue defects and exposed deep structures, functional limb salvage can be obtained by such a combined approached using distal bypass and free flap in conjunction with an experienced plastic-reconstructive surgeon.[16,17] Such procedures can either be performed combined in one setting, or staged with the revascularization and debridement performed first, followed by free flap coverage 1–3 weeks later. In our experience, patients requiring these reconstructions, frequently include diabetics with end-stage renal failure. The technique is also applicable to other patients with severe atherosclerotic disease who develop osteomyelitis or nonhealing bony lesions after fractures. We limit such lower extremity free-tissue transfers in combination with distal limb-salvage bypass grafts to ambulatory patients with sufficiently high functional capacity.

Considerable clinical judgement is required in deciding who would do better with a primary amputation and a prosthesis, and who would be a better candidate for a free flap. In appropriately selected patients, the benefits of revascularization and free-tissue transfer are substantial, and this option should be considered in patients with complex lower extremity wounds involving exposed bone or tendon, particularly deep heel ulcers.

CONCLUSIONS

In summary, reoperative distal bypass can be extremely challenging. In particular, when ipsilateral greater saphenous vein is absent, even primary operations can prove difficult. The techniques discussed herein should arm the vascular surgeon appropriately when entering combat with a recurrently ischemic limb. The following general principles should be applied whenever possible.

1 Avoid reopening previously explored arteries for proximal or distal anastomosis. Expose virgin territory if the extent of hemodynamically significant occlusive disease permits.
2 Familiarize yourself with alternate surgical approaches, such as the lateral and medial deep femoral artery exposures, the posterior and lateral popliteal artery approaches, and posterior exposure of the popliteal, infrageniculate and distal peroneal arteries.
3 Prudently utilize contralateral greater saphenous vein when available.
4 Avoid the use of mediocre or suboptimal vein conduits – take the necessary time to harvest additional vein if required to optimize conduit quality.
5 Profundaplasty and proximal endarterectomy of the SFA are extremely valuable adjunctive measures.
6 Perform completion angiography and duplex scanning of complex reconstructions – the best time to identify a problem or conduit defect is while you are still in the operating room.
7 Consider tunneling redo bypasses subcutaneously beneath intact skin. This maneuver renders postoperative surveillance and revision much easier.
8 Selected patients with extensive gangrene and/or exposed calcaneus may also require free-tissue transfer.

REFERENCES

1 Edwards JM, Taylor LM, Porter JM. Treatment of failed lower extremity bypass with new autogenous vein bypass. *J Vasc Surg* 1990; **11**: 132–45.
2 Whittemore AD, Clowes AW, Couch NP, Mannick JA. Secondary femoropopliteal reconstruction. *Ann Surg* 1981; **193**: 35–42.
3 Gentile AT, Lee RW, Moneta GC, Taylor LM Jr, Edwards JM, Porter JM. Results of bypasses to the popliteal and tibial arteries with alternative sources of autogenous vein. *J Vasc Surg* 1996; **23**: 272–80.
4 Belkin M, Donaldson MC, Whittemore AD *et al*. Observations on the use of thrombolytic agents for thrombotic occlusion of infrainguinal vein grafts. *J Vasc Surg* 1990; **11**: 289–96.
5 Sullivan KL, Gardiner GA Jr, Kandarpa K *et al*. Efficacy of thrombolysis in infrainguinal bypass grafts. *Circulation* Suppl I 1991; **83**: I99–I105.
6 DeMaioribus CA, Mills JL, Fujitani RM, Taylor JM, Joseph AE. A reevaluation of intraarterial thrombolytic therapy for acute lower extremity ischemia. *J Vasc Surg* 1993; **17**: 888–95.
7 Faries PL, Arora S, Pomposelli FB, Puling M, Smakowski P *et al*. The use of arm vein in lower extremity revascularizations: Results of 520 procedures performed over 8 years. *J Vasc Surg* 2000; **31(1)**: 50–9.
8 Ouriel K. The posterior approach to popliteal–crural bypass. *J Vasc Surg* 1994; **19**: 74–80.
9 Nunez AA, Veith FJ, Collier P *et al*. Direct approaches to the distal portions of the profunda femoris artery for limb salvage bypasses. *J Vasc Surg* 1988; **8**: 576–81.
10 Mills JL, Taylor JM, Fujitani RM. The role of the deep femoral artery as an inflow site for infrainguinal revascularization. *J Vasc Surg* 1993; **18**: 416–23.
11 Stabile BE, Wilson SE. The profunda femoris-popliteal artery bypass. *Arch Surg* 1977; **112**: 913–18.
12 Farley JJ, Kiser JC, Hitchcock CR. Profunda femoris-popliteal shunt. *Ann Surg* 1964; **160**: 23–5.
13 Gentile AT, Berman SS, Reinke KR *et al*. A regional pedal ischemia scoring system for decision analysis in patients with heel ulceration. *Am J Surg* 1998; **176**: 109–14.
14 Gooden MA, Gentile AT, Mills JL *et al*. Free tissue transfer to extend the limits of limb salvage for lower extremity tissue loss. *Am J Surg* 1997; **174**: 644–9.
15 Gooden MA, Gentile AT, Demas CP, Berman SS, Mills JL. Salvage of femoropopliteal bypass graft complicated by interval gangrene and vein graft blowout using a flow-through radial forearm fasciocutaneous free flap. *J Vasc Surg* 1997; **26**: 711–4.
16 Cronenwett JL, McDonald MD, Zwolak RM *et al*. Limb salvage despite extensive tissue loss: free tissue transfer combined with distal revascularization. *Arch Surg* 1989; **124**: 609–15.
17 Greenwald LL, Comerota AJ, Mitra A, Grosh JD, White JV. Free vascularized tissue transfer for limb salvage in peripheral vascular disease. *Ann Vasc Surg* 1990; **4**: 244–54.

11

Intraoperative graft assessment: angioscopy/duplex scan/angiography

ALEX WESTERBAND AND JOSEPH L MILLS

INTRODUCTION

Approximately 20–30 per cent of infrainguinal bypass grafts require revision within 18 months following implantation.[1-3] Early (<30 days) graft failure is commonly attributed to technical and judgmental errors. However, it appears likely that many bypass failures that occur from 1 to 18 months postoperatively result from the progression of a pre-existing defect unrecognized or ignored at the initial operation.[4] It has become clear that the incidence of early graft failure could potentially be reduced by the use of different methods of intraoperative graft assessment that allow the detection and correction of lesions which will later threaten graft patency. Among the available modalities, angioscopy, duplex scanning and completion angiography are the most commonly used in vascular surgical practice today.

INTRAOPERATIVE GRAFT ASSESSMENT BY ANGIOSCOPY

Endoscopy in the vascular system was introduced in the early part of this century by Cutler[5] but it was not until the 1960s that a strong interest in this technology began to emerge.[6,7] In 1977 Towne and Bernhard published a report on the use of vascular endoscopy during various arterial reconstructions.[8] Since then, significant improvements have occurred in the quality of the equipment; we now have small-diameter fiberoptic angioscopes – as small as 2.0 mm – which provide a three-dimensional image of the vessel lumen and a videoadapter, which offers improved resolution and magnification capability. This improvement in equipment has been accompanied by an increase in the use of angioscopy for diagnostic and therapeutic purposes. Angioscopy has numerous potential applications in lower extremity arterial reconstruction, the most important of which is thorough assessment of conduit quality.

It has been established that the presence of pre-existing pathology within a vein conduit can diminish subsequent vein graft patency. Panetta and colleagues reported a 40 per cent decrease in patency rate at 30 months when the transplanted greater saphenous vein had pre-existing intrinsic pathology.[9] Intrinsic vein lesions are especially common in arm vein conduits, perhaps due to their previous use for intravenous access and blood withdrawal. Stonebridge et al. identified intraluminal abnormalities in 74 per cent of arm veins prior to their use as infrainguinal bypass grafts;[10] correction of these abnormalities resulted in a 1-month patency rate of 100 per cent. Angioscopy has proved to be a sensitive and accurate method to identify intraluminal venous disease.[11] It can be used for retrograde in situ vein inspection, or on the back table in preparation for a reversed saphenous vein graft or a translocated vein graft. The in situ inspection is more commonly preferred since it allows visualization of the venous conduit through small limited incisions and, when segments are noted to be severely diseased and unusable, they are left in place, avoiding the need for extended skin incisions and theoretically decreasing the risk of wound complications.

For in situ retrograde vein inspection a small skin incision is performed over the distal segment of the vein and the vein is exposed. Then a small venotomy is performed, the angioscope is inserted through an irrigation sheath; a methodical inspection of the vein is accomplished, abnormalities when detected are correspondingly noted. When angioscopy is conducted in the upper extremities to evaluate the quality of the arm veins as possible alternative conduits, a proximal tourniquet allows one to limit the volume of irrigation fluid used.

When inspection is performed angioscopically on the back table, the angioscope is inserted through the irrigation sheath via the distal end, after all side branches have been ligated and the proximal segment occluded.

Angioscopy allows the detection of thrombus within the conduit, sclerotic and calcified segments, transluminal bands or strands, areas of focal stenosis or complete occlusion with recanalized segments. It may fail to detect abnormalities associated with normal-appearing intima, such as varicose veins or thick-walled veins.

Results

In a recent prospective study of the value of prebypass saphenous vein angioscopy, Sales et al.[12] identified seven abnormal veins among 32 greater saphenous vein conduits examined; despite correction of the abnormalities, only one of the angioscopically abnormal vein grafts remained patent at 12 months. This report confirms that pre-existing intrinsic vein disease has a significant negative impact on the patency rate of arterial reconstructions. Marcaccio et al.,[13] in a retrospective series of infrainguinal bypass grafts performed with arm vein conduits and routine intraoperative angioscopic assessment, found intraluminal disease in 71 of 113 arm veins (62.8 per cent) harvested for use as bypass conduits. The most common abnormality encountered was previous thrombosis (54 per cent). Angioscopy was used to assist in the correction of 95.8 per cent of all vein abnormalities and the repair was judged to be satisfactory in 66.1 per cent of the cases. The 1-month patency rate in angioscopically normal and successfully repaired grafts was 95.5 per cent; the remaining group in which the graft was considered to be of inferior quality even after repair had a 1-month patency rate of only 70 per cent. However, patency rates did not significantly differ at 1-year follow-up. Wilson et al.[14] prospectively compared angioscopic findings and graft outcome in 52 cases, and found

significant correlations between the presence of abnormalities at angioscopy and an unfavorable outcome.

These reports emphasize the sensitivity of angioscopy as a method of detecting the presence of intraluminal disease in venous conduits prior to their use for peripheral arterial bypass. Angioscopy may also assist in the correction of encountered anomalies.

Long-term prospective studies are still lacking to determine whether or not the use of angioscopy for initial assessment of the quality of the vein is associated with an increased long-term patency rate when compared to long-term results obtained without the use of angioscopy.

Angioscopy is being used by many centers today as an adjunct to monitor critical portions of the reconstruction for in situ bypass operations. Reports proposing several advantages of this technique have been published.[15–25] Angioscopy allows the performance of valvulotomy under direct vision, identifying incomplete valve lysis, residual competent valve leaflets and perhaps reducing the risk of valvulotomy-induced injury.[21] It also helps to identify side branches, arteriovenous communications and assists in the occlusion of venous tributaries.[26–28] The ultimate results are a decrease in morbidity associated with wound complications, the incidence of which varies from 17 to 44 per cent in large series.[29–31] As a method of intraoperative assessment for all vein grafts, whether in situ, reverse, translocated or composite grafts, angioscopy allows a complete inspection of proximal and distal anastomoses, reveals the presence of misplaced sutures, intimal flaps, thrombotic and platelet debris, and atherosclerotic plaques near the anastomosis.

Despite these theoretical advantages, the utility of angioscopy in routine infrainguinal arterial reconstructions remains unproven. Those favoring its routine use claim that early patency rate is improved (Table 11.1).

However, multiple groups have reported excellent early vein graft patency without angioscopy and the impact of angioscopy on long-term patency rate has not been established. In some institutions, its value has been recognized mainly as an adjunct for in situ bypass, as a way to decrease morbidity[24] and length of stay,[23,24] but an improved patency rate has not been demonstrated.[22,24] The additional volume of fluid infused does not appear to create any hemodynamic derangement when minimized and taken into account by the anesthesiologist.

Table 11.1 *Early patency following intraoperative angioscopy*

Author	Number of patients	Angioscopic/number of defects	1-month patency (%)
Miller et al.[32]	128	32	99.1
Harward et al.[25]	50	12	100
Clair et al.[33]	32	—	90.3

Concerns about intimal damage due to angioscopy are controversial.[34]

Limitations of angioscopy

Angioscopy does not provide any hemodynamic information; despite the availability of small diameter angioscopes, it also fails to provide a good assessment of the run-off vessels, particularly the infrapopliteal arteries. Whenever a reassessment of the quality of the run-off vessel is essential, angioscopy needs to be supplemented with a completion arteriogram.

INTRAOPERATIVE GRAFT ASSESSMENT BY DUPLEX SCAN

Despite several advantages, angioscopy shares one of the major limitations of angiography in that both provide anatomic information only without important physiologic data. Among the different methods allowing an hemodynamic assessment are the following.

- Continuous wave Doppler instruments are very useful but are mainly sensitive to changes in the peak systolic frequency; such changes signal the presence of major technical defects; but other less severe defects such as intimal flaps may go unnoticed.[35]
- Pulse Doppler spectral analysis is more sensitive for assessing residual flow disturbances following arterial reconstructions and has been found to have a negative predictive value of 100 per cent.[36] Minor flow disturbances are revealed by an increase in the spectral width (spectral broadening) in late systole. This great sensitivity is responsible for its lack of specificity. Also, pulsed Doppler flow analysis cannot provide any anatomical data. On the other hand, B-mode imaging ultrasonography has been shown to have a high level of accuracy – 96 per cent in Sigel's series[37] – in detecting vascular defects intraoperatively, but it does not provide hemodynamic information.
- More recently, the advantages of combining both B-mode imaging and pulsed Doppler spectral analysis in a single tool, the duplex scan, have been recognized. The addition of color-flow imaging provides greater accuracy, sensitivity and speeds up the examination.

Duplex scanners consist of a high-resolution imaging transducer (7.5–10 MHz) combined with a pulse-gated Doppler velocimeter (5.0–7.5 MHz); the Doppler signals are analysed by fast Fourier spectral analysis. The addition of imaging capability allows precise placement of a single-pulsed wave sample volume and accurate assessment of the flow disturbance caused by any defect identified on the B-mode image. With color-flow imaging, each digitized sample volume is assigned a color based on velocity and direction of flow. Color saturation is proportional to the Doppler shift, which in turn depends on the red blood cell velocity and the angle of Doppler beam insonation. Localized areas of decreased color saturation are associated with increased red cell velocity and therefore stenosis.[38]

Important technical points critical for an accurate intraoperative graft assessment by duplex scan are summarized in Table 11.2.

Since Duplex scanning provides both anatomic and physiologic data, it can be very useful for the intraoperative assessment of infrainguinal reconstructions. Abnormal graft hemodynamics include a peak systolic velocity less than 45 cm/s or greater than 50 per cent increase in peak systolic frequency with spectral broadening at the site of a presumed defect. Duplex scanning allows one to localize the region of interest with the B-mode imaging and to identify the presence of a structural defect along the graft or at its anastomoses. The absence of diastolic flow with or without the presence of a systolic thumping signal can also be demonstrated using continuous-wave Doppler analysis and this usually indicates inadequate run-off or distal occlusion. An arteriogram is then indicated to assess the anatomy of the distal vessels and identify the presumed defect.

Table 11.2 *Critical components of intraoperative duplex imaging*

Proper acoustic coupling (saline, gel, gel with plastic sleeve)
60° Doppler angle of insonation
Center stream localization of the pulsed Doppler sample volume
Use of the highest frequency probe possible for both imaging and flow assessment
Analysis of waveform characteristics, systolic and diastolic components of the flow cycle
Measurement of peak systolic flow velocity
Performance of augmentation maneuvers (flow should increase in response to pharmacological vasodilation with papaverine)

Limitations of duplex scanning

- As indicated above, duplex scanning only indirectly assesses the distal run-off and an arteriogram may be indicated to provide such information.
- Contrary to *in situ* vein grafts, which can be examined in their entirety, and defects such as retained valve leaflets and arteriovenous fistulae identified and corrected, reverse vein conduits are more difficult to image intraoperatively when they have been tunneled anatomically.

- Duplex scanning is also operator dependent, and requires skills and experience for correct interpretation of data. Intraoperative duplex skills are more difficult and tedious to acquire than those required for arteriography or angioscopy.
- Mismatch between the diameter of the graft and the outflow vessel can result in elevated flow velocities with spectral broadening in the area just distal to the anastomosis; in the absence of any obvious B-mode defect, an arteriogram may then be necessary to evaluate the distal anastomosis.

In summary, duplex scanning appears to be a very useful tool for intraoperative graft assessment because of its ability to provide both important anatomic and hemodynamic information; it allows early detection of even minor defects and their close surveillance postoperatively for progression.[39] However, it may not always provide all the information needed, particularly in the assessment of the run-off vessels, where it should be combined with arteriography.

INTRAOPERATIVE GRAFT ASSESSMENT BY ANGIOGRAPHY

Arteriography has long been the gold standard in intraoperative graft assessment following infrainguinal bypass graft procedures; its value as an important method to detect technical defects following lower extremity vascular reconstructions is universally recognized. In the 1960s, Renwick et al.[40] reported their experience with completion angiography, and noted that 27 per cent of reconstructions revealed defects requiring correction, despite a normal appearance by simple visual inspection and external palpation. The 2-week primary patency rate in this group was 100 per cent compared to 72 per cent in a control group in which the study was not performed. Such a high incidence of recognized defects has become rare today and now averages 5–9 per cent.[40–43] Mills et al.[44] in a prospective study of the value of routine completion angiography evaluated 214 consecutive infrainguinal bypass grafts and found significant technical problems requiring revision in 18 grafts (8 per cent); the 30-day primary patency was 99 per cent for femoropopliteal grafts and 93 per cent for femorodistal grafts; secondary patency was 100 per cent and 96 per cent respectively. The authors concluded that routine completion arteriography is an 'excellent method of ensuring the intraoperative technical adequacy of infrainguinal bypass'.[44] Intraoperative angiography allows the detection of anatomical defects, such as proximal or distal anastomotic stenoses as well as midgraft valvular or branch ligature stenoses, graft kinks or twists. After in situ saphenous vein bypass grafting, it also allows the detection of residual arteriovenous fistulae but is less sensitive in the detection of retained valve cusps. The results of the prospective study reported by Mills and co-workers[44] have shown a sensitivity of 90 per cent and a specificity of 98 per cent for reverse vein grafts. However, angiography has its limitations: like angioscopy it does not provide any hemodynamic information; false-positive arteriograms may occur due to spasm; false-negative ones also occur due to improper contrast density, timing and failure to obtain multiple projections. White et al.[45] in a preliminary study comparing angiographic and angioscopic findings in the same group of patients found a false-negative rate of 12.5 per cent and a false-positive rate of 8 per cent in the angiography group. The status of intraoperative angiography as the gold standard is being challenged by proponents of angioscopy and duplex scanning. We have identified the advantages and limitations of each of the available methods; these are summarized in Table 11.3. Controversy remains regarding which method to use. Miller et al.[32] conducted a prospective study comparing angioscopy and angiography: 32 corrective interventions were deemed necessary in the completion angioscopy group and only seven in the completion angiography group. However, although angioscopy appeared to be more sensitive than angiography by revealing more technical defects, no statistical improvement in the propor-

Table 11.3 *Comparison between angioscopy, duplex scanning and completion angiography*

Methods	Advantages	Disadvantages
Angioscopy	Accurate and complete information on the quality of the conduit	Quality of the run-off not appreciated
	May allow endovascular correction of defects	Relative risk of fluid overload
Duplex scanning	Provides both hemodynamic and anatomic information	Quality of the run-off not always appreciated
	Allows grading of the physiologic significance of a minor defect	Requires experience for correct interpretation
Completion angiography	Best to evaluate run-off vessels	No hemodynamic information
	Good anatomic information on the graft itself	Less sensitive than angioscopy for detection of intraluminal defects
		Risk of dye-induced injury

Table 11.4 *Proposed indications for use of angioscopy, duplex scan and/or completion angiography*

Procedures	Recommendations
Routine femoropopliteal bypass (*in situ*, RSVG)	Completion arteriogram alone
Routine femorodistal bypass (*in situ* or RSVG)	Arteriogram + either angioscopy or duplex scan
Complex reconstructions (use of alternate veins, spliced veins), reoperative leg bypass	All three methods

RSVG = reverse saphenous vein graft.

tion of failures could be demonstrated when the grafts were monitored by angioscopy as compared to angiographic monitoring. This seems to suggest that some minor defects probably do not need to be corrected and a better definition of a minor defect versus a significant defect is necessary. Duplex criteria could possibly help to classify these lesions more accurately than either angioscopy or angiography. In another prospective comparison of completion angiography and angioscopy by Baxter *et al.*,[46] completion arteriography was specific (95 per cent) but only moderately sensitive (67 per cent) compared with angioscopy. Another prospective study reported by Waters *et al.*[47] compared angioscopy, duplex scan and angiography, and found angioscopy to be the most sensitive, followed by angiography. This study suggests a higher sensitivity of angioscopy; however, the sensitivity rate with duplex scanning can be extremely variable depending upon the experience of the operator.

CONCLUSIONS

This review has allowed us to derive interesting observations regarding the use of angioscopy, duplex scanning and completion angiography, and leads to reasonable suggestions for their respective use. A summary of their indications and applications in routine clinical practice appears in Table 11.4.

We currently believe that in a routine femoropopliteal bypass graft using a saphenous vein conduit, which appears to be of good quality, the excellent patency rate generally observed (1-month primary patency rate 99 per cent, secondary patency rate 100 per cent)[44] does not justify the added costs of either angioscopy or a duplex scan, and completion angiography alone to verify the adequacy of the distal anastomosis and run-off vessels may be all that is needed. In routine femorodistal bypasses, we again recommend the routine use of completion arteriogram combined with either angioscopy or duplex scanning to evaluate graft anatomy. In those particular instances of complex reconstructions involving the use of alternate veins or spliced veins, the three methods appear to be complementary to each other. By providing accurate hemodynamic information duplex

scanning may allow better grading and categorization of minor defects previously identified intraoperatively by angioscopy or angiography. With the exception of the use of angioscopy for arm vein evaluation, none of these techniques has been convincingly demonstrated to improve graft patency or reduce the subsequent incidence of graft revision.

REFERENCES

1 Grigg MJ, Nicolaides AN, Wolfe JHN. Femorodistal vein bypass graft stenoses. *Br J Surg* 1988; **75**: 737–40.
2 Mills JL. Mechanisms of vein graft failure: the location, distribution and characteristics of lesions that predispose to graft failure. *Semin Vasc Surg* 1993; **6**: 78–91.
3 Mills JL, Fujitani RM, Taylor SM. The characteristics and anatomic distribution of lesions that cause reverse vein graft failure: a five year prospective study. *J Vasc Surg* 1993; **17**: 195–206.
4 Mills JL, Gahtan V, Bandyk DF, Esses GE. The origin of infrainguinal vein graft stenosis: a prospective study based on duplex surveillance. *J Vasc Surg* 1995; **21**: 16–25.
5 Cutler EC, Levine A, Beck CS. The surgical treatment of mitral stenosis: Experimental and clinical studies. *Arch Surg* 1924; **9**: 689–821.
6 Greenstone SM, Shore JM, Heringman EC *et al*. Arterial endoscopy (Arterioscopy). *Arch Surg* 1966; **93**: 811–12
7 Vollmar JF: Die Gefabendoskopie: Ein neuer Weg der intraoperativen Gefabdiagnostik. *Endoscopy* 1969; **1**: 141–4.
8 Towne JB, Bernhard VM Vascular endoscopy: Useful tool or intraoperative toy? *Surgery* 1977; **82**: 415–9.
9 Panetta TF, Marin ML Veith FJ *et al*. Unsuspected preexisting saphenous disease: an unrecognized cause of vein bypass failure. *J Vasc Surg* 1992; **15**: 102–12.
10 Stonebridge PA, Miller A, Tsoukas A *et al*. Angioscopy of arm veins infrainguinal bypass grafts. *Ann Vasc Surg* 1991; **5**: 170–5.
11 Sales CM, Marin ML, Veith FJ *et al*. Saphenous vein angioscopy: a valuable method to detect unsuspected venous disease. *J Vasc Surg* 1993; **18**: 198–206.
12 Sales CM, Goldsmith J, Veith FJ. Prospective study of the value of prebypass saphenous vein angioscopy. *Am J Surg* 1995; **170**: 106–8.

13 Marcaccio EJ, Miller A, Tannenbaum GA *et al.* Angioscopically directed interventions improve arm vein bypass grafts. *J Vasc Surg* 1993; **17**: 994–1004.

14 Wilson YG, Davies AH, Currie IC *et al.* Angioscopy for quality control of saphenous vein during bypass grafting. *Eur J Vasc Endovasc Surg* 1996; **11**: 12–18.

15 Grundfest WS, Litvack F, Sherman T *et al.* Delineation of peripheral and coronary detail by intraoperative angioscopy. *Ann Surg* 1985; **202**: 394–400.

16 Seeger JM, Abela GS. Angioscopy as an adjunct to arterial reconstructive surgery: a preliminary report. *J Vasc Surg* 1986; **4**: 315–20.

17 Fleisher HL, Thompson BW, McCowan TC *et al.* Angioscopically monitored saphenous vein valvulotomy. *J Vasc Surg* 1986; **4**: 360–4.

18 Matsumoto T, Hashizume M, Yang Y *et al.* Direct vision valvulotomy in in situ venous bypass. *Surg Gynecol Obstet* 1987; **165**: 362–64.

19 Miller A, Campbell DR, Gibbons GW *et al.* Routine intraoperative angioscopy in lower extremity revascularization. *Arch Surg* 1989; **124**: 604–8.

20 Donaldson MC, Mannick JA, Whittemore AD. Femoro-distal bypass with in situ greater saphenous vein. Long-term results using the Mills valvulotome. *Ann Surg* 1991; **213**: 457–65.

21 Miller A, Stonebridge PA, Tsoukas AI *et al.* Angioscopically directed valvulotomy: a new valvulotome and technique. *J Vasc Surg* 1991; **13**: 813–21.

22 Woelfle KD, Bruijnen H, Zuegel N *et al.* Technique and results of vascular endoscopy in arterial and venous reconstructions. *Ann Vasc Surg* 1992; **6**: 347–56.

23 Davies AH, Magee TR, Thompson JF *et al.* Preliminary experience of angioscopy in femorodistal bypass. *Ann Royal Coll Surg Engl* 1993; **75**: 178–80.

24 Maini BS, Andrews L, Salimi T *et al.* A modified, angioscopically assisted technique for in situ saphenous vein bypass: impact on patency, complications and length of stay. *J Vasc Surg* 1993; **17**: 1041–9.

25 Harward TRS, Govostis DM, Rosenthal QJ *et al.* Impact of angioscopy on infrainguinal graft patency. *Am J Surg* 1994; **168**: 107–10.

26 Rosenthal D, Herring MB, O'Donovan TJ *et al.* Endovascular infrainguinal in situ saphenous vein bypass. A multicenter preliminary report. *J Vasc Surg* 1992; **16**: 453–8.

27 Rosenthal D, Dickson C, Rodriguez FJ *et al.* Infrainguinal endovascular in situ saphenous vein bypass: Ongoing results. *J Vasc Surg* 1994; **20**: 389–95.

28 Cikrit DF, Dalsing MC, Lalka SG *et al.* Early results of endovascular-assisted in situ saphenous vein bypass grafting. *J Vasc Surg* 1994; **19**: 778–87.

29 Wengrovitz M, Atnip RG, Gifford RRM *et al.* Wound complications of autogenous subcutaneous infrainguinal arterial bypass surgery: predisposing factors and management. *J Vasc Surg* 1990; **11**: 156–63.

30 Schwartz ME, Harrington EB, Schanzer H. Wound complications after in situ bypass. *J Vasc Surg* 1988; **7**: 802–7.

31 Reifsnyder T, Bandyk D, Seabrook G *et al.* Wound complications of the in situ saphenous vein bypass technique. *J Vasc Surg* 1992; **15**: 843–50.

32 Miller A, Marcaccio EJ, Tannenbaum GA *et al.* Comparison of angioscopy and angiography for monitoring infrainguinal bypass vein grafts: results of a prospective randomized trial. *J Vasc Surg* 1993; **17**: 382–98.

33 Clair DG, Golden MA, Mannick JA *et al.* Randomized prospective prospective study of angioscopically assisted in situ saphenous vein grafting. *J Vasc Surg* 1994; **19**: 992–1000.

34 Lee G, Beerline D, Lee MH *et al.* Hazards of angioscopic examination: documentation of damage to the arterial intima. *Am Heart J* 1988; **116**: 1530–6.

35 Spencer TD, Goldman MH, Hyslop JW *et al.* Intraoperative assessment of in situ saphenous vein bypass with continuous-wave Doppler probe. *Surgery* 1984; **96**: 874–7.

36 Bandyk DF, Jorgensen RA, Towne JB. Intraoperative assessment of in situ saphenous vein arterial grafts using pulsed doppler spectral analysis. *Arch Surg* 1986; **121**: 292–9.

37 Sigel B, Coelho JCU, Flanigan P *et al.* Detection of vascular defects during operation by imaging ultrasound. *Ann Surg* 1982; **196**: 473–80.

38 Mills JL, Bandyk DF. Intraoperative use of ultrasound. In: Jamieson CW, Yao JST eds *Rob and Smith's operative surgery*. London: Chapman and Hall, 1994: 5–10.

39 Bandyk DF, Mills JL, Galitan V *et al.* Intraoperative duplex scanning of arterial reconstructions: fate of repaired and unrepaired defects. *J Vasc Surg* 1994; **20**: 426–33.

40 Renwick S, Royle JP, Martin P. Operative angiography after femoropopliteal reconstructions – its influence on early failure rate. *Brit J Surg* 1968; **55**: 134–6.

41 Brewster DC, LaSalle AJ, Robinson JG *et al.* Femoropopliteal graft failures. Clinical consequences and success of secondary reconstructions. *Arch Surg* 1983; **118**: 1043–7.

42 Shoenfeld NA, O'Donnell TF, Bush HL *et al.* The management of early in situ saphenous vein bypass occlusions. *Arch Surg* 1987; **122**: 871–5.

43 Leather RP, Shah DM, Chang BB *et al.* Resurrection of the in situ saphenous vein bypass. 1,000 cases later. *Ann Surg* 1988; **208**: 435–42.

44 Mills JL, Fujitani RH, Taylor SM. Contribution of routine intraoperative completion arteriography to early infrainguinal bypass patency. *Am J Surg* 1992; **164**: 506–11.

45 White GH, White RA, Kopchok GE *et al.* Intraoperative video angioscopy compared with arteriography during peripheral vascular operations. *J Vasc Surg* 1987; **6**: 488–95.

46 Baxter BT, Rizzo RJ, Flinn WR *et al.* A comparative study of intraoperative angioscopy and completion arteriography following femorodistal bypass. *Arch Surg* 1990; **125**: 997–1002.

47 Waters MA, Musson A, Magnant JG *et al.* A blinded comparison of angiography, angioscopy and duplex scanning in the intraoperative evaluation of in situ saphenous vein bypass grafts. *J Vasc Surg* 1992; **15**: 121–9.

12

Expected outcome: early results, life table patency, limb salvage

RONALD L DALMAN

INTRODUCTION

The last half century has witnessed significant advances in the care and outcome of patients with all aspects of peripheral vascular disease, including lower extremity revascularization procedures and limb salvage. Despite such advances, outcome standards for lower extremity revascularization remain undefined. This lack of standardization is due in part to rapid and continuing improvements in surgical technique, technology, vascular imaging modalities and anesthetic care; a continuous process of improvement which frustrates attempts to define and update standards at any given moment. Also persistent ambiguities regarding the definition of procedural success remain unresolved. Unlike carotid endarterectomy, where neurologic and cardiovascular outcome can be measured with a degree of precision, comorbid variables, such as wound size, intercurrent soft-tissue or bone infections and preoperative and postoperative ambulatory status all complicate and obscure outcome assessment following lower extremity arterial reconstructive surgery.

Recognizing these difficulties, surgeons traditionally have emphasized graft patency and complete wound healing or limb salvage as measurable, hard endpoints following limb revascularization. The goal of lower limb revascularization is ultimately to return the patient to ambulation and/or self-sufficient living. Gibbons and associates recently attempted to assess improvement in quality of life indicators, such as improved activities of daily living, mental well-being and vitality in 156 patients who underwent limb revascularization during 1 year. Despite achieving enviable patency results (92 per cent primary and 95 per cent secondary at 6 months), and significant improvements in pain and walking distance, only 47 per cent of respondents reported feeling 'back to normal' six months after their procedure, and 10 per cent more patients were using devices to assist walking than before their surgery.[1] Clearly, despite patent grafts, many patients do not feel substantially better following limb revascularization procedures. This fact deserves much further study, especially in regards to quality of life goals for managed care plans and capitated care reimbursement scenarios.[2] Without patent grafts, limbs salvage is in doubt. However, graft patency alone is not necessarily sufficient to provide complete healing and recovery for patients with severe peripheral vascular occlusive disease.

Most patients report substantial improvement in walking distance and healing of ischemic ulcers following successful limb revascularization. In most scenarios of limb ischemia and surgical therapy, clinical experience is the surest guide to predicting functional outcome. For example, in the claudicator with absent pedal pulses on physical examination, pulse restoration portends substantial improvement in walking distance. Similarly, in the patient with ischemic rest pain, incremental augmentation of pedal blood flow as determined by an increased ankle pressure should provide substantial symptomatic relief. Using increased ankle blood pressure or the derivative ankle–brachial index to predict outcome precisely is often unreliable because the ultimate goal of limb revascularization is increased limb or pedal perfusion, of which pressure is an indirect measure. Presumably, some minimum flow volume (ml/min) or tissue perfusion rate (ml/min per g) is required to heal wounds, and that volume or rate is related to the size of the wound, degree of tissue viability, percentage oxygen saturation of hemoglobin, percent carboxyhemoglobin, etc. Preliminary work using cine phase-contrast magnetic resonance flow-volume imaging is promising, but even this method of flow quantification is limited by the extremely low volumes present in patients with severe peripheral vascular occlusive disease, and marked intra- and interpatient variability in flow due to limb resistance, temperature and cardiac output considerations.[3]

Graft patency and limb salvage define results of most surgical series. From the inception and popularization of limb revascularization procedures in the late 1950s and early 1960s through the mid-1980s, the quality of reports concerning outcome following these procedures was inconsistent. Indications, severity of ischemia, description of procedures, definitions of success and methods of reporting postoperative follow-up varied widely, relegating the value of even the most influential surgical reports to 'anecdotal' status. Without standards or uniformly accepted definitions, few if any conclusions could be drawn from the increasing world-wide experience with limb salvage. In an effort to improve the quality of results reporting, the Ad Hoc Committee on Reporting Standards, of the Societies of Vascular Surgery/North American Chapter, International Society for Cardiovascular Surgery, led by Robert B. Rutherford, took up the challenge of establishing benchmarks for indications and outcome. Their report, published in 1986, is both a clear and compelling plea for standardization, and provides a practical and resilient template for reporting results. These proposals have survived the test of time[4] and are currently referenced by editors from nearly all major journals publishing such reports.

REPORTING STANDARDS

Foreshadowing the concerns of Gibbons[1] and others, Rutherford and his colleagues acknowledged at the time that emphasizing patency as the primary endpoint of reconstructive procedures was insufficient:

> Although patency is accepted as the ultimate criterion of success when results of arterial reconstruction are reported, this is primarily because it is a discrete and comparable end point. However, situations exist in which patency does not necessarily mean success … such situations (where graft patency does not result in wound healing or relief of symptoms) may be termed 'hemodynamic failures'. Similarly … if a bypass graft performed for 'limb salvage' occludes but the limb is no longer threatened (is this a failure?) … suffice it to say that clear definitions of patency, foot salvage, and/or 'significant' clinical improvement are needed to serve as ultimate measures of success, and reporting the rate of other criteria in addition to patency will provide greater perspective and better grounds for comparison.[5] [parentheses added]

Categories for chronic limb ischemia adopted by the Ad Hoc Committee are listed in Table 12.1. The suggested outcome scale following intervention is summarized in Fig. 12.1.[4]

Publication and subsequent acceptance of these criteria ushered in a new era of results reporting in lower extremity arterial reconstructive surgery. More recently, Rutherford has revised and extended these criteria specifically to include catheter-based or interventional vascular procedures, in a well-intentioned effort to provide a level playing field in results reporting and

Table 12.1 *Clinical categories of chronic limb ischemia*

Grade	Category	Clinical description	Objective criteria
0	0	Asymptomatic, no hemodynamically significant occlusive disease	Normal treadmill/stress test
I	1,2,3	Mild, moderate and severe claudication, respectively	Mild – completes treadmill exercise test, AP after exercise <50 mmHg, but >25 mmHg less than BP Moderate – between categories 1 and 3 Severe – cannot complete treadmill, exercise and AP after exercise <50 mmHg
II	4	Ischemic rest pain	Resting AP <40 mm Hg, flat or barely pulsatile ankle or metatarsal PVR; TP <30 mmHg
III	5,6	Minor tissue loss – nonhealing ulcer, focal gangrene with diffuse pedal ischemia Major tissue loss – extending above TM level, functional foot no longer salvageable	Resting AP <60 mmHg, ankle or metatarsal PVR flat or barely pulsatile; TP <40 mmHg Same as category 5

AP = ankle pressure, BP = blood pressure, PVR = pulse volume recording, TM = transmetatarsal, TP = toe pressure.

+3   Markedly improved: symptoms gone or markedly improved, ABI increased to more than 0.90.

+2   Moderately improved: still symptomatic but at least single category improvement; ABI increased by more than 0.10 but not normalized.

+1   Minimally improved: greater than 0.10 increase in ABI but no categorical improvement, or vice versa (i.e. upward categorical shift without an increase in ABI of more than 0.10).

0   No change: no categorical shift and less than 0.10 change in ABI.

−1   Mildly worse: no categorical shift but ABI decreased more than 0.10.

−2   Moderately worse: one category worse or unexpected minor amputation.

−3   Markedly worse: more than one category worse or unexpected major amputation.

Figure 12.1 *Outcome scale following intervention for chronic limb ischemia. ABI = ankle–brachial index.*

compare outcomes based on results, not on the method of intervention employed.[6] An updated version of the original Ad Hoc Committee recommendations is also anticipated.[7]

If graft patency is to be considered the primary endpoint for limb bypass series, the method of patency determination must be objective and reproducible. This proof must be positive, that is, the absence of negative data does not equate to affirmation of patency. Rutherford and co-authors in their original 1986 report[4] listed five acceptable methods of patency determination, including the following:

1   Arteriography or other established imaging technique (including but not limited to digital subtraction arteriography, ultrasound, radionuclide or magnetic resonance imaging).

2   Maintenance of achieved improvement in the appropriate segmental limb pressure index (at least 0.10 above the preoperative index and no more than 0.10 less than the maximum postoperative index).

3   Maintenance of a plethysmographic tracing or oscillometric reading distal to the reconstruction, which is significantly greater in magnitude than the preoperative value. (This is acceptable *only* when accurate pressures cannot be measured, as with calcific arteries in a diabetic patient.)

4   The presence of a palpable pulse, or the recording of a biphasic or triphasic Doppler wave form at two points directly over a *superficially* placed graft.

5   Direct observation of patency at reoperation or during a post-mortem examination.

Since that time, significant advances in imaging techniques, including color and power duplex Doppler imaging, magnetic resonance arteriography and now three-dimensional duplex Doppler imaging have made objective determination of patency easier, safer and much more accurate. Also, widespread adoption of duplex graft surveillance protocols for clinical follow-up, discussed in detail elsewhere in this text, have made many of the controversies surrounding what test or testing method represents sufficient proof of patency moot.

Other patency considerations relevant to the issue of reporting standards include the definitions of primary, primary assisted and secondary patency. If additional surgery is required to preserve patency, is the graft in fact still considered 'patent'? Following the recommendations of Ad Hoc Committee of the Joint Vascular Societies, the graft is considered to be patent if

'it has had uninterrupted patency with either no procedure performed on it, or a procedure performed such as transluminal dilation or proximal or distal extension to the graft, to deal with disease progression in the adjacent native vessel. Thus the only exceptions that do not qualify the graft for primary patency are procedures performed for disease beyond the graft and its two anastomoses. Dilations or minor revisions performed for stenoses, dilations, or other structural defects *before* occlusion do not constitute exceptions as they are intended to prevent eventual graft failure'.[4]

The widespread use of postoperative graft surveillance has significantly increased the number of grafts which are revised while still patent, owing to lesions or areas of graft stenosis identified during direct graft imaging. At the time of the report of the Ad Hoc Committee, such surveillance was not commonly performed. In an effort to distinguish between grafts that are revised prior to occlusion from grafts which have occluded and require thrombectomy as well as revision, the term 'primary assisted patency' has gained popularity. Generally, the phrase is taken to refer to grafts that are patent when revised, as compared to secondary patency, which indicates graft occlusion. In the pregraft surveillance era, such a distinction was rarely necessary, as relatively few failing grafts were identified prior to occlusion. However, the original committee did not make this distinction and no formal definition of the term 'assisted primary patency' is provided in the original Rutherford report.[4] Along these same lines, should a graft become completely occluded, and subsequently replaced, the term 'patency' no longer pertains to the original graft, and the second or 'redo' graft then becomes the index graft.

Determining both primary and secondary patency for lower extremity arterial reconstructive surgery is essential for results reporting. Primary patency provides insight regarding the natural history of the procedure, and the comparison of primary and secondary patency provides insight into the resilience and ultimate clinical utility of the graft. Results are to be reported in the life table format.[8,9] This method, originally popularized for the reporting of trials of cancer therapy, has become, in the years since the Committee's report, familiar to most if not all vascular surgeons. Life table or actuarial reporting minimizes the statistical inefficiencies inherent in rolling enrollment throughout the period of a clinical trial, and provides accountancy methods for tabulating graft failure, death or termination. While providing a simple and reliable method of following results, life table reporting *per se* does not insure accurate results. Practices, such as 'front loading' of a life table, or the selective rather than uniform inclusion of all study participants enrolled on an 'intention to treat' basis can seriously compromise the validity of the results, while appearing to uphold reporting conventions. Similarly, as has become apparent with increasing experience, certain phenomena such as high cohort mortality during the early or middle interval follow-up can skew results. Despite these and other previously identified limitations,[10] use of the life table is mandatory for the expression of results in all large series of arterial reconstructive procedures submitted for publication in the *Journal of Vascular Surgery* and similar publications. The method of construction of life tables, and their conventions and interpretation are thoroughly reviewed in the report of the Ad Hoc Committee.[4] All comparisons of life table estimates must be performed using the log-rank test. Errors can be introduced when patencies are compared at specific intervals with the standard errors. The simple log rank test compares two or more life tables over the entire period of observation.

Reports comparing outcome, especially between different classes of procedures in different groups of patients are difficult to interpret when significant co-morbidities are not tabulated and reported. In attempting to provide indices for intergroup comparison, the Ad Hoc Committee suggested a severity scale for commonly identified co-morbid variables in these patients, including diabetes, hypertension, tobacco use, hyperlipidemia, etc.[4] Although current reports of arterial reconstructive procedures tabulate the presence of such variables, the use of severity scales for standardization has not been widely adopted, and is not currently generally required for publication of results. This failure to standardize the severity of patient disease continues to limit the comparability of these reports. As noted recently by Rutherford, '... proper comparison of outcomes goes much farther than standard reporting practices, as essential as these are. It requires not only reporting outcomes in a standard fashion *but including comparable data on all factors known to affect those outcomes*' (original italics).[7] Similarly, a proposed scale for severity of arteriographic run-off was introduced in the original Ad Hoc Committee report, and has met with even less enthusiasm and rarely appears or is referenced in contemporary articles on this subject. With newer imaging modalities, the assessment of 'run-off' *per se* is no longer limited to the luminal imaging provided via arteriography, and

presumably newer more physiologic imaging and flow quantification methods will allow more accurate and specific criteria to develop.

Finally, several other terms used in reports of limb revascularization procedures are defined by the Ad Hoc Committee, and their use in such reports should strictly adhere to the agreed-upon meaning. A 'primary operation' is the first operation of a certain class performed on a specific arterial segment. Should the procedure fail, a 'secondary operation' is performed within the exact same segment. Procedures performed due to a lack of desired outcome, despite continued patency or technical success of the primary procedure, are considered sequential primary procedures. A 'principal' procedure constitutes the procedure thought most likely to effect the desired hemodynamic result. An 'adjunctive' procedure is performed to modify or augment the principal procedure. An 'ancillary' procedure is a procedure necessary to support the performance of the principal procedure but which is not directly related to the hemodynamic or functional result. The example of an adjunctive procedure cited by the Ad Hoc Committee is an intraoperative arteriogram.[4]

'Elective' procedures are performed on a routine, scheduled basis at the discretion of the patient and surgeon. The term 'urgent' refers to procedures that are performed with the absolute minimum preparatory time following the decision to operate. 'Emergency' operations are performed as soon as possible, usually because of an immediate threat to limb or life. A 4-hour time limit between evaluation and intervention is suggested to define the term 'emergency'.[4] A 'reconstructive procedure' is one that

> is performed to remove an obstructive or aneurysmal lesion involving the arterial wall and/or to restore pulsatile flow beyond the involved arterial segment. Included in this category are bypass grafts, interposition grafts, resection and anastomosis, endarterectomy, or surgical angioplasty with and without patch graft.

In distinction, a 'restorative' procedure is one in which the native conduit is preserved and luminal patency is achieved via removal of intraluminal obstructions. These procedures include thrombectomy, embolectomy, intra-arterial thrombolysis, and transluminal dilation. 'Non-reconstructive' procedures are performed to improve or to protect blood flow without arterial reconstruction or intervention. These procedures include fasciotomy, sympathectomy and relief of external compression. 'Ablative' procedures are 'procedures designed to remove non-viable or diseased material (tissue or graft) or that interrupt flow in patent vessels. These procedures include major or minor amputations, debridement or removal of an infected graft, and arterial ligation'.[4]

In 1991 we completed an exhaustive review of the previous decades reported experience with lower extremity arterial reconstructive surgery.[11] Thirteen of the 45 references were published prior to the 1986 Rutherford report, but the remainder were chosen specifically because they used accepted reporting methods. The references incorporated in the following tables substantially represent the range of results reported in the decade of the 1980s, a time when lower extremity arterial reconstructive surgery came of age.

INTERPRETATION OF TABLES AND OUTCOME DATA

Tables 12.2–12.6 were constructed by using the weighted averages of the series based on the number of patients reported in each interval. As such, they represent a form of 'meta-analysis'. Since 1991, several important changes in practice standards have modified the results reported in these series. Secondary patency as such was reported only for *in situ* grafts in the pregraft surveillance era, due to the tendency of these grafts to retain patent side branches despite angiographic intraoperative assessment. More recent surgical series including data on graft surveillance now provide secondary patency data for all types of procedures, including reversed saphenous vein, reflecting the influence of surveillance on daily practice. Results have improved accordingly. Nehler and associ-

ates recently reported assisted primary patencies of original reversed saphenous vein grafts revised for stenotic lesions of 99 per cent, 96 per cent and 92 per cent at 1, 3 and 5 years, respectively. Limb salvage was 99 per cent, 97 per cent and 97 per cent at the same intervals.[12] As noted by Peter Fry in his commentary on these results,

> this achievement ... demonstrates in graphic detail what could have been achieved in the past when we were all reporting 60 per cent and 70 per cent primary cumulative patency, if we had at that time the ability to perform the kind of graft surveillance that can be practiced today, particularly with the addition of duplex scanning.[12]

Reflecting a trend that was already accelerating in 1990, prosthetic bypass procedures in the lower extremities continue to decline and are now limited to the popliteal artery above the knee. Quinones-Baldrich and associates at UCLA continue to support a policy of primary prosthetic above-knee procedures, followed by autogenous conduit when graft failures occur.[13] In many areas of the USA, few if any prosthetic bypass conduits are used in any infrainguinal position. Most influential centers have adopted all-autogenous policies regarding infrainguinal graft conduits, although recent series suggest that composite grafts including multiple pieces of arm or saphenous vein do not perform up to the standard of intact ipsilateral saphenous veins.[14] Initially thought to represent a biologic alternative to polytetrafluoroethylene

Table 12.2 *Above-knee femoropopliteal grafts*

Primary patency[a]	1 month	6 months	1 year	2 years	3 years	4 years
Reverse saphenous vein	99	91	84	82	73	69
Arm vein	99		82	65	60	60
Human umbilical vein	95	90	82	82	70	70
Polytetrafluoroethylene (PTFE)		89	79	74	66	60

[a] All patencies are expressed as percentages; all series published since 1981.

Table 12.3 *Below-knee femoropopliteal grafts*

	1 month	6 months	1 year	2 years	3 years	4 years
Patency[a]						
Primary						
Reverse saphenous vein	98	90	84	79	78	77
In situ vein bypass	95	87	80	76	73	68
Secondary						
In situ vein bypass	97	96	96	89	86	81
Arm vein	97		83	83	73	70
Human umbilical vein	88	82	77	70	61	60
PTFE	96	80	68	61	44	40
Limb salvage						
Reverse saphenous vein	100	92	90	88	86	75
In situ vein bypass	97	96	94	84	83	

[a] All patencies are expressed as percentages; all series published since 1981.

Table 12.4 *Infrapopliteal grafts*

	1 month	6 months	1 year	2 years	3 years	4 years
Patency[a]						
Primary						
Reverse saphenous vein	92	81	77	70	66	62
In situ vein bypass	94	84	82	76	74	68
Secondary						
Reverse saphenous vein	93	89	84	80	78	76
In situ vein bypass	95	90	89	87	84	81
Arm vein	94		73	62	58	
Human umbilical vein	80	65	52	46	40	37
PTFE	89	58	46	32		21
Limb salvage						
Reverse saphenous vein	95	88	85	83	82	82
In situ vein bypass	96		91	88	83	83
PTFE		76	68	60	56	48

[a] All patencies are expressed as percentages; all series published since 1981.

Table 12.5 *At or below-ankle grafts*

Patency[a]	1 month	6 months	1 year	2 years	3 years
Primary					
Reverse saphenous vein	95	85	81		
Secondary					
Reverse saphenous vein	96	90	85	81	76
In situ vein bypass	93	93	92	82	72
Foot salvage	99	94	93	87	84

[a] All patencies are expressed as percentages; all series published since 1981.

Table 12.6 *Miscellaneous data*

Patency[a]	1 month	6 months	1 year	2 years	3 years	4 years	5 years
Grafts with proximal anastomosis at the common femoral artery							
Primary	93	83	80	78	78	78	
Secondary	95	91	86	82	80	80	
Grafts with proximal anastomosis distal to the common femoral artery							
Primary	97	89	83	79	75	74	73
Secondary	100	96	90	86	80		
Reoperation							
All grafts[b]		90	80	65	55	45	
Primary autogenous vein	96	82	79	71	62	57	57
Primary PTFE	100	62	42	28			34
All autogenous grafts							
Patients with diabetes mellitus			90		82		77
Patients without diabetes mellitus			88		78		72
Foot salvage after grafting							
Patients with diabetes mellitus			87		85		
Patients without diabetes mellitus			96		93		
Common femoral endarterectomy and superficial femoral endarterectomy		86	78	73	70		
Common femoral endarterectomy	97		97	97	97	94	
Survival with claudication							88
Survival with bypass for limb salvage	97	97	92	86	76	68	64

[a] All patencies are expressed as percentages; all series published since 1981.
[b] All grafts, all conduits, irrespective of number of operations required to maintain patency.

(PTFE), available evidence concerning the performance of cryopreserved vein grafts does not support their preferential use to PTFE, except in situations where compromised wound sterility or frank sepsis would make selection of a prosthetic graft ill-advised.[15]

Substantially extended experience with pedal bypass procedures, primarily performed in diabetic patients has been reported by Logerfo and associates in Boston.[16] Many if not most contemporary series now report a significant number of such procedures, in striking contrast to our report of 1991, when only three references reporting such procedures were available. Based on the advocacy of the Boston group, the perception of the diabetic patient as a poor operative candidate due to the presence of 'small vessel disease' has evolved into the recognition that preserved plantar or dorsal pedal arteries are frequently present and represent excellent run-off beds. Concerns regarding the appropriate role of limb revascularization surgery in older patients have tempered enthusiasm regarding such procedures as well. Despite the obvious drawbacks associated with amputation, many surgeons have been reluctant to consider infrainguinal revascularization procedures for patients in their eighth and ninth decades. However, growing experience with safe and effective procedures in these patients, as recently reported by Nehler and associates[17] suggests that considerations of age as the sole or most significant determinant of operative candidacy are not supported by available experience.

In conclusion, current outcome standards following lower extremity revascularization represent the evolution of surgical skill, imaging technology, standards of anesthetic care, and the adaptation of rigorous reporting standards for patency, limb salvage and survival. The ultimate outcome indicators, including blood flow augmentation, precise wound healing and quality of life indices are as of yet undeveloped. Only by adherence to precise reporting standards can objective determinations of outcome and comparison of techniques be accomplished. Outcome data are increasingly relevant in the era of managed care, when health maintenance organizations and other providers are examining all aspects of charges and costs, and the effectiveness and durability of any form of intervention is becoming paramount. Indeed, the decade-old attempt to standardize outcome, developed at a time when controversies were limited primarily to the primacy of autogenous or venous conduit, is paying handsome dividends in the minimalist medical environment of the 1990s. Continued progress in the outcome of limb salvage procedures is dependent on rigorous and rigid adherence to accepted reporting standards.

REFERENCES

1 Gibbons GW, Burgess AM, Guadagnoli E *et al*. Return to well being and function after infrainguinal revascularization. *J Vasc Surg* 1995; **21**: 35–45.

2 Hertzer NR. Presidential address: Outcome assessment in vascular surgery – Results mean everything. *J Vasc Surg* 1995; **21**: 6–14.

3 Debatin IF, Dalman RL, Herflcens RJ, Harris EJ, Pelc NJ. Phase contrast MRI assessment of pedal blood flow. *Eur Radiol* 1995; **5**: 36–42.

4 Rutherford RB, Flanigan DP, Gupta SK *et al*. Suggested standards for reports dealing with lower extremity ischemia. *J Vasc Surg* 1986; **4**: 80–94.

5 Rutherford RB, Flanigan DP, Gupta SK *et al*. Suggested standards for reports dealing with lower extremity ischemia. *J Vasc Surg* 1986; **4**: 83.

6 Ahn SS, Rutherford RB, Becker GJ *et al*. Reporting standards for lower extremity arterial endovascular procedures. *J Vasc Surg* 1993; **17**: 1103–7.

7 Rutherford RB. Presidential address: Vascular surgery – comparing outcomes. *J Vasc Surg* 1996; **23**: 5–17.

8 Peto R, Pike MC, Armiage P *et al*. Design and analysis of randomized trials requiring prolonged observations of each patient. I. Introduction and design. *Br J Cancer* 1976; **34**: 585–612.

9 Peto R, Pike MC, Armiage P *et al*. Design and analysis of randomized trials requiring prolonged observations of each patient. II. Analysis and examples. *Br J Cancer* **35**: 1–39.

10 Underwood CG, Charlesworth D. Uses and abuses of life table analysis in vascular surgery. *Br J Surg* 1984; **71**: 495–8.

11 Dalman RL, Taylor LM Jr. Basic data related to infrainguinal revascularization procedures. In: Porter JM, Taylor LM Jr eds *Basic data underlying clinical decision making in vascular surgery*. St Louis: Quality Medical Publishing, Inc., 1994.

12 Nehler MR, Moneta GL, Yeager RA *et al*. Surgical treatment of threatened reversed infrainguinal vein grafts. *J Vasc Surg* 1994; **20**: 558–63.

13 Quinones-Baldrich WJ, Prego AA, Ucelay-Gomez R *et al*. Long term results of infrainguinal revascularization with polytetrafluoroethylene: a ten-year experience. *J Vasc Surg* 1992; **16**: 209–17.

14 Holzenbein TJ, Pomposelli FB Jr., Miller A *et al*. Results of a policy with arm veins used as the first alternative to an unavailable ipsilateral greater saphenous vein for infrainguinal bypass. *J Vasc Surg* 1996; **23**: 130–40.

15 Walker PJ, Mitchell RS, McFadden PM *et al*. Early experience with cryopreserved saphenous vein allografts as a conduit for complex limb salvage procedures. *J Vasc Surg* 1993; **18**: 561–8.

16 Pomposelli FB Jr., Maraccio EJ, Gibbons GW *et al*. Dorsalis pedis arterial bypass; durable limb salvage for foot ischemia in patients with diabetes mellitus. *J Vasc Surg* 1995; **21**: 375–84.

17 Nehler MR, Moneta GL, Edwards JM *et al*. Surgery for chronic LE ischemia in patients eighty or more years of age: operative results and assessment of post-operative independence. *J Vasc Surg* 1993; **18**: 618–24.

13

Pathobiology, detection and treatment of vein graft stenosis

JOSEPH L MILLS AND CHRISTOPHER L WIXON

INTRINSIC STENOSES

Intrinsic stenoses develop and threaten patency in 25–30 per cent of infrainguinal autogenous grafts placed for the treatment of chronic lower extremity occlusive disease. In order to optimize limb-salvage rates, the vascular surgeon must be ever-vigilant against the insidious development of such defects by performing graft surveillance. When lesions reach hemodynamic significance, one must humbly acknowledge the graft imperfection and rescue the failing conduit.

Myointimal hyperplasia was first suggested by Alexis Carrel in 1906, when he described, 'a glistening thickened surface covering the anastomotic suture several days after construction of an arterial anastomosis'.[1] The significance of this observation, however, was not recognized for more than 60 years, when the first reports appeared in the literature implicating myointimal hyperplasia as the cause of failure of an autogenous bypass.[2,3] This suspicion was elegantly confirmed in a landmark clinical study by Szilagyi, who demonstrated by serial angiography the development and progression of such intrinsic structural defects in nearly one-third of 377 patients in whom lower extremity vein conduits had been implanted.[4]

Since the report of Szilagyi, significant progress has been made in screening methods to detect lower extremity bypass graft stenosis and the duplex scanner has replaced more invasive methods. Unfortunately, similar progress in the treatment of such lesions has not been

achieved. Currently, the mainstay of treatment is surgical excision with graft interposition or patch angioplasty. Recent enthusiasm for catheter-based therapies has been met with mixed reviews and the promise of local brachytherapy has yet to be fulfilled. When these therapies are viewed in the context of the recent quantum leaps made in the field of vascular biology, they appear remarkably primitive. As such, a brief consideration of the pathobiology of intimal hyperplasia is pertinent prior to discussing methods of detection and treatment of vein graft lesions.

PATHOBIOLOGY OF INTIMAL HYPERPLASIA

Arterialization and myointimal hyperplasia

Since the 1930s, the medial smooth muscle cell has been recognized as the dominant cell of myointimal hyperplasia.[5–7] During embryogenesis, the vascular smooth muscle cell possesses a cellular ultrastructure similar to the fibroblast: an extensive rough endoplasmic reticulum, a prominent Golgi complex and few contractile elements.[8,9] These cells proliferate and lay down the extracellular matrix proteins that provide the necessary scaffolding upon which the vessel develops into its mature form.[10] At the conclusion of the developmental phase, the phenotypically synthetic (immature) vascular smooth muscle cells lose their synthetic organelles and acquire a highly organized pattern of contractile myofilaments.[8,9] These contractile (mature) smooth muscle cells are arranged in concentric layers within a matrix of connective tissue in the media and are the dominant phenotype found in the media of a healthy artery and vein. The intima of the vessel consists of a single layer of endothelial cells resting on a thin basal lamina. These endothelial cells respond to mechanical, chemical and humoral changes, and act as mediators of underlying smooth muscle cells by releasing growth-promoting and inhibitory factors.

The governing theory of vein graft remodeling and intimal hyperplasia after injury may hinge on the ability of the vascular smooth muscle cell (SMC) to shift back and forth between the contractile and synthetic states (Fig. 13.1). This process has been characterized as *phenotypic modulation* and occurs in response to an alteration in the smooth muscle cell milieu (e.g. varying shear stress, loss of contact inhibition, changing basement membrane composition, influence of cytokines).[11] Smooth muscle cell phenotypic modulation is fundamentally important and occurs as a normal component of vascular healing after a graded injury (Table 13.1).

Like the phases of wound healing, the phases of vessel healing have been well described (at least in animal models), and occur in an orderly process with hyperacute, acute and chronic phases.[12] The *hyperacute phase* begins shortly after injury and consists of endothelial denudation, mural aggregation of platelets and release of multiple trophic factors. These intimal changes signal a subpopulation of underlying medial smooth muscle cells to transform from the quiescent contractile phenotype to the immature, synthetic phenotype. The *acute phase* lasts from hours to 6–12 weeks, and is characterized by organization of thrombus in the vessel lumen, regrowth of endothelial cells and release of various cytokines (trophic and inhibitory). In this same interval, changes also occur in the vessel wall and include medial smooth muscle cell migration across the internal elastic lamina, intense smooth muscle cell proliferation and continued synthesis of growth regulators. In addition, there appears to be infiltration of leucocytes in this acute phase. During the *chronic phase*, which lasts weeks to months, re-endothelialization of the vessel lumen occurs with reduced levels of intimal smooth muscle cell proliferation but persistent synthesis of extracellular matrix proteins by the smooth muscle cells.

The sequence of vascular injury, followed by smooth muscle cell phenotypic modulation, migration from the media to the intima, proliferation and deposition of extracellular matrix proteins characterizes the process of vein graft adaptation to arterialization and myointimal hyperplasia (Figs 13.2 and 13.3).

What remains unclear, however, is whether the area of stenosis, associated with focal myointimal hyperplasia, represents an abnormal response to a graded vascular injury (keloid theory), or whether the process represents the normal reparative or wound healing process in a region of excessive injury.[13] Many previous reports have failed to differentiate between the normal reparative process occurring after vascular interventions, and the pathologic process that results in progressive myointimal hyperplasia and the development of flow reducing stenoses. It is important to note that most vein grafts, despite their long length, develop only solitary stenoses at focal sites either adjacent to the anastomoses or at valve sites. Thus the process of arterialization itself does not seem sufficient to cause pathologic lesions and other processes must contribute, such as hemodynamic factors, valve sites, pre-existing conduit abnormalities or nonjudicious vein harvest technique.

Table 13.1 *Grades of arterial injury*

Grade I	Injury occurs as a result of changing mural shear stress and results in only functional alteration of endothelial and smooth muscle cells
Grade II	Injury represents endothelial denudation without damage to the underlying media (occurs with arterialization of a vein graft)
Grade III	Injury involves endothelial denudation and extensive intimal and medial injury (occurs following endarterectomy, angioplasty, areas of valve lysis and perianastomotic regions)

Signaling

The literature is replete with reports describing stimuli for vascular smooth muscle cell activation. Potential mechanisms include loss of the inhibitory effects of the endothelium, the local production of growth factors, platelet degranulation and loss of contact inhibition. Although the precise mechanisms and factors responsible for the induction of smooth muscle cell activation and suppression are incompletely understood in humans, they remain critical to our understanding of

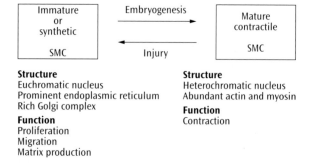

Figure 13.1 *Smooth muscle cell phenotypic modulation.*

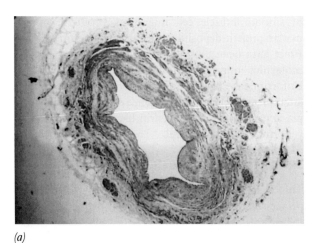
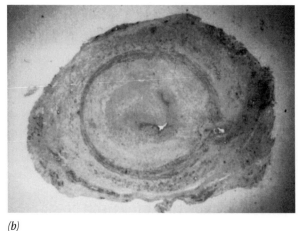

(a)   *(b)*

Figure 13.2 *(a) Hematoxylin and eosin (H&E) stain of a normal saphenous vein prior to implantation into the arterial circulation. There is moderate medial thickening present in this vein, a typical finding in grossly normal saphenous veins obtained from older patients used for bypass. (b) H&E stain of a cross-section obtained from a human vein graft stenosis. Note the extremely small, crescentic, residual lumen in the center of the specimen and the exuberant myointimal thickening resulting in pathologic vein graft stenosis. This figure also appears in the colour plate section.*

myointimal hyperplasia. While an extensive discussion of the proposed mechanisms that signal myointimal hyperplasia is beyond the scope of this chapter, a basic understanding of the trophic and inhibitory growth factors is necessary prior to understanding the basis of potentially novel treatment approaches. Important trophic and inhibiting growth factors include those shown in Table 13.2

In vitro and *in vivo* studies in both humans and animals confirm the importance of a number of cell types – and their products – in the process of arterialization and the development of myointimal hyperplasia.[14] These include the platelet, macrophage, endothelial cell, fibroblasts and the smooth muscle cell.

Table 13.2 *Important trophic and inhibiting growth factors*

Trophic growth factors	Inhibitory factors
Platelet-derived growth factor (PDGF)	Nitric oxide (EDRF)
Insulin-like growth factor-1 (IGF-1)	Heparan sulfates
Fibroblast growth factor (FGF)	Transforming growth factor-β (TGF-β)

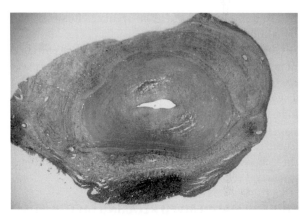

Figure 13.3 *Pentochrome stain of a cross-section of vein graft stenosis specimen showing very narrow lumen and exuberant extracellular matrix deposition resulting in pathologic vein graft stenosis. This focal lesion was detected by duplex surveillance 6 months following graft implantation. This figure also appears in the colour plate section.*

PLATELET-DERIVED GROWTH FACTOR (PDGF)

This is a growth promoter that is produced in several isoforms by vascular smooth muscle cells, endothelial cells and activated platelets.[15] The isoform secreted by the platelet (PDGF-BB) appears to have the highest affiliation for the smooth muscle cell and is therefore of primary importance.[16] PDGF serves both as a chemoattractant and a mitogen for smooth muscle cells and fibroblasts, and *in vivo* infusion of PDGF-BB has resulted in accelerated smooth muscle cell migration.[17] Likewise, application of anti-PDGF antibodies in a porcine model of balloon angioplasty demonstrated a 40 per cent reduction in intimal thickening.[18] This observation has led to the possible clinical application of monoclonal platelet glycoprotein blocking agents, the GPIIb-IIIa inhibitors, which are now in clinical use following percutaneous coronary balloon angioplasty. Studies indicate their use reduces the incidence of early failure after coronary angioplasty and stenting, but it is not clear that this approach reduces the incidence of intermediate and long-term restenosis.[19]

INSULIN-LIKE GROWTH FACTOR-1 (IGF-1)

Expression of the IGF-1 gene in the vascular smooth muscle cell increases almost tenfold within 1 week after vessel injury.[20] IGF-1 has several effects and appears to amplify the effect of PDGF on smooth muscle cell proliferation as well as to stimulate the maturation of collagen fibers by augmenting the production of hydroxyproline.[21]

FIBROBLAST GROWTH FACTORS (FGF)

These are a group of heparin-binding factors synthesized by both the vascular smooth muscle cell and the endothelial cell, and stored in the extracellular matrix.[22] After vessel injury, basic FGF (bFGF) is released and initiates proliferation of both endothelial and smooth muscle cells. This factor also is important in the regulation of extracellular matrix deposition. Infusion of bFGF in animal models results in increased intimal hyperplasia and bFGF receptors appear to be up-regulated following balloon injury.[23,24]

Our group has demonstrated increased concentration of macrophages in areas of focal myointimal hyperplasia harvested from human infrainguinal bypass grafts.[25] These cells synthesize and release a large number of biologically potent molecules including interleukins, adhesive glycoproteins, prostaglandins and leukotrienes. These substances are formed from arachidonic acid via the cyclooxygenase and lipoxygenase pathways, and play important roles in inflammatory states.

ENDOTHELIAL-DERIVED RELAXING FACTOR (EDRF)

Perhaps the most well-recognized cytokine is the growth-inhibitor, EDRF. We now recognize this compound to be synonymous with nitric oxide. Nitric oxide is synthesized from the conversion of L-arginine to citrulline by either constituent or inducible nitric oxide synthase (c-NOS and I-NOS). Under normal conditions, tonic release of nitric oxide from the endothelial cell offers several inhibitory effects: vascular smooth muscle relaxation, inhibition of platelet aggregation, and inhibition smooth muscle cell proliferation. Following endothelial cell damage, these tonic inhibitory effects may be lost and indirectly lead to smooth muscle cell proliferation and intimal hyperplasia. Oral administration of L-arginine has demonstrated a more rapid restoration of endothelial-dependent relaxation, which can be completely antagonized by the NOS-antagonist, L-NAME (N^G-nitro- L-arginine methyl ester).[26,27]

HEPARAN SULFATES

These are synthesized in the endothelial cells, localized on the cell surface membranes and are known inhibitors of smooth muscle cell migration, proliferation and matrix protein deposition. Several mechanisms for this effect have been proposed which suggest that heparin molecules oppose the mitogenic effects of FGF.[28] Unfortunately, despite this theoretical activity, clinical attempts to decrease the incidence of myointimal hyperplasia using heparin or heparin-like molecules have not yet proven clinically useful.

TRANSFORMING GROWTH FACTOR-β (TGF-β)

This is activated from its latent form by plasmin, and provides negative feedback inhibition by inducing plasminogen activator inhibitor. TGF-β is interesting in that it is reported to possess both a trophic and inhibitory effect. *In vitro*, it has been shown to inhibit smooth muscle cell migration and proliferation, but appears to stimulate the production and stabilization of matrix proteins.[29] Hence, TGF-β may play an important role during the chronic phase of vessel healing.

Many other cytokines are proposed to exert either trophic or inhibitory effects on the vascular smooth muscle cell. These include vasoactive peptides (catecholamines and angiotensin II), products of inflammation (tumor necrosis factor, interleukins), matrix proteins (fibronectin, laminin) and polyamines. Indeed, smooth muscle cell activation remains a highly complex and controversial topic. In addition to smooth muscle cell activation and proliferation, the control and regulation of matrix deposition is critically important.[30] Despite 30 years of intense basic science research, the clinical goal of preventing intimal hyperplasia remains elusive. A multitude of agents have been suggested, including antiplatelet agents, anti-inflammatory agents, antioxidants, calcium channel blockers, anticoagulants, gene therapy, as well as more recently antisense oligonucleotides. To date, none of these therapies has significantly reduced the development of clinically significant intimal hyperplasia. The clinician, despite abundant scientific knowledge, is thus left with the burdensome chore of identifying grafts at risk for the development of myointimal hyperplasia, grading the severity of such lesions and intervening prior to the occurrence of vein graft occlusion.

SIGNIFICANCE OF VEIN GRAFT STENOSIS

Concerns over limited resources have caused healthcare providers and third-party payers to evaluate the durability of specific interventional and surgical procedures more critically. These issues will gain further importance as the aging population places increasing financial demands on the available resources. When such issues are considered in the context of myointimal hyperplasia after vascular intervention, there is certainly ample cause for concern. Following angioplasty, the restenosis rate is

Colour plates

These illustrations also appear in the text in black and white

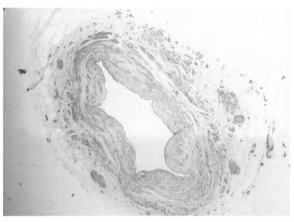
(a)

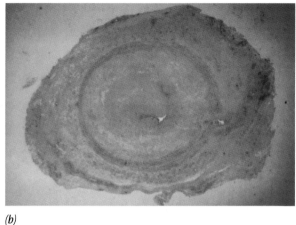
(b)

Plate 1 *(Figure 13.2) (a) Hematoxylin and eosin (H&E) stain of a normal saphenous vein prior to implantation into the arterial circulation. There is moderate medial thickening present in this vein, a typical finding in grossly normal saphenous veins obtained from older patients used for bypass. (b) H&E stain of a cross-section obtained from a human vein graft stenosis. Note the extremely small, crescentic, residual lumen in the center of the specimen and the exuberant myointimal thickening resulting in pathologic vein graft stenosis.*

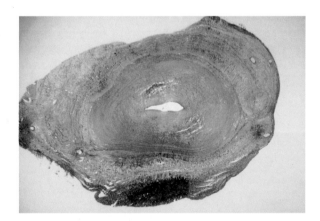

Plate 2 *(Figure 13.3) Pentochrome stain of a cross-section of vein graft stenosis specimen showing very narrow lumen and exuberant extracellular matrix deposition resulting in pathologic vein graft stenosis. This focal lesion was detected by duplex surveillance 6 months following graft implantation.*

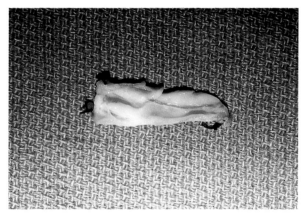

Plate 3 *(Figure 13.4) Longitudinally opened section of abnormal saphenous vein segment identified during intraoperative vein graft preparation. Sclerotic valve leaflets with a strand of hemosiderin deposition are noted, probably due to previous localized thrombophlebitis which later recanalized. This segment of vein was identified by observing segmental lack of distension in an otherwise normal-appearing conduit.*

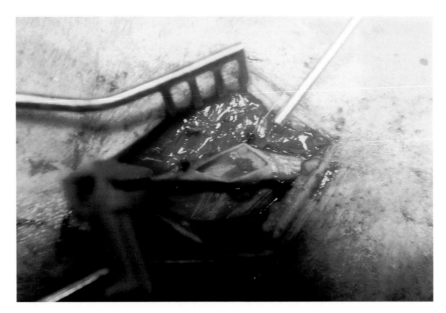

Plate 4 *(Figure 13.5) This patient developed hemodynamic failure of a femorotibial bypass graft 48 hours after surgery. The patient was returned to the operating room and intraoperative arteriography demonstrated a filling defect in the mid-graft. The lesion was exposed through a short longitudinal incision and the flow disturbance was identified by hand-held Doppler. The vein was opened longitudinally and extensive platelet deposition was identified at the site of an otherwise normal valve leaflet. The valve leaflets were excised, a vein patch angioplasty performed and the patient was anticoagulated.*

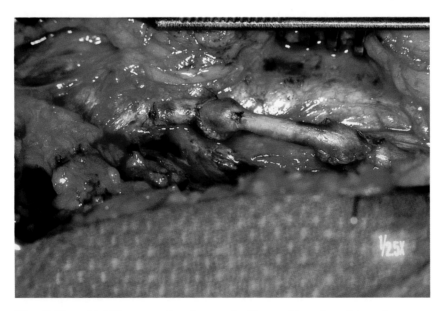

Plate 5 *(Figure 13.10) Intraoperative photograph of interposition vein graft to replace a longer segment graft stenosis. Anastomoses are spatulated to prevent napkin-ring-like restenosis.*

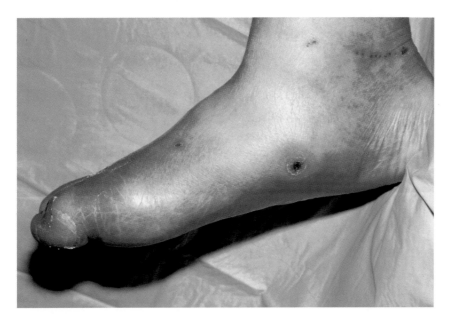

Plate 6 *(Figure 14.2) Charcot foot deformity with mid-foot collapse.*

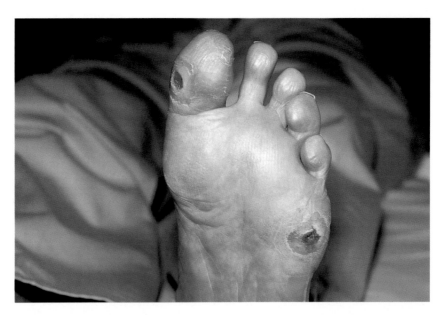

Plate 7 *(Figure 14.4) Neuropathic ulcers at pressure points of the first interphalangeal and fifth metatarsophalangeal joints.*

as high as 30–50 per cent within 6 months to a year, particularly in the coronary circulation. Lower rates of restenosis, ranging from 20 to 30 per cent appear to occur after placement of autogenous vein grafts for lower extremity arterial occlusive disease over a 2–3-year period following implantation.[31–33]

Without question, the most significant advance in vascular diagnostic imaging in the last quarter century has been the development of the duplex scanner. It has become the most effective screening test for carotid occlusive disease, and in many centers serves as the sole routine preoperative study for the evaluation of patients with carotid artery stenosis. Duplex scanning has also had a significant impact on postoperative surveillance of infrainguinal vein grafts.[34–40]

Early failure (<30 days) after infrainguinal bypass has generally been attributed to technical or judgmental error, intermediate failure (30 days to 3 years) ascribed to myointimal hyperplasia and late failure (>3 years) has been attributed to recurrent atherosclerosis.[31] In an important study, Szilagyi and associates noted that grafts at risk could be identified by following the progression of focal regions of stenosis using serial angiography.[4] Certain fibrotic, intrinsic graft lesions tended to progress to hemodynamic significance and ultimately cause graft thrombosis. Long-term studies following infrainguinal vein bypass demonstrate that at least 60 per cent of all failures are due to intrinsic graft stenosis within the conduit or its anastomoses.[41,42] A smaller, but significant percentage of grafts develop progressive inflow or outflow disease which may lead to altered graft hemodynamics, low flow velocities and ultimate bypass graft thrombosis. Prior to the advent of the duplex scanner, however, the only way to identify these lesions was by serial arteriography. Unfortunately, routine arteriography was too invasive and expensive to qualify as an effective screening tool, and the first reports of noninvasive methods using duplex surveillance did not appear until the mid-1980s. Subsequently, the application of duplex scanning rapidly evolved into the gold standard for postoperative surveillance.

The efficacy of duplex surveillance is based on the following premises:

1 vein graft failure most often results from the development of intrinsic graft stenosis;
2 high-grade vein graft stenosis leads to graft thrombosis if the lesion is not revised;
3 vein graft stenosis is frequently clinically silent and not reliably detectable prior to the onset of graft occlusion by either history, physical examination or simple noninvasive study;
4 vein graft stenosis and low flow states can be accurately identified, graded and monitored for progression by duplex surveillance;
5 prophylactic revision of patent, but failing vein grafts yields results greatly superior to those obtained following either thrombolysis or thrombectomy and revision of occluded vein grafts;
6 vein graft patency and limb salvage rates are significantly improved by a program of postoperative duplex surveillance.

Although duplex surveillance of infrainguinal bypass grafts has become widely accepted and likely improves the primary assisted patency rates of infrainguinal bypass grafts by 15–20 per cent,[32,36,39] the optimal frequency and intensity of graft surveillance remains controversial. Several authors have advocated that routine surveillance be discontinued after 1 year,[43–45] while others recommend that graft surveillance be continued indefinitely.[46,47] Convincing data now exist to support meticulous, long-term postoperative duplex surveillance of both reversed vein and *in situ* conduits following infrainguinal revascularization.[48,49] There are no existing data to support duplex surveillance of nonautogenous prosthetic grafts, however.

INCIDENCE OF POSTOPERATIVE GRAFT STENOSIS

Over a decade of experience with postoperative vein graft surveillance currently exists. The incidence of duplex-identified graft stenosis varies from 12 to 37 per cent, with the precise figure depending on the threshold criteria used to define graft stenosis (Table 13.3). Of the stenoses identified in these studies, the majority developed within the first year of implantation. Nevertheless, after this early peak in graft stenosis there is an ongoing persistent, although lower rate of graft stenosis, which mandates lifelong graft surveillance.[47] Finally, the natural course of vein graft stenosis is clearly evident from the data in Table 13.3; the majority of grafts bearing high-grade stenosis (>70 per cent) eventually occlude.

There is now substantial evidence suggesting that vein grafts that thrombose prior to a surgical revision have significantly reduced cumulative patency (Table 13.4. See p. 121). The reason for this is multifactorial but is almost certainly related to the endothelial damage resulting from the thrombotic event itself.

DETECTION AND GRADING OF GRAFT STENOSIS

It is our opinion that graft surveillance consists of multiple components. We presently obtain a graft surveillance study within the first 1–2 weeks after graft implantation, repeat a study 6 weeks postoperatively and then obtain studies every 3 months for the first year and every 6 months thereafter. After the third year, studies are obtained annually.[56] A complete graft surveillance study

Table 13.3 *Time course and natural history of vein grafts stenoses*

Author	Number of grafts with stenoses/total grafts (mean follow-up)	Time course of identification of stenosis	Outcome
Grigg (1988)[34]	19/75 (1 year)	89% within 6 months	65% of grafts with stenoses occluded versus 7% of nondiseased grafts
Moody (1990)[35]	22/80 (13 months)	94% within 6 months	22.7% of grafts with stenoses occluded 6.9% of nondiseased grafts occluded
Buth (1991)[36]	43/116 (2 years)	81% within 1 year	47% of grafts with stenoses occluded 0% of nondiseased grafts occluded
Nielsen (1993)[37]	15/16 (3 months)		63% of grafts with stenoses occluded 6% of nondiseased grafts occluded
Idu (1993)[38]	58/201 (21 months)	21% within 3 months 28% 3–6 months 6% 6–12 months	39% of grafts with stenoses occluded
Mattos (1993)[39]	62/170 (39 months)	77% within first year 95% within first 2 years	26% of grafts with stenoses occluded 9% of nondiseased grafts occluded

should consist of the following. (1) The ankle–brachial index pressures are measured. In the absence of calcified vessels, hemodynamically significant improvement and normal hemodynamics should be expected. In addition toe pressures are frequently obtained, especially if the ankle pressures are unreliable due to medial calcinosis. (2) The adjacent inflow artery, the entire graft and its anastomosis, and the adjacent outflow artery are scanned in their entirety with color flow duplex surveillance. Depending on the depth of the graft, longitudinal color Doppler imaging of the complete reconstruction should be performed with either a 5.0 or 7.5 MHz linear array probe. Representative center stream velocity spectra should be recorded at multiple graft segments with careful examination of the anastomotic regions of the vein graft. Velocity spectra measurements should be made at a Doppler angle of 60 or less. If a focal color flow disturbance (i.e. mosaic color pattern) or 'flow jet' is noted at any site, careful interrogation with measurement of peak systolic velocity (V_p) and velocity ratio (V_r) should be performed. A V_p that exceeds 150 cm/s and a V_r greater than 1.5 are abnormal. These sites should be noted on early postoperative flow scans and followed by detailed surveillance.[40] It is our opinion, supported by data from other centers, that early postoperative scans are extremely important because they allow the stratification of vein grafts into high- and low-risk groups.[56] If a graft harbors a detectable lesion within the first 3 months, there is a 45 per cent requirement for subsequent graft revision. These lesions are frequently rapidly progressive and need close follow-up. If the early graft scan is abnormal, we would follow this graft every 6 weeks until either the lesion resolves, which occurs approximately 30 per cent of the time, the lesion stabilizes (20 per cent), or the lesion progresses to require

revision (40–50 per cent). Multiple criteria have been described for grading vein graft stenosis.[32,33,35,53,56–60] We believe the simplest utilize the velocity ratio and the peak systolic velocity. A velocity ratio greater than 1.5 is abnormal. Generally, lesions with a velocity ratio of greater than 3.5 or a peak systolic velocity greater than 300 cm/s should be repaired.[61]

In addition to measurements of peak systolic velocity and velocity ratios, careful analysis of duplex-derived graft waveforms, as well as assessments of global flow velocity are important. If the graft waveforms are triphasic, we generally follow identified lesions associated with flow disturbances. In fact, we have observed a modest number of lesions that approach threshold criteria for repair based on V_p and V_r measurements. Nevertheless, if the waveforms remain triphasic and the ankle brachial index normal, we have followed these lesions closely and have been rewarded on occasion with regression of a lesion that would have otherwise met criteria for repair.

After infrainguinal bypass surgery, a spectrum of clinically unsuspected abnormalities may be present in the conduit. These include retained valves, fibrotic valves, or stenotic or sclerotic vein segments. In addition, there may be lesions in the adjacent arteries, such as clamp injury or endarterectomy endpoint problems, or anastomotic defects associated with intimal lesions or suture stenosis. All these may reduce graft flow and precipitate graft thrombosis, or they may act as a nidus for the development of progressive intimal hyperplasia. It is our opinion that serial postoperative duplex surveillance allows one to detect and monitor such lesions and follow them for progression. Meticulous surveillance is important early because these early-appearing lesions are often rapidly progressive and will lead to early graft occlusion in the first 3–6 months if not repaired.[56,60,62–64]

Table 13.4 *Outcome of graft revision preceded by graft occlusion*

Author	Number of failed grafts	Outcome
Whittemore (1981)[50]	109	19% cumulative patency at 5 years
Sladen (1981)[51]	13	23% cumulative patency at 1 year 46% amputation rate
Cohen (1986)[52]	25	28% cumulative patency at 5 years
Green (1986)[53]	75	33% cumulative patency at 1 year 26% cumulative patency at 3 years
Graor (1988)[54]	60	20% cumulative patency at 1 year
Belkin (1990)[55]	22	37% cumulative patency at 1 year
Donaldson (1992)[42]	40	23% cumulative patency at 3 years 22% cumulative patency at 2 years

Vein graft stenoses and their associated risk of graft occlusion can be stratified in the following manner (Table 13.5). The highest risk group for graft occlusion (Category I) is characterized by a V_r greater than 3.5 and/or a V_p greater than 300 cm/s associated with a diminution of distal graft flow velocity (i.e. low flow graft) such that the distal graft flow is less than 45 cm/s as well as ankle–brachial diminution exceeding 0.15. These lesions are high grade and associated with low graft flows. These patients should be admitted to the hospital, heparinized and the lesion promptly repaired. Category II are lesions with high V_p values (greater than 300 cm/s) and V_r values of greater than 3.5, but with normal graft flow velocities and normal ankle–brachial pressure measurements. If the graft waveforms were previously triphasic and have become abnormal or certainly if there is any drop in ankle–brachial indices indicating hemodynamic significance, we would recommend repair. In carefully selected patients with borderline velocities for repair in whom the graft waveforms are still triphasic and the ankle–brachial indices have not changed, we perform serial scans every 4–6 weeks until hemodynamic deterioration is detected. Category III grafts exhibit lesions with V_p values between 150 and 300 cm/s and V_r values less than 3 and are monitored with 6-weekly graft surveillance studies to rule out progression. In our experience, approximately half of these lesions will stabilize or resolve, thus close follow-up avoids unnecessary arteriography and unnecessary revision surgery. However, in approximately 40 per cent of patients with such lesions, progression will occur and require repair. Category IV is the lowest risk group and it includes patients who have normal ankle–brachial indices, and no lesions on graft duplex surveillance and normal waveforms. The incidence of graft occlusion in patients with such studies is less than 2 per cent over a 6–12 month period.[53,56]

Table 13.5

Category	High velocity criteria	Low velocity criteria	Δ ABI
Category I (highest risk)	V_p >300 cm/s or V_r >3.5	GFV < 45 cm/s or	> 0.15
Category II (high risk)	V_p >300 cm/sec or V_r >3.5	GFV > 45 cm/s and	< 0.15
Category III (intermediate risk)	150 < V_p >300 cm/s and/or V_r >2.0	GFV > 45 cm/s and	< 0. 15
Category IV (low risk)	V_p < 150 cm/s	GFV > 45 cm/s and	<0. 15

ABI = ankle–brachial index, GFV = graft flow velocity. Δ = change in ABI.

DISTRIBUTION OF GRAFT LESIONS AND RECOMMENDATIONS FOR REPAIR

Sixty to seventy per cent of vein graft failures in the first 5 postoperative years occur due to intrinsic graft stenosis. We generally favor operative revision of these lesions, particularly if they occur within the first 1–2 years postoperatively. We have not been impressed with the long-term results of balloon angioplasty.[52,65,66] Focal fibrotic circumferential lesions require excision and can be handled with interposition vein graft replacement when they are in the mid-graft. Selected mid-graft lesions can be treated with excision of the fibrotic valve leaflet and vein patch angioplasty. Although controversial,[67] in our experience, nearly all mid-graft lesions represent retained or sclerotic valve leaflets.[31] Focal juxta anastomotic lesions usually occur on the venous side of either the distal or proximal anastomosis, and occur with nearly equal frequency at either end of the vein, whether it is used reversed or *in situ*. These lesions usually require resection and replacement either with a vein graft interposition, or the graft can be reimplanted into an alternate inflow site. For example, if the stenosis occurs at the origin of a common femoral to distal bypass graft, the vein can often be mobilized distal to the stenosis and anastomosed to the deep femoral artery, thus sparing the need for further conduit. It is extremely important to document that the repair has restored normal graft hemodynamics either with intraoperative duplex scanning or by completion arteriogram of the repair, as well as a complete evaluation of the rest of the conduit to make sure no additional lesions are present. The presence of a high-grade stenosis, especially in the proximal graft, will frequently mask the presence of other lesions by duplex scanning. Approximately 80 per cent of graft stenoses are solitary, but 20 per cent are associated with synchronous or metachronous lesions; therefore the entire conduit should be evaluated. If a focal lesion has been followed in the vein graft and has progressed to the point where it requires repair, it is acceptable to repair the lesion without preoperative arteriography. However, the entire conduit requires evaluation at the time of graft revision to be sure no other lesions are present. If there is any question about inflow, outflow or multiple graft lesions, preoperative arteriography should be performed.

A successful repair of a graft stenosis restores normal graft flow velocities and normal hemodynamics, and improves the ankle–brachial index if this was abnormal preoperatively. In addition, successful revision operations result in excellent 5-year patency with multiple reports yielding assisted primary patency of over 80 per cent at 5 years.[46,68,69] That is, successfully revised failing grafts approach the patency of unrevised grafts which never developed a lesion. Only one prospective randomized trial[70] has documented that femoral–popliteal or crural vein graft patency is improved by intensive surveillance. However, multiple clinical studies attest to excellent assisted primary patency rates that are vastly superior to reports published prior to the advent of duplex surveillance. It is our current opinion that it would be unethical to subject patients to further randomized prospective trials of vein graft surveillance since there are abundant natural history studies and a prospective randomized trial does exist in literature. It is interesting to note, however, that the prospective randomized trial[70] and all clinical experience indicates that routine surveillance of prosthetic bypass grafts is not beneficial.

NATURAL HISTORY OF VEIN GRAFT LESIONS

Significant natural history data are available that document the graft-threatening potential of high-grade fibrotic graft strictures, as was initially suggested by Szilagyi's serial arteriographic study.[4] Idu, Buth *et al.* demonstrated that all grafts with duplex-detected stenoses greater than 70 per cent diameter reduction occluded if not repaired.[33,38] We presently recommend that all vein grafts be subjected to postoperative graft surveillance. Postoperative graft surveillance includes scanning the adjacent inflow and outflow arteries as well as the entire graft conduit, searching for focal flow abnormalities, documenting global and distal graft flow velocity, analysis of duplex derived Doppler waveforms, ankle–brachial index and frequently toe pressure measurement. Criteria for repair are in evolution, but generally patients who have a significant change in ankle–brachial index, develop a focal V_p of greater than 300 cm/s or a V_r greater than 3.5, and reduce their distal graft flow to less 45 cm/s, if such distal graft flow was normal previously, should be considered for repair. Isolated lesions may be repaired based on duplex scanning only but intraoperative examination of the entire conduit is mandatory if preoperative arteriography is not performed. Early graft scans are critically important. It is well documented that approximately 30 per cent of grafts have abnormalities within them that are either present at the time of graft implantation or develop very early after surgery.[56] It is our impression that early-appearing graft stenoses are much more likely to be malignant and should be monitored closely.[60–64] Nearly half of these lesions will result in progressive, severe hemodynamic abnormalities requiring graft revision. If early graft scans are normal, the incidence of subsequent graft stenosis is lower. After 1 year the intensity of graft surveillance is reduced from every 3 months to every 6 months, and after 3 years, we reduce it to an annual study.

It is also important to note that certain graft configurations are at higher risk for stenosis. A vein graft performed with high-quality greater saphenous vein using either the reversed or *in situ* configuration appears to be at the lowest risk of subsequent graft stenosis. The highest risk grafts include alternate conduits, such as arm vein, spliced lesser and greater saphenous veins, as well as all redo or reoperative distal bypass grafts. It is our practice to perform reoperative surgery by tunneling the alternate vein graft subcutaneously, thus rendering postoperative graft surveillance much easier and allowing ready revision if required, since the graft is superficial. At least 30–40 per cent of arm vein conduits harbor valve or short segment sclerotic defects, which, if unidentified or unrepaired, will result in intermediate term graft occlusion.

TREATMENT OF SPECIFIC GRAFT-THREATENING LESIONS

Pre-existing vein conduit defects

Prevention and treatment of vein graft stenosis begin in the operating room at the time of the primary leg bypass operation. It is very important when the surgeon prepares the vein for implantation, that any significant defects in the vein conduit itself are detected, repaired or replaced at the time of the initial bypass operation. Generally, areas of focal sclerosis in the vein will be identified by careful palpation and observation of lack of distensibility. Figure 13.4 illustrates a segment of vein excised from an otherwise apparently normal vein which contained thickened valve leaflets with a reddish-brown string of hemosiderin deposition, likely resulting from a previous episode of thrombophlebitis. The remainder of the vein distended quite adequately and the vein itself irrigated reasonably well, but this short segment failed to dilate. It was therefore excised and split open revealing a

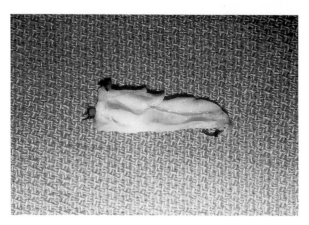

Figure 13.4 *Longitudinally opened section of abnormal saphenous vein segment identified during intraoperative vein graft preparation. Sclerotic valve leaflets with a strand of hemosiderin deposition are noted, probably due to previous localized thrombophlebitis which later recanalized. This segment of vein was identified by observing segmental lack of distension in an otherwise normal-appearing conduit. This figure also appears in the colour plate section.*

significant conduit abnormality. Such lesions can be subtle, but can generally be detected by careful observation and gentle palpation.

Occasionally, in the early postoperative period, a valvular lesion or subtle technical defect will result in platelet deposition and reduce distal graft flow, which can be detected either clinically or by duplex surveillance. Figure 13.5 demonstrates platelet deposition at the site of an apparently normal valve leaflet that resulted in a failing femoral tibial reversed vein bypass graft in the early postoperative period. If this lesion had not been detected, the graft would undoubtedly have thrombosed. Cases such as these in which extensive platelet deposition

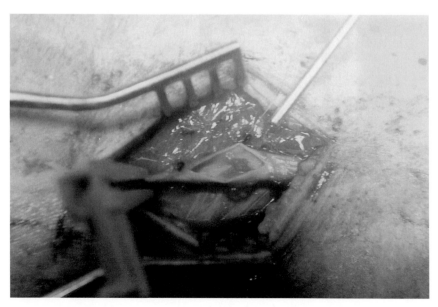

Figure 13.5 *This patient developed hemodynamic failure of a femorotibial bypass graft 48 hours after surgery. The patient was returned to the operating room and intraoperative arteriography demonstrated a filling defect in the mid-graft. The lesion was exposed through a short longitudinal incision and the flow disturbance was identified by hand-held Doppler. The vein was opened longitudinally and extensive platelet deposition was identified at the site of an otherwise normal valve leaflet. The valve leaflets were excised, a vein patch angioplasty performed and the patient was anticoagulated. This figure also appears in the colour plate section.*

develops early on valve lesions lend support to the theory that platelet aggregation and release of platelet-derived growth factors are important in the development of graft lesions.[15,16]

Progressive postoperative vein graft stenosis

Rarely, grafts develop diffuse, extensive, long segment narrowing (<3–5 per cent).[41] If recurrent limb ischemia is present, the entire conduit will require replacement. However, over 80 per cent of graft lesions are single and focal. We have categorized these focal lesions into juxta-anastomotic and midgraft lesions.[31] Juxta-anastomotic lesions occur with nearly equal frequency at both the distal and proximal ends of the vein graft, predominantly on the vein side of the arterial to vein graft anastomosis. These lesions may result from relative size discrepancies between the donor artery and recipient vein, or from flow and shear stress abnormalities in the area of the anastomosis, but their typical location strongly suggests a hemodynamic cause.

Figure 13.6 demonstrates a focal proximal juxta-anastomotic stenosis at the origin of a superficial femoral to posterior tibial bypass graft which was detected by duplex surveillance six months postoperatively. Such a lesion could be repaired by interposition vein grafting, vein patch angioplasty, or proximal anastomotic translocation (Fig. 13.7). The latter procedure is especially useful in situations of limited available vein conduit, when the primary graft originated from the common femoral artery, and when the profunda femoris artery is a large caliber inflow conduit free of lesions. Figure 13.8 is an arteriogram obtained intraoperatively following a proximal anastomotic translocation for a focal high-grade proximal graft stenosis. Although proximal anastomotic graft

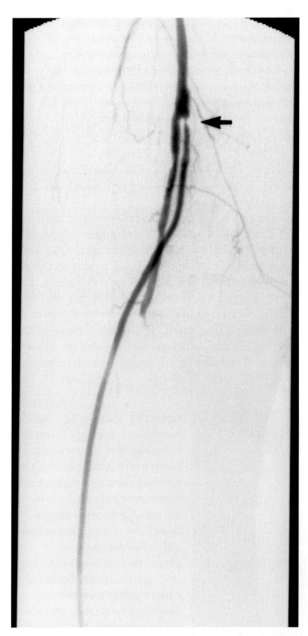

Figure 13.6 *Conventional arteriogram demonstrating a typical, tight, focal, proximal juxta-anastomotic vein graft stenosis (arrow) detected by duplex surveillance 6 months after graft implantation.*

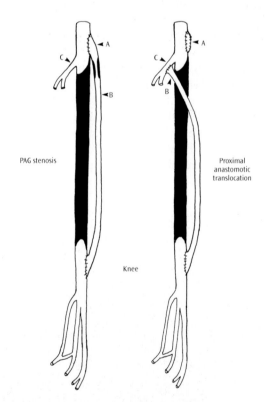

Figure 13.7 *The technique of proximal anastomotic translocation applicable in patients with disease-free deep femoral arteries and proximal (PAG) focal high-grade graft stenosis. The graft may be transected below the site of the stenosis, mobilized and reanastomosed to the deep femoral artery, sparing the need to harvest additional conduit.*

lesions are usually short and focal, they can occur over a longer segment (Fig. 13.9) and in such cases require vein graft interposition (Fig. 13.10). Mid-graft or graft body lesions are frequently focal, and seem to develop almost exclusively at valve sites (Fig. 13.11), whether the vein is used *in situ*, nonreversed or reversed. Such mid-graft lesions in the lower thigh or calf segment of the vein can frequently be repaired with either vein patch angioplasty or interposition vein grafting (Fig. 13.12). After exposure of the stenosis and systemic heparinization, repair is performed using distal exsanguination with an Esmarch bandage and proximal tourniquet control, thus limiting the extent of required dissection and obviating the need to place clamps on the vein graft.

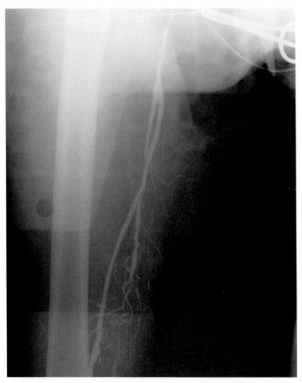

Figure 13.8 *Intraoperative arteriogram obtained following proximal transanastomotic location of a vein graft from the common femoral to the deep femoral artery. The anastomosis is widely patent and free of defects.*

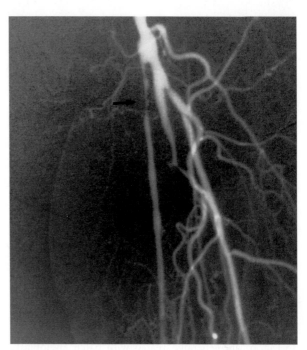

Figure 13.9 *Occasional proximal graft lesions are longer and more diffuse (arrow). Such lesions are generally best treated with interposition vein grafting.*

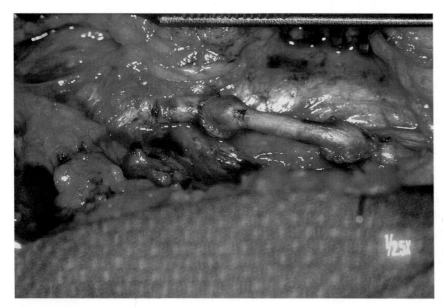

Figure 13.10 *Intraoperative photograph of interposition vein graft to replace a longer segment graft stenosis. Anastomoses are spatulated to prevent napkin-ring-like restenosis. This figure also appears in the colour plate section.*

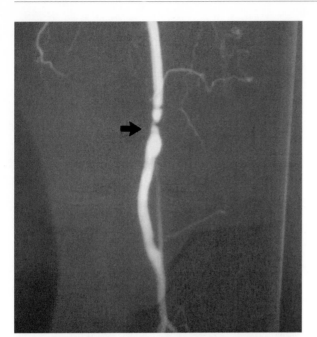

Figure 13.11 *Arteriogram demonstrating a complex, focal mid-graft stenosis occurring at a valve site (arrow). The lesion was associated with a fibrotic valve leaflet. The lesion is well proximal to a widely patent distal anastomosis to the below knee popliteal artery.*

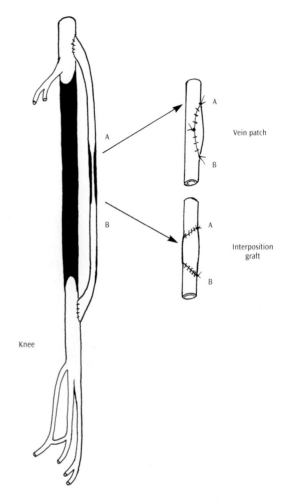

Figure 13.12 *Mid-graft lesions are best treated either with vein patch angioplasty or interposition vein grafting depending on their length and the degree of fibrosis involved.*

Distal juxta-anastomotic vein graft lesions, (Fig. 13.13a, b) are generally treated with patch angioplasty or short segment interposition vein grafting depending on their length. Such lesions are also frequently best approached with distal exsanguination and tourniquet control. A focal popliteal fossa lesion, such as that demonstrated in Fig. 13.13 can be expeditiously exposed via a posterior approach, avoiding dissection in a scarred medial field.

Progression of outflow native arterial disease

Finally, lesions may develop in the graft run-off in the native arterial tree beyond the distal graft anastomosis[71] either alone or in conjunction with a distal anastomotic stenosis. Such lesions can be treated with a jump or sequential graft (Fig. 13.14a. See p. 126). Figure 13.14b demonstrates an *in situ* femoral to below-knee popliteal artery bypass, which developed a high-grade outflow stenosis in the proximal anterior tibial artery 1 year following implantation. This lesion was treated with proximal tourniquet technique and a sequential graft was originated from the patent *in situ* bypass graft, tunneled through the interosseous membrane and anastomosed to the proximal anterior tibial artery (Fig. 13.14c).

Rarely, outflow arteries below a patent, otherwise functional, graft free of lesions can develop high-grade progressive atherosclerosis, which results in a graft with low flow velocity and recurrent ischemia of the foot. These lesions can sometimes be treated with distal anastomotic translocation or target artery relocation. Figure 13.15, (see p. 127), demonstrates such a scenario, in which a patent graft was hemodynamically failing due to progressive disease in the plantar arteries. The anastomosis was relocated to a more proximal peroneal vessel with restoration of normal hemodynamics.

Progression of inflow disease

Inflow disease may develop proximal to an otherwise normally functioning vein graft.[72] In fact, we have identified patent vein grafts distal to a total inflow artery occlusion. Such patients may present with recurrent

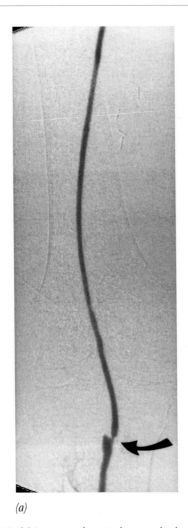

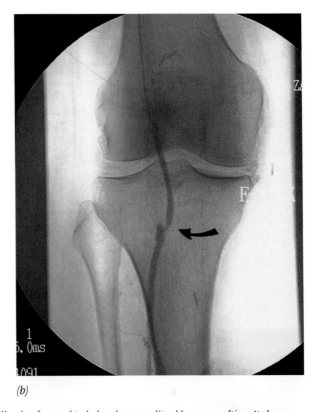

(a)   (b)

Figure 13.13 *(a) Postoperative arteriogram obtained 6 months following femoral to below-knee popliteal bypass grafting. It shows a widely patent graft down to the level of the distal anastomosis at which site (arrow) a very high grade stenosis has developed. (b) Magnified view of high-grade distal juxta-anastomotic vein graft artery anastomosis (arrow). Such lesions can be readily approached posteriorly avoiding dissection through a medial field scarred by previous operation.*

claudication or rest pain, and a diminished or absent femoral pulse. Duplex scans in such cases will identify a patent vein graft with low flow velocities (<45 cm/s) and biphasic or monophasic waveforms. Appropriate inflow reconstruction (iliac percutaneous transluminal angioplasty, endarterectomy, axillofemoral bypass, aortofemoral bypass or femoral femoral bypass) will restore normal hemodynamics. Autogenous vein grafts that are free of intrinsic defects are extremely tolerant of low flow states and will frequently remain patent in such circumstances of poor inflow due to inflow disease progression, providing the alert surgeon with the opportunity to address the inflow lesion prior to graft occlusion and profound limb ischemia.

As is clear from the examples presented, early and late appearing graft lesions can tax the ingenuity and strain the perseverance of the most capable vascular surgeon. We hope the techniques presented herein render the treatment of such lesions more successful. Our strong preference is to repair vein graft lesions operatively as the results of percutaneous transluminal angioplasty have generally been quite poor. The one exception may be in patients who develop late-appearing graft lesions more than $1\frac{1}{2}$–2 years following graft placement. These lesions appear to behave differently from early-appearing lesions, and occasional focal midgraft lesions in such patients may lend themselves to percutaneous transluminal angioplasty. If this procedure is selected, hemodynamic success must be documented by duplex surveillance, and close postangioplasty surveillance is necessary to be certain the lesion does not recur.

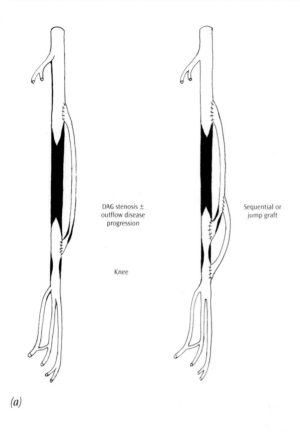

DAG stenosis ± outflow disease progression

Knee

Sequential or jump graft

(a)

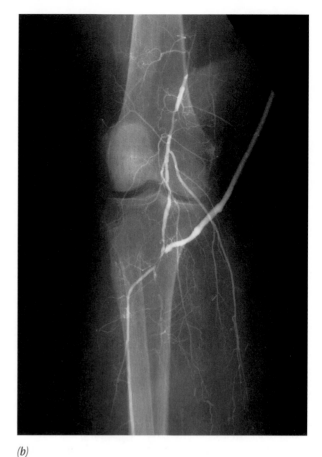

(b)

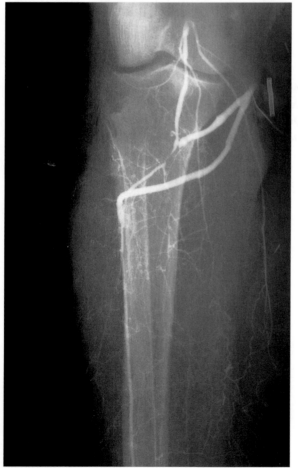

(c)

Figure 13.14 *(a) Grafts may develop intrinsic lesions at the outflow distal artery graft (DAG) anastomosis or in the outflow vessels beyond the anastomosis as shown in this diagram. Such lesions can be treated with sequential or jump grafts. (b) Arteriogram obtained 1 year following femoral to distal below knee popliteal in situ bypass. A pre-occlusive high-grade stenosis is present in the proximal anterior tibial artery just beyond the distal anastomosis. (c) This lesion was treated with a jump graft from the previously patent in situ bypass to the proximal anterior tibial artery, tunneled through the interosseous membrane.*

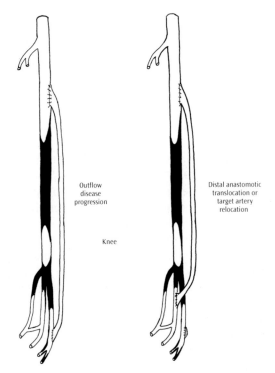

Figure 13.15 *In rare instances, marked atherosclerotic outflow disease progression beyond the distal anastomosis in the native arterial tree may reduce graft flow and result in recurrent foot ischemia or a hemodynamically threatened graft. On occasion, such patent grafts can be reanastomosed to an alternate target artery, such as the peroneal artery shown here, with restoration of normal hemodynamics.*

REFERENCES

1 Carrel A, Guthrie CC. Anastomosis of blood vessels by the patching method and transplantation of the kidney. *JAMA* 1906; **47**: 1648–50.

2 Grondin CM, Meere C, Castonguay Y, Lepage G, Grondin P. Progressive and late obstruction of an aorto-coronary venous bypass graft. *Circulation* 1971; **43**: 698–702.

3 Breslau RC, DeWeese JA. Successful endophlebectomy of autogenous venous bypass graft. *Ann Surg* 1965; **162**: 251–4.

4 Szilagyi DE, Elliot JP, Hageman JH *et al*. Biologic fate of autogenous vein implants as arterial substitutes: clinical angiographic, and histo-pathologic observations in femoro-popliteal operations for atherosclerosis. *Ann Surg* 1973; **178**: 232–46.

5 Stchelkounoff I. L'intima des petites arteres et des veines et le mesenchyme vasculaire. *Arch Anat Microsc Morphol Experimentalles* 1936; **32**: 139–94.

6 Webster WS, Bishop SP, Greer JC. Experimental aortic intimal thickening. Morphology and source of intimal cells. *Am J Pathol* 1974; **76**: 245–4.

7 Spaet TH, Stemerman MB, Veith FJ, Lejnieks I. Intimal injury and regrowth in the rabbit aorta. Medial smooth muscle cells as a source of neointima. *Circ Res* 1975; **36**: 58–70.

8 Gerrity RG, Cliff WJ. The aortic tunica media of the developing rat. Quantitative stereologic and biochemical analysis. *Lab Invest* 1975; **32**: 585–600.

9 Nakamura H. Electron microscopic study of the prenatal development of the thoracic aorta in the rat. *Am J Anat* 1988; **181**: 406–18.

10 Ross R, Klebanoff SJ. The smooth muscle cell. In vivo synthesis of connective tissue proteins. *J Cell Biol* 1971; **50**: 159–71.

11 Chamley-Campbell J, Campbell GR, Ross R. The smooth muscle cell in culture. *Physiol Rev* 1979; **59**: 1–61.

12 Davies MG, Hagen P. Pathobiology of intimal hyperplasia. *Br J Surg* 1994; **81**: 1254–69.

13 Geary RL, Nikkar SJ, Wagner WD *et al*. Wound healing: a paradigm for lumen narrowing after arterial reconstruction. *J Vasc Surg* 1998; **27**: 96–108.

14 Westerband A, Mills JL, Marek JM *et al*. Immunocytochemical determination of cell type and proliferation rate in human vein graft stenoses. *J Vasc Surg* 1997; **25**: 64–73.

15 Ross R. Platelet derived growth factor. *Lancet* 1989; **1**(8648): 1179–82.

16 Bowen-Pope DF, Hart CE, Seifert RA. Sera and conditioned media contain different isoforms of platelet-derived growth factor (PDGF) which bind to different classes of PDGF receptor. *J Biol Chem* 1989; **264**: 2502–8.

17 Jawien A. Bowen-Pope DF, Lindner V, Schwartz SM, Clowes AW. Platelet-derived growth factor promotes smooth muscle migration and intimal thickening in a rat model of balloon angioplasty. *J Clin Invest* 1992; **89**: 507–11.

18 Ferns GA, Raines EW, Sprugel KH, Motani AS, Reidy MA, Ross R. Inhibition of neointimal smooth muscle accumulation after angioplasty by an antibody to PDGF. *Science* 1991; **253**: 1129–32.

19 Dangas G. Colombo A. Platelet glycoprotein IIb/IIIa antagonists in percutaneous coronary revascularization. *Am Heart J* 1999; **138**(1 Pt 2): S16–23.

20 Cercek B, Fishbein MC, Forrester JS, Helfant RH, Fagin JA. Induction of insulin-like growth factor I messenger RNA in rat aorta after balloon denudation. *Circ Res* 1990, **66**: 1755–60.

21 Lynch SE, Colvin RB, Antoniades HN. Growth factors in wound healing. Single and synergistic effects on partial thickness porcine skin wounds. *J Clin Invest* 1989; **84**: 640–6.

22 Klagsbrun M, Edelman ER. Biological and biochemical properties of fibroblast growth factors. Implications for the pathogenesis of atherosclerosis. *Arteriosclerosis* 1989; **9**: 269–78.

23 Casscells W, Lappi DA, Shrivastav S *et al*, Regulation of fibroblast growth factor system in vascular injury. *Circulation* 1992; **86**(Suppl I): 184.

24 Lindner V, Majack RA, Reidy MA. Basic fibroblast growth

factor stimulates endothelial regrowth and proliferation in denuded arteries. *J Clin Invest* 1990; **85**: 2004–8.

25 Westerband A, Mills JL, Hunter GC, Gentile AT, Ihnat D, Heimark RL. Topography of cell replication in human vein graft stenoses. *Circulation* 1999; **98**(19 Suppl): II325–9.

26 McNamara DB, Bedi B, Aurora H *et al*. L-Arginine inhibits balloon catheter-induced intimal hyperplasia. *Biochem Biophys Res Commun* 1993; **193**: 291–6.

27 Tarry WC, Makhoul RG. Nitric oxide precursor speeds the recovery of endothelial-dependent vasorelaxation and reduces intimal hyperplasia after endothelial injury. *Surg Forum* 1993; **44**: 384–7.

28 Clowes AW, Karnovsky MJ. Suppression by heparin of smooth muscle cell proliferation in injured arteries. *Nature* 1977; **265**: 625–6.

29 Li Z, Alavi M, Wasty F, Ismail N, Moore S. Collagen biosynthesis by neointimal smooth muscle cells *in vitro*. *FASEB J* 1993; **7**: A791.

30 Gentile AW, Mills JL, Westerband A *et al*. Characterization of cellular density and determination of neointimal extracellular matrix constituents in human lower extremity vein graft stenosis. *Cardiovasc Surg* 1999; **7**(4): 464–9.

31 Mills JL. Mechanisms of vein graft failure: The location, distribution and characteristics of lesions that predispose to graft failure. *Semin Vasc Surg* 1993; **6**(2): 78–91.

32 Giannoukas AD, Androulakis AE, Labropoulos N, Wolfe JHN. The role of surveillance after ingrainguinal bypass grafting. *Eur J Vasc Endovasc* 1996; **11**: 279–89.

33 Idu MM, Truyen E, Buth J. Surveillance of lower extremity vein grafts. *Eur J Vasc Surg* 1992; **6**: 456–62.

34 Grigg MJ, Nicolaides AN, Wolfe JHN. Detection and grading of femorodistal vein graft stenoses: Duplex measurements compared with angiography. *J Vasc Surg* 1988; **8**: 661–6.

35 Moody P, Gould DA, Harris PL. Vein graft surveillance improves patency in femoropopliteal bypass. *Eur J Vasc Surg* 1990; **4**: 117–121.

36 Buth J, Disselhoff B, Sommeling C, Stam L. Colour-flow duplex criteria for grading stenosis in infrainguinal vein grafts. *J Vasc Surg* 1991; **14**: 716–28.

37 Nielsen TG, Von Jessen F, Schroeder TV. Earlier experiences with duplex scanning of fernoropopliteal vein grafts. *Ugeskr-Laeger* 1993; **155**: 881–4.

38 Idu MM, Blankenstein JD, DeGier P, Truyen E, Buth J. Impact of colour-flow duplex surveillance program on infrainguinal vein graft patency: A five year experience. *J Vasc Surg* 1993; **17**: 42–53.

39 Mattos MA, van Bemmelen PS, Hodgson KJ, Ramsey DE, Barkmeier LD, Sumner DS. Does detection of stenoses identified with color duplex scanning improve infrainguinal graft patency? *J Vasc Surg* 1993; **17**: 54–66.

40 Bandyk DF. Essentials of graft surveillance. *Semin Vasc Surg* 1993; **6**: 92–102.

41 Mills JL, Fujitani RM, Taylor SM. The characteristics and anatomic distribution of lesions that cause reversed vein graft failure: a five year prospective study. *J Vasc Surg* 1993; **17**: 195–206.

42 Donaldson MG, Mannick JA, Whittemore AD. Causes of primary graft failure after in situ saphenous vein bypass grafting. *J Vasc Surg* 1992; **15**: 113–20.

43 Taylor PR, Wolfe JHN, Tyrrell MR *et al*. Graft stenosis – justification for 1-year surveillance. *Br J Surg* 1990; **77**: 1125–8.

44 Moody P, Gould DA, Harris PL. Vein graft surveillance improves patency in femoro popliteal bypass. *Eur J Vasc Surg* 1990; **4**: 117–21.

45 Harris PL. Vein graft surveillance – all part of the service. *Br J Surg* 1992; **79**: 97–8.

46 Bergamini TM, George SM, Massey HT *et al*. Intensive surveillance of femoropopliteal–tibial autogenous vein bypasses improves long-term graft patency and limb salvage. *Ann Surg* 1995; **221**: 507–18.

47 Passman MA, Moneta GL, Nehler MR *et al*. Do normal early color-flow duplex surveillance examination results of infrainguinal vein grafts preclude the need for late graft revision? *J Vasc Surg* 1995; **22**: 476–84.

48 Ihnat DM, Mills JL, Dawson DL *et al*. The correlation of early flow disturbances with the development of infrainguinal graft stenosis: a 10-year study of 341 autogenous vein grafts. *J Vasc Surg* 1999; **30**: 8–15.

49 Erickson CA, Towne JB, Seabrook GR *et al*. Ongoing vascular laboratory surveillance essential to maximize long-term in situ saphenous vein bypass patency. *J Vasc Surg* 1996; **23**: 18–27.

50 Whittemore AD, Clowes AW, Couch NP, Mannick JA. Secondary femoropopliteal reconstruction. *Ann Surg* 1981; **193**: 35–42.

51 Sladen JG, Gilmour JL. Vein graft stenosis: characteristics and effect of treatment. *Am J Surg* 1981; **141**: 549–553.

52 Cohen JR, Mannick JA, Couch NP, Whittemore AD. Recognition and management of impending vein graft failure. Importance for long term patency. *Arch Surg* 1986; **121**: 758–9.

53 Green RM, McNamara J, Ouriel K, DeWeese JA. Comparison of infrainguinal graft surveillance techniques. *J Vasc Surg* 1990; **11**: 207–15.

54 Graor RA, Risius B, Young JR *et al*. Thrombolysis of peripheral arterial bypass grafts: Surgical thrombectomy compared with thrombolysis. A preliminary report. *J Vasc Surg* 1988; **7**: 347–55.

55 Belkin M, Donaldson MC, Whittemore AD *et al*. Observations on the use of thrombolytic agents for thrombotic occlusion of infrainguinal vein grafts. *J Vasc Surg* 1990; **11**: 289–96.

56 Mills JL, Bandyk DF, Gahtan V *et al*. The origin of infrainguinal vein graft stenosis: a prospective study based on duplex surveillance. *J Vasc Surg* 1995; **21**: 16–25.

57 Gahtan V, Payne LP, Roper LD *et al*. Duplex criteria for predicting progression of vein graft lesions: Which stenoses can be followed? *J Vasc Technol* 1995; **19**: 211–15.

58 Papanicolaou G, Zierler RE, Beach KW *et al*. Hemodynamic parameters of failing infrainguinal bypass grafts. *Am J Surg* 1995; **169**: 238–44.

59 Sladen JG, Reid JDS, Cooperberg PL *et al*. Color flow duplex

screening of infrainguinal bypass grafts combining low- and high-velocity criteria. *Am J Surg* 1989; **158**: 107–12.

60 Caps, MT, Cantwell-Gab K, Bergelin RO, Strandness DE. Vein graft lesions: time of onset and rate of progression. *J Vasc Surg* 1995; **22**: 466–75.

61 Westerband A, Mills JL, Kistler S *et al*. Prospective validation of threshold criteria for intervention in infrainguinal vein grafts undergoing duplex surveillance. *Ann Vasc Surg* 1997; **11**: 44–8.

62 Wilson YG, Davies AH, Currie IC *et al*. The value of pre-discharge duplex scanning in infrainguinal graft surveillance. *Eur J Vasc Endovasc Surg* 1995; **10**: 237–42.

63 Nielsen TO. Natural history of infrainguinal vein bypass stenoses: early lesions increase the risk of thrombosis. *Eur J Vasc Endovasc Surg* 1996; **12**: 60–4.

64 Olojuba DH, McCarthy MJ, Naylor AN, Bell PRF, London NJM. At what peak velocity ratio value should duplex-detected infrainguinal vein graft stenoses be revised? *Eur J Vasc Endovasc Surg* 1998; **15**: 258–60.

65 Dunlap P, Hartshorne T, Bolia A, Bell PRF, London NJM. The long term outcome of infrainguinal vein graft surveillance. *Eur J Vasc Endovasc Surg* 1995; **10**: 352–5.

66 Perler BA, Osterman FA, Mitchell SE *et al*. Balloon dilatation versus surgical revision of infrainguinal autogenous vein graft stenosis. Long-term follow-up. *J Cardiovasc Surg* 1990; **31**: 656–61.

67 Moody AP, Edwards PR, Harns PL. The aetiology of vein graft stricture: a prospective marker study. *Eur J Vasc Surg* 1992; **6**: 509–11.

68 Bandyk DF, Schmitt DD, Seabrook GR *et al*. Monitoring functional patency of in-situ saphenous vein bypasses: the impact of a surveillance protocol and elective revision. *J Vasc Surg* 1989; **9**: 286–96.

69 Nehler MR, Moneta GL, Yeager RA. Surgical treatment of threatened reversed infrainguinal vein grafts. *J Vasc Surg* 1994; **20**: 558–65.

70 Lundell A, Lindblad B, Berquist D *et al*. Femoropopliteal-crural graft patency is improved by ABI intensive surveillance program: a prospective randomized study. *J Vasc Surg* 1995; **21**: 26–34.

71 Veith FJ, Weiser RK, Gupta SK. Diagnosis and management of failing lower extremity arterial reconstruction prior to graft occlusion. *J Cardiovasc Surg* 1984; **25**: 381–4.

72 Taylor SM, Mills JL, Fujitani RM *et al*. Does arterial inflow failure cause distal vein graft thrombosis. *Ann Vasc Surg* 1991; **8**: 92–8.

14

Foot complications in diabetics

JOHN D HUGHES AND JOSEPH L MILLS

INTRODUCTION

Foot complications in diabetics are a major healthcare issue. There are over 14 million people with diabetes in the USA. Each year, approximately 2.5 per cent of diabetics will develop a foot ulcer, accounting for the major cause of hospitalization of this population.[1] Although only approximately 5 per cent of the population has diabetes, this group accounts for half of all amputations performed in the USA. Foot ulceration is also associated with an increased risk of death in diabetics.[2]

PATHOPHYSIOLOGY

The predisposition of diabetics to the development of foot ulceration is related to many factors, the most important of which are peripheral neuropathy and atherosclerosis. These two complications allow even minor trauma to develop into open lesions. Generally, ulcers do not occur spontaneously but begin secondary to trauma, which may frequently be trivial and often unnoticed by the patient. Other factors associated with foot complications include smoking, glucose control, albuminuria, microangiopathy, limited joint mobility and immunosuppression.[1,3,4]

Diabetic neuropathy is a common underlying complication contributing to foot ulceration. Advanced neuropathy has been found to be present in nearly all diabetics with peripheral vascular disease and foot ulcers.[5] The precise etiology of neuropathy is unknown, although it has been associated with hyperglycemia and microangiopathy. Thickening of the basement membrane of nutrient vessels to the nerves may interfere with their metabolism, resulting in dysfunction and injury.

Byproducts of glucose metabolism also may accumulate within the nerve, adversely affecting its function. Neuropathy affects three nerve types: sensory, motor, and autonomic. Each of these alone, and in combination, can contribute to the development of skin ulceration.

Sensory neuropathy renders the diabetic vulnerable to ulceration through minor trauma, such as puncture, blunt pressure shear, abrasion or minor laceration. Callus may act as a foreign body over a bony prominence and result in a subdermal hematoma, with subsequent breakdown of overlying tissue. Whereas this type of trauma would be readily recognized by pain or discomfort in the sensate foot, the patient with insensate neuropathy receives no warning. The trauma may continue, with recognition and treatment being delayed until an open lesion has developed, possibly complicated with infection.

Muscle weakness resulting from motor neuropathy disproportionately affects the intrinsic flexor muscles of the foot, leaving the extensors relatively unopposed. This has the effect of changing the conformation of the foot, creating the 'intrinsic minus' foot. Lumbrical muscle weakness results in the extension of the toes at the metatarsophalangeal joint and flexion at the first interphalangeal joint, creating a claw deformity (Fig. 14.1). This imbalance leads to abnormal dynamic plantar pressure points over the metatarsal heads,[6] especially of the 1st, 4th and 5th digits, and the tips of the toes. Such motor deformity, in combination with sensory neuropathy, predisposes the tissue overlying these bony pressure points to ulceration from repetitive trauma. Muscle and ligament weakness also contributes to loss of the arch and subsequent mid-foot collapse, with a resultant Charcot foot deformity (Figs 14.2 and 14.3). This situation likewise creates abnormal pressure points and allows formation of ulcers in the mid-foot overlying misplaced tarsal bones. Finally, the deformities of the foot create a gait disturbance, which again may predispose to abnormal pressure points.

Autonomic neuropathy results in loss of sympathetic function, in turn leading to the development of dry skin, which is prone to fissuring and increased susceptibility to minor trauma. In turn, this may open a pathway for bacterial infection to develop.

Ischemia due to atherosclerosis contributes to 38–52 per cent of foot ulcers developing in diabetics. Histologically, atherosclerosis in the diabetic is indistinguishable from that of nondiabetics. The pathophysiology is felt to be the same. Endothelial injury is followed

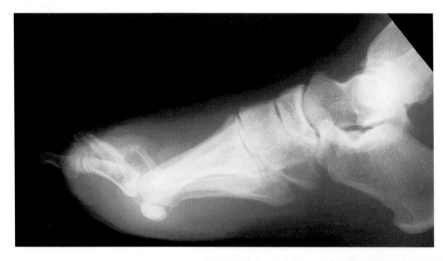

Figure 14.1 *Plain foot radiograph demonstrating the effects of motor neuropathy, with metatarsophalangeal joint extension and first interphalangeal joint flexion.*

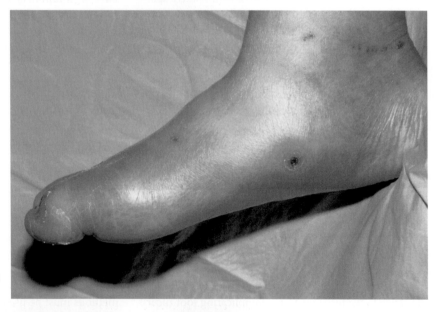

Figure 14.2 *Charcot foot deformity with mid-foot collapse. This figure also appears in the colour plate section.*

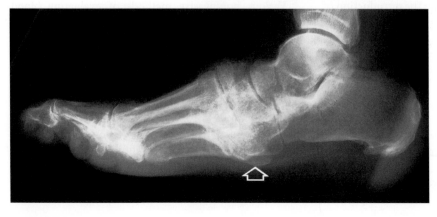

Figure 14.3 *Radiograph of the foot shown in Fig. 14.2. Notice the protruding first cuneiform (arrow) underlying the ulcer depicted in Fig. 14.2*

by platelet aggregation, white blood cell infiltration, fatty deposition and smooth muscle proliferation, which leads to an occlusive plaque. Arteries in diabetics do have an increased tendency to develop medial calcification, a finding frequently noted on plain radiographs. Although this calcification may render the vessels incompressible, potentially impairing noninvasive diagnostic tests and operative procedures, it is not necessarily associated with obstruction.

There are notable differences in both the onset and the distribution of atherosclerosis between diabetics and nondiabetics. Diabetics tend to have earlier onset of atherosclerosis, the reasons for which are not clear. More than 50 per cent of diabetics have obvious atherosclerotic cardiovascular disease within 15 years of the onset of diabetes, and are 20 times more likely to have significant lower extremity arterial disease than nondiabetics. The other risk factors for developing atherosclerosis, i.e. hypertension, hyperlipidemia and smoking, are similar to those for the nondiabetic population. Although vascular disease in diabetics may affect the same large arteries as nondiabetics, such as the aorta, iliacs and superficial femoral vessels, there is a predilection for more pronounced involvement of the infrageniculate popliteal artery and the tibial vessels, with relative sparing of the vessels of the foot. The popular misconception of a unique form of microangiopathy, or 'small vessel disease', as a cause of ischemic ulcers has fallen into disfavor. Multiple studies have failed to demonstrate differences in occlusive arteriolar disease between those with and without diabetes.[7] In addition, blood flow studies in diabetics who have had leg revascularization demonstrate no differences in response to papaverine, indicating unimpaired ability of the arterioles to dilate.

Albuminuria resulting from nephropathy has been associated with the development of foot ulcers in Type II diabetics.[4] This also correlates with a higher frequency of retinopathy. These conditions may be associated with the duration of disease.

Diabetes affects the immune system, impairing leukocyte adhesion, chemotaxis, phagocytosis, release of tissue factors and the inflammatory response to injury. These factors result in delayed wound healing and decreased resistance to bacterial invasion, complicating foot ulceration. Infection generally begins after the introduction of bacteria through the ulceration or a puncture. Infectious complications manifest in a clinical spectrum ranging from superficial cellulitis to osteomyelitis and deep space abscess, and frequently involve several different organisms.

EVALUATION

As with almost all diseases, the evaluation of diabetics with foot lesions begins with the history and physical examination. As diabetes affects multiple systems, it is important to determine the extent of disease in other systems, in addition to those relating to the affected extremity: especially the cardiac and renal systems. Angina, previous myocardial infarction and heart failure may influence the treatment of the ulcerated foot. Likewise, the degree of diabetic nephropathy may direct the method of workup for vascular compromise. Important points in the history pertaining to the foot include previous ulcerations, trauma, such as puncture, burns, abrasions, lacerations, injury with nail clipping, and a change in footwear. These inquiries provide clues to the etiology and duration of the injury, and may influence treatment, as well as suggest ways to prevent recurrences in the future.

On physical examination, particular notice must be taken of the location of the lesions, the extent of sensory loss, the presence of foot deformity and evidence of ischemia. Ulcers involving the plantar surface of the foot are usually neuropathic, resulting from loss of protective sensation as well as foot deformity (Fig. 14.4). Lesions located at the tips of the toes, along the nails and in the web spaces are more often ischemic. Heel ulcers may be decubitus (and neuropathic) or ischemic, but frequently have a component of both. Purulence, crepitus and inflammatory changes are indicative of infection. However, due to white blood cell impairment, the lack of visible signs of inflammation does not rule out infection. The presence of visible or palpable bone in the depth of the wound signals a high likelihood of osteomyelitis. The majority of diabetics with foot ulcers will demonstrate some loss of temperature (small fiber), vibratory (large fiber) and pressure sensation.[8] Vibratory, monofilament and deep tendon reflex tests may document neuropathy. The absence of an Achilles tendon reflex and lack of sensation to the 5.07 monofilament fiber has been found to be a significant predictor of foot ulceration.[9] The vascular status of the extremity should be assessed in all diabetics with foot lesions, even in the presence of neuropathy. Eighty per cent of diabetics with vascular disease will also have neuropathy. The presence of palpable pulses is generally indicative of circulation sufficient for healing. If foot pulses are absent, additional testing methods must be used to assess extremity perfusion.

Various noninvasive methods of evaluating blood flow to the foot have been described. The most commonly used method is Doppler-derived pressure measurement. Ankle pressures may help assess the circulation but are not applicable in at least 20 per cent of patients, owing to the presence of incompressible calcified vessels. With compressible vessels, an ankle pressure of 80 mmHg or less has been associated with poor healing of ulcers, or local amputations. Toe pressure measurements are often of benefit in evaluating patients with calcified vessels. The digital arteries are not as frequently involved with medial calcification as more proximal vessels, and therefore may be compressible when

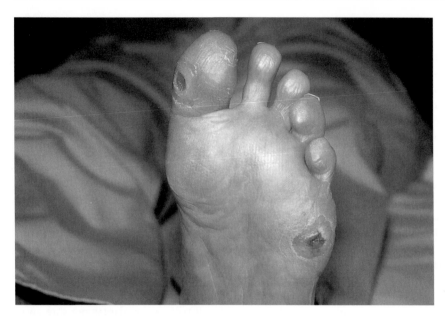

Figure 14.4 *Neuropathic ulcers at pressure points of the first interphalangeal and fifth metatarsophalangeal joints. This figure also appears in the colour plate section.*

the femoral and tibial vessels are not. Generally, a toe pressure exceeding 40 mmHg is indicative of adequate blood flow to allow healing of a local amputation or ulcer. Other methods of evaluation include transcutaneous oxygen measurements ($TcPO_2$). A $TcPO_2$ level of 30 mmHg or greater is suggestive of adequate circulation.[10] If these evaluations indicate inadequate circulation for healing, further testing should be performed to determine the anatomy and to plan an appropriate revascularization procedure. A variety of tests are available, each with its own strengths and weaknesses. Duplex scanning is a safe, noninvasive visualization method, which is accurate in identifying and grading the severity of arterial stenosis, and determining vessel patency. There are virtually no side effects. It is operator dependent, and complete studies with detailed lower extremity artery mapping may be difficult and time consuming. Although it is increasingly relied upon for evaluation, most surgeons do not plan an operation based solely upon duplex-derived information alone.

Other, relatively noninvasive imaging tests, include magnetic resonance angiography (MRA) and computed tomography (CT) angiography. MRA uses no nephrotoxic contrast agents and may be formulated to provide an image similar to conventional angiograms. It also may be helpful in identifying vessels in the distal leg or foot, which may not be visualized with conventional angiography, due to sluggish flow. The drawbacks of this method are that it is heavily dependent on computer software, not universally available and has a tendency to overestimate the degree of stenosis. CT angiography requires intravenously administered contrast. Advantages include avoidance of an arterial cannulation, visualization of nonvascular structures and computer enhanced views of the vessels. Disadvantages consist of nephrotoxicity from contrast media and operator dependence. This method is

more commonly used in imaging the aorta and branches, and currently has limited applicability in the leg. Conventional and intra-arterial digital angiography are the most common methods of evaluating the vascular anatomy when planning an intervention. Advantages include general availability and familiarity. Angiography provides an image which is relatively accurate and easy to interpret. It may be extended to evaluate the aorta and both legs, or limited to the involved extremity. The extent of study may be influenced by pulse examination, noninvasive tests and the required contrast load. Because of the pattern of arterial occlusion in diabetics, detailed views of the infrageniculate circulation and the pedal arteries are essential. Proximal occlusion of all trifurcation vessels does not necessarily mean there are no patent distal arteries. The peroneal artery as well as the pedal arteries are frequently spared and may serve as suitable target vessels for distal revascularization. Lateral foot views are extremely useful in identifying these vessels. The disadvantages of angiography include potential nephrotoxicity, the complications associated with arterial cannulation and occasionally nonvisualization of patent distal vessels due to sluggish flow.

When evaluating diabetic foot problems it is important to detect any underlying infection, since this may dramatically alter treatment. A thorough physical examination, including probing of the ulcer for bone, and routine foot films are usually sufficient. In difficult or equivocal cases, further imaging methods may be helpful. Plain foot radiographs to look for soft-tissue gas and osteomyelitis should be performed in all patients. Although plain film has relatively low sensitivity for osteomyelitis the specificity is over 90 per cent, and therefore is helpful if positive. MRI studies to detect infection, especially of the bone, have been found to have sensitivity of approximately 90 per cent, with specificity ranging from 71 to 100 per cent.[11–13] This study also gives additional information about deep-seated abscess, effusion and bone edema. Bone scans have been less useful, with sensitivity and specificity of only 50–60 per cent.

The majority of diabetic foot infections are polymicrobial. When deep tissue cultures are obtained and subjected to careful microbiological techniques, a mean of 3.2 organisms can be identified from a typical foot infection. Superficial wound cultures are not recommended since they frequently reflect surface contaminants from the skin and do not represent the true pathogens causing the infection. To increase the accuracy of cultures, the specimen must be taken from deep in the wound, an operative specimen, aspirate of bullae or abscess, or surgically excised bone. Specimens of the foot lesions should be sent for aerobic and anaerobic cultures. The most common aerobes include *Staphylococcus* species (*aureus* and *epidermidis*) and *Streptococcus*. *Enterococcus* and *Proteus* species are also relatively common. Anaerobes most frequently involve *Peptostreptococcus* and *Bacteroides* species.

TREATMENT

Diabetic foot care begins with ulcer prevention. Foremost, the patient should be thoroughly educated in the causes and potential serious consequences of ulcer formation, and about proper foot care. This includes careful daily examination of the feet for blisters, cuts or cracks, sores or discoloration. If the patient has poor vision, a family member or friend may help. The feet should be washed with warm water, checking the temperature with the fingers, not the foot, since neuropathy may decrease temperature sensation. The feet should be dried gently and a moisturizing lotion applied to avoid skin cracking. Patients should not walk barefoot, but wear socks and comfortable shoes. Shoes should be soft at the time of purchase, avoiding those which are stiff and in need of breaking in. The insides of the shoes must be checked prior to putting them on, to be sure there are no foreign bodies or irregularities inside which could traumatize the foot. Toenails are trimmed straight across to avoid ingrown nails, and smoothed with a file. If the nails are thickened or abnormal, trimming should be performed by a healthcare professional. Hot water bottles, heating pads and sun tanning must be avoided due to blunted protective sensation and the risk of burn. The assistance of a podiatrist and orthotics specialist, preferably as part of a team approach to the care of such patients, is essential to proper patient management.

Treatment of an established ulcer is to a large extent dependent on the etiology of the ulcer and whether infection is present. Since neuropathic ulcers usually result from pressure abnormalities, efforts are generally directed toward pressure redistribution. The most con-

servative method is total non-weight bearing. This effectively relieves pressure on the plantar surface, but has the obvious drawback of immobilization and is not usually necessary in uncomplicated ulcers. Patients with normal peripheral pulses and early neuropathic, noninfected ulcers may be effectively treated as outpatients. There is evidence that debridement of callus and necrotic tissue as an outpatient will improve the healing rate.[14] Shoe inserts or soft plastic liners may help relieve pressure on bony prominences. Some patients will benefit from special extra-depth deep-box shoes. Those with more severe bony deformities, such as mid-foot collapse, may require molded shoes. Total contact casting and boot casts have been used with success in patients with acute Charcot's arthropathy and noncomplicated neuropathic ulceration.[15–17] Contact casting involves a cast molded to the lower leg and foot, providing a walking heel, using minimal padding.[18] This method serves to provide support for the foot and redistribute the plantar pressure away from the ulcer, while allowing continued ambulation. If these methods do not effectively relieve the pain of arthopathy and stabilize the deformity of a Charcot's joint, further reconstructive procedures may be necessary, e.g. reduction and fusion of affected joints using internal fixation.[19] Metatarsal head resection is another method of pressure point reduction, which will frequently allow ulcer healing without significantly increasing the pressure on the remaining metatarsal heads.[20]

Infected ulcers are treated emergently with hospitalization. Parenteral broad spectrum antibiotics and aggressive debridement and drainage of fluid collections are essential to maximize limb salvage.[21,22] If the patient is frankly septic, and has fasciitis, it may be necessary to perform an open amputation at the ankle or higher to control the infection. Otherwise, local debridement should be carried out in the operating room under anesthesia with proper lighting and good surgical instruments. All necrotic tissue must be debrided back to viable tissue and all infected spaces should be drained without regard for anatomic landmarks. Plantar fasciitis, which may present only with erythema on the sole of the foot, must not be left undrained. A long vertical incision of the plantar surface of the foot will allow adequate visualization and drainage of this space. If the wound is adequately vascularized, it may then be treated in open fashion, and allowed to close by secondary intention, or possibly require a skin graft or flap for coverage. Open treatment generally consists of wet-to-wet or wet-to-dry dressings using normal saline moistened gauze, and changed every 8–12 hours.

Foot lesions with an ischemic component generally must be managed with intent to revascularize the extremity, otherwise healing will not take place. This requires complete hemodynamic vascular anatomy assessment as described above, including angiography. Owing to the typical diabetic atherosclerotic disease pattern of tibial obstruction with relative sparing of the pedal vessels, distal bypasses are commonly required. Graft origin is determined by the disease location, which frequently permits an inflow site in the distal superficial femoral or popliteal artery. There are reports of improved patency rates for these short grafts,[23,24] in addition to requiring less vein length. Best results are experienced when using vein conduit, usually the greater saphenous. Equally good patency rates are reported with reversed and *in situ* vein conduit. If greater saphenous vein is not available or inadequate, acceptable alternative vein conduits include lesser saphenous, cephalic and basilic vein, which frequently must be spliced. Infrainguinal bypass success rates in diabetic patients are similar to those in nondiabetics, with 1-year graft patency rates of 80–90 per cent, and 5-year graft patency rates of 50–80 per cent.[25] Synthetic bypass conduit performs poorly below the knee. For this reason, it is not frequently used unless there is no adequate vein available. Improved results with below-knee prosthetic grafts have been reported when combined with vein angioplasty at the distal anastamosis, such as a Taylor patch or Miller cuff. Percutaneous angioplasty may occasionally be helpful, but owing to the severe, long segment nature of occlusive disease of the tibial vessels in the majority of these patients, surgical bypass is generally required for revascularization.

Microvascular free flaps are occasionally necessary for coverage of larger lesions, especially those involving the Achilles tendon and the heel.[26,27] The inflow for the flap may be based upon an existing bypass graft or done simultaneously with vascular bypass if the native circulation is not satisfactory.

REFERENCES

1 Moss SE, Klein R, Klein B. The prevalence and incidence of lower extremity amputation on a diabetic population. *Arch Intern Med* 1992; **152**: 610–16.

2 Boyko EJ, Ahroni JH, Smith DG, Davignonu D. Increased mortality associated with diabetic foot ulcer. *Diabet Med* 1996; **13**(11): 967–72.

3 Shaw EJ, Boulton AJM. The pathogenesis of diabetic foot problems. *Diabetes* 1997; **46**(Suppl 2): S58–S61.

4 Zander E, Heinke P, Gottschling D, Zander G, Strese J, Herfurth S, Michaelis D. Increased prevalence of elevated urinary albumin excretion rate in type 2 diabetic patients suffering from ischemic foot lesions. *Exp Clin Endocrinol Diabetes*. 1997; **105**(Suppl 2): 51–3.

5 Hoeldtke RD, Davis KM, Hshieh PB, Gaspar SR, Dworkin GE. Are there two types of diabetic foot ulcers? *Journal of Diabetes and its Complications* 1994; **8**(2): 117–25.

6 Stess RM, Jensen SR, Mirmiran R. The role of dynamic plantar pressures in diabetic foot ulcers. *Diabetes Care* 1997; **20**(5): 855–8.

7 LoGerfo FW, Coffman JD. Vascular and microvascular disease of the foot in diabetics. *N Engl J Med* 1984; **311**(25): 1615–19.

8 Sosenko JM, Kato M, Soto R, Bild DE. Comparison of quantitative sensory – threshold measures for their association with foot ulceration in diabetic patients. *Diabetes Care* 1990; **13**: 1057–61.

9 McNeely MJ, Boyko EJ, Ahroni JH *et al*. The independent contributions of diabetic neuropathy and vasculopathy in foot ulceration. *Diabetes Care* l995; **18**(2): 216–19.

10 Ballard JL, Eke CC, Bunt TJ, Killeen JD. A prospective evaluation of transcutaneous oxygen measurements in the management of diabetic foot problems. *J Vasc Surg* 1995; **22**(4): 485–92.

11 Cook TA, Rahim N, Simpson HC, Galland RB. Magnetic resonance imaging in the management of diabetic foot infection. *Br J Surg* 1996; **83**(2): 245–8.

12 Croll SD, Nicholas GG, Osborne MA, Wasser TE, Jones S. The role of magnetic resonance imaging in the diagnosis of osteomyelitis in diabetic foot infections. *J Vasc Surg* 1996; **24**(2): 266–70.

13 Craig JG, Amin MB, Wu K *et al*. Osteomyelitis of the diabetic foot: MR imaging – pathologic correlation. *Radiology* 1997; **203**(3): 849–55.

14 Steed DL, Donohoe D, Webster MW, Lindsley L. Effect of extensive debridement and treatment on the healing of diabetic foot ulcers. Diabetic Ulcer Study Group. *J Am Coll Surg* 1996; **183**(1): 61–4.

15 Lavery LA, Armstrong DG, Walker SC. Healing rates of diabetic foot ulcers associated with midfoot fracture due to Charcot's arthropathy. *Diabet Med* 1997; **14**(1): 46–9.

16 Armstrong DG, Todd WF, Lavery LA, Harkless LB, Bushman TR. The natural history of acute Charcot's arthropathy in a diabetic foot specialty clinic. *J Am Podiat Med Assoc* 1997; **87**(6): 272–8.

17 McGill M, Collins P, Bolton T, Yue DK. Management of neuropathic ulceration. *J Wound Care* 1996; **5**(2): 52–4.

18 Caputo GM, Cavanagh PR, Ulbrecht JS, Gibbons GW, Karchmer AW. Assessment and management of foot disease in patients with diabetes. *N Engl J Med* 1994; **331**(13): 854–60.

19 Early JS, Hasen ST. Surgical reconstruction of the diabetic foot: a salvage approach for midfoot collapse. *Foot Ankle Int* 1996; **17**: 325–30.

20 Patel VG, Wieman TJ. Effect of metatarsal head resection for diabetic foot ulcers on the dynamic plantar pressure distribution. *Am J Surg* 1994; **167**(3): 297–301.

21 Smith AJ, Daniels T, Bohnen JM. Soft tissue infections and the diabetic foot. *Am J Surg* 1996; **172**(6A): 7S–12S.

22 Tan JS, Friedman NM, Hazelton-Miller C, Flanagan JP, File TM Jr. Can aggressive treatment of diabetic foot infections reduce the need for above-ankle amputation? *Clin Infect Dis* 1996; **23**(2): 286–91.

23 Mohan CR, Hoballah JJ, Martinasevic M *et al*. Revascularization of the ischemic diabetic foot using popliteal artery inflow. *Int Angiol* 1996; **15**(2): 138–43.

24 Mills JL, Gahtan V, Fujitani RM, Taylor SM, Bandyk DF. The utility and durability of vein bypass grafts originating from the popliteal artery for limb salvage. *Am J Surg* 1997; **168**: 646–51.

25 Stonebridge PA, Murie JA. Infrainguinal revascularization in the diabetic patient. *Br J Surg* 1993; **80**: 1237–41.

26 Karp NS, Kasabian AK, Siebert JW, Eidelman Y, Colen S. Microvascular free-flap salvage of the diabetic foot: A 5 year experience. *Plastic Reconstruct Surg* 1994; **94**(6): 834–40.

27 Gooden MA, Gentile AT, Mills JL *et al*. Free tissue transfer to extend the limits of limb salvage for lower extremity tissue loss. *Am J Surg* 1997; **174**: 644–9.

Index